Decision Making in
INFERTILITY

Decision Making in INFERTILITY

Editors

Apoorva Pallam Reddy
MS DNB OBG Diploma in Gyne Endoscopy Fellowship in Reproductive Medicine
Medical Director
Phoenix Speciality Clinic
Bengaluru, Karnataka, India

Rajeev Agarwal MD (Manipal)
Consultant Gynecologist
Infertility Specialist and Laparoscopic Surgeon
Medical Director
Care IVF
Kolkata, West Bengal, India

Foreword
Jaideep Malhotra

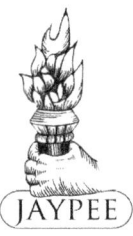

JAYPEE BROTHERS MEDICAL PUBLISHERS
The Health Sciences Publisher
New Delhi | London | Panama

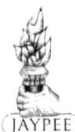 **Jaypee Brothers Medical Publishers (P) Ltd**

Headquarters
Jaypee Brothers Medical Publishers (P) Ltd
4838/24, Ansari Road, Daryaganj
New Delhi 110 002, India
Phone: +91-11-43574357
Fax: +91-11-43574314
Email: jaypee@jaypeebrothers.com

Overseas Offices

J.P. Medical Ltd
83 Victoria Street, London
SW1H 0HW (UK)
Phone: +44 20 3170 8910
Fax: +44 (0)20 3008 6180
Email: info@jpmedpub.com

Jaypee-Highlights Medical Publishers Inc
City of Knowledge, Bld. 235, 2nd Floor
Clayton, Panama City, Panama
Phone: +1 507-301-0496
Fax: +1 507-301-0499
Email: cservice@jphmedical.com

Jaypee Brothers Medical Publishers (P) Ltd
Bhotahity, Kathmandu, Nepal
Phone: +977-9741283608
Email: kathmandu@jaypeebrothers.com

Website: www.jaypeebrothers.com
Website: www.jaypeedigital.com

© 2020, Jaypee Brothers Medical Publishers

The views and opinions expressed in this book are solely those of the original contributor(s)/author(s) and do not necessarily represent those of editor(s) of the book.

All rights reserved. No part of this publication may be reproduced, stored or transmitted in any form or by any means, electronic, mechanical, photocopying, recording or otherwise, without the prior permission in writing of the publishers.

All brand names and product names used in this book are trade names, service marks, trademarks or registered trademarks of their respective owners. The publisher is not associated with any product or vendor mentioned in this book.

Medical knowledge and practice change constantly. This book is designed to provide accurate, authoritative information about the subject matter in question. However, readers are advised to check the most current information available on procedures included and check information from the manufacturer of each product to be administered, to verify the recommended dose, formula, method and duration of administration, adverse effects and contraindications. It is the responsibility of the practitioner to take all appropriate safety precautions. Neither the publisher nor the author(s)/editor(s) assume any liability for any injury and/or damage to persons or property arising from or related to use of material in this book.

This book is sold on the understanding that the publisher is not engaged in providing professional medical services. If such advice or services are required, the services of a competent medical professional should be sought.

Every effort has been made where necessary to contact holders of copyright to obtain permission to reproduce copyright material. If any have been inadvertently overlooked, the publisher will be pleased to make the necessary arrangements at the first opportunity. The **CD/DVD-ROM** (if any) provided in the sealed envelope with this book is complimentary and free of cost. **Not meant for sale.**

Inquiries for bulk sales may be solicited at: jaypee@jaypeebrothers.com

Decision Making in Infertility

First Edition: **2020**

ISBN: 978-93-88958-94-3

Dedicated to
*Our parents for giving us the freedom to dream passionately and
our spouses for supporting us in achieving those dreams.*

Phone: 23014481

Congress Parliamentary Party

Sonia Gandhi
Chairperson

September 11, 2019

Dear Dr Yasodhara,

Thank you for your letter of 7th September 2019 along with a copy of the book "Decision Making in Infertility" brought out by your daughter, Dr Apoorva Pallam Reddy. I appreciate the gesture.

With good wishes,

Yours sincerely,

Dr P Yasodhara
Sri Durga Hospital
15/266, Brindavanam
Nellore 524 001
Andhra Pradesh

Contributors

Aarti Deendayal MS
Senior Consultant and Fertility Specialist
Mamta Fertility Hospital
Hyderabad, Telangana, India

Aditi Kanungo MBBS MS
Fertility Consultant
Care IVF
Kolkata, West Bengal, India

Aditya Khurd
DNB Fellowship in Reproductive Medicine (Bengaluru)
Fellowship in Minimal Access Surgery (Kochi)
Consultant
Khurd Fertility, Endoscopy and IVF Center
Pune, Maharashtra, India

Anjali M MS
Associate Professor
Department of Obstetrics and Gynecology
Kasturba Medical College, Manipal Academy of Higher Education
Manipal, Karnataka, India

Ankita Kaushal
MBBS MS (Obs & Gyne) FRM Fellow in Reproductive Medicine
Scientific Director
Dr Ankita's Fertility Centre
Mumbai, Maharashtra, India

Anshu Jindal MD DNB MNAMS FICMCH
Consultant
Jindal Hospital and Infertility Centre
Meerut, Uttar Pradesh, India

Anurag Mallick MS Diploma in Gyne Endoscopy
Calcutta Medical Research Institute
Kolkata, West Bengal, India

Aparna MCH
Resident
Amrita Institute of Medical Sciences (AIMS)
Kochi, Kerala, India

Apoorva Pallam Reddy
MS DNB OBG Diploma in Gyne Endoscopy
Fellowship in Reproductive Medicine
Medical Director
Phoenix Speciality Clinic
Bengaluru, Karnataka, India

Aruna Siddharth DGO
Consultant
Phoenix Speciality Clinic
Bengaluru, Karnataka, India

Ashish Kale MD DNB MNAMS FICOG FICS
Director
Ashakiran Hospitals and Asha IVF Centers
Pune, Maharashtra, India

Ashwini Kale DNB OG
Consultant
Dr Ashish Kale's IVF Centre
Pune, Maharashtra, India

Astha Ubeja MD
Consultant
Prakash Hospital and Research Centre
Khandwa, Madhya Pradesh, India

Aswathy Kumaran MS DNB FNB
Assistant Professor
Department of Obstetrics and Gynecology
Kasturba Medical College, Manipal Academy of Higher Education
Manipal, Karnataka, India

Basab Mukherjee
MD MRCOG (UK) FRCOG FICOG
Consultant
Aashirbad Clinic
Kolkata, West Bengal, India

Bebu Seema Pandey
MD FICOG FRM Dip USG Fellow in Laparoscopy-Hysteroscopy
Director
Seema Hospital and Eva Fertility Clinic and IVF Centre
Azamgarh, Uttar Pradesh, India

Bhaskar Pal MD DGO DNB MRCOG
Consultant
Medstar Clinic
Kolkata, West Bengal, India

Bhavana Mittal DNB FNB MNAMS FICOG
Director
Shivam IVF Centre
Delhi, India

Bimal John MS Dip MIS FMAS
Director—Minimally Invasive Gynecology and Program Head
Assisted Reproduction Unit
Credence Hospital and Credence Specialty Clinics
Thiruvananthapuram, Kerala, India

Biswanath Ghosh Dastidar MS (Obs & Gyne)
IVF Consultant
Ghosh Dastidar Institute
Kolkata, West Bengal, India

Chaitanya Nagori DGO DNB
Director and Consultant
Dr Nagori's Institute for Infertility and IVF
Ahmedabad, Gujarat, India

Chand Mohammad MSc Biotech
Embryologist
Rainbow IVF, Agra, Uttar Pradesh, India

Chetan Kaur Ruprai MBBS MRCOG Dip MedEd
Consultant
Department of Obstetrics and Gynecology
Calderdale and Huddersfield NHS Foundation Trust
Huddersfield, UK

Damodar MBBS MD
Associate Director and Senior Consultant
Damodar Rao Hospital
Coimbatore, Tamil Nadu, India

Diksha Goswami MD FNB (Rep Med) DNB MRCOG FICOG
Director
IVF Centre, Pushpanjali Multispeciality Hospital
Agra, Uttar Pradesh, India

Divyashree PS MS DNB (Obs & Gyne) FNB (Rep Med) PGDMLE
Clinical Director
Milann JP Nagar
Bengaluru, Karnataka, India

Dorothy P Ghosh MBBS DNB
Consultant
Care IVF
Kolkata, West Bengal, India

Fessy Louise T DGO DNB FAGE MNAMS DPS MICOG FICOG
Consultant
Amrita Fertility Centre
Kochi, Kerala, India

Hema Desai MS
Consultant and Fertility Specialist
Mamta Fertility Hospital
Hyderabad, Telangana, India

Hrishikesh Pai MD FCPS FICOG MSc (USA)
Consultant Gynaecologist and IVF Specialist
Lilavati Hospital, Mumbai
Fortis Hospital, New Delhi, Gurugram, Noida, Faridabad
DY Patil Hospital
Mumbai, Maharashtra, India

Indranil Dutta
MS Dip Advanced Endoscopic Gyne Surgery
Fellowship in Laparoscopy Fellowship in USG
Fellow in Gynecology Fellowship in Infertility
Senior Assistant Professor
IQ and NH Medical College, Durgapur
Consultant
GICE Nursing Home
Kalyani, West Bengal, India

Jaideep Malhotra MD
Consultant
Rainbow Hospital
Agra, Uttar Pradesh, India

Jaydeep Tank MD DNB DGO FCPS MICOG
Consultant Obstetrician, Gynecologist, Fertility Care Physician
Ashwini Maternity and Surgical Hospital, Center for Endoscopy
and Assisted Reproduction, Mumbai
Jupiter Hospital
Mumbai, Maharashtra, India

Jiteeka Thakkar DGO DFP
Infertility Specialist and Laparoscopic Surgeon
Kadia Polyclinic
Mumbai, Maharashtra, India

Kamini Patel MBBS DICOG DGO
CEO and IVF Specialist
Vani IVF Centre
Ahmedabad, Gujarat, India

Kanti Bansal MD DGO FICOG
IVF and Infertility Specialist
Safal Fertility Foundation and Bansal Hospital
Ahmedabad, Gujarat, India

Kartika D Kumar
CIMAR Fertility Center, A Unit of Edappal Hospitals Pvt Ltd
Kochi, Kerala, India

Kathyaini VS DGO Fellowship in Reproductive Medicine
Consultant IVF Specialist
Apollo Fertility
Bengaluru, Karnataka, India

Kavitha Gautham MS DRM FICOG FIMGA
Consultant
Bloom Fertility and Healthcare
Chennai, Tamil Nadu, India

Kedar Ganla MD DNB FCPS DGO DFP
Consultant Fertility Physician, Scientific Director
Ankoor Fertility Clinic
Mumbai, Maharashtra, India

Keshav Malhotra MBBS MCE
Director
Rainbow IVF
Agra, Uttar Pradesh, India

Kishore Pandit DGO Dip Endoscopy Fellow (IVF)
Consultant
Lifeline Hospital
Pune, Maharashtra, India

KK Gopinathan MBBS MS (Obs & Gyne)
Senior Consultant and Scientific Director
CIMAR Fertility Center, A Unit of Edappal Hospitals Pvt Ltd
Kochi, Kerala, India

Contributors

Kundan Ingale DGO DNB Fellow in Endoscopy
Infertility Specialist
Nirmiti Clinic
Pune, Maharashtra, India

Malvika Sabarwal DGO FICOG Dip Gyne Endoscopic Surgery
Senior Consultant
Apollo Spectra Hospitals
New Delhi, India

Meenu Agarwal
DNB DGO Dip Endoscopic Surgery and ART (Germany)
Fellowship in Endometriosis Surgery (Austria)
Bachelor in Gynecological Endoscopy (European Board Certified)
National Director—Clinical Board
Morpheus IVF
Pune, Maharashtra, India

Meenu Batra
DMRD Fellowship Training in Obstetric Ultrasound and
Basics of Fetal Medicine (Mediscan, Chennai)
Consultant Radiologist
CIMAR Fertility Center, A Unit of Edappal Hospitals Pvt Ltd
Kochi, Kerala, India

Meenu Handa MS (Obs & Gyne) DNB Fellow Reproductive
Medicine Unit Head
Fortis Bloom IVF Centre
Gurugram, Haryana, India

Mithila Mahesh MS OBG
Consultant Gynecologist
Sri Durga Hospital and IVF Center
Nellore, Andhra Pradesh, India

Molina Patel MD
Consultant
Akanksha Hospital
Gujarat, India

Mrugesh Patel MBBS DGO Dip Endoscopy (Germany)
Director
Mother Care Endoscopy Center
Mehsana, Gujarat, India

Nandita Palshetkar MD FPPS
Director
Bloom IVF, Mumbai
Consultant
Lilavati Hospital and Fortis Hospital
Mumbai, Maharashtra, India

Narendra Malhotra
MBBS MD FICMCH FICOG FICMU FRSH FRCOG FMAS ASFIAPM
Rainbow IVF, Agra, Uttar Pradesh, India
Past President FOGSI, ISAR

Nayana Patel MD (Obs & Gyne)
Consulting Obstetrics and Gynecologist, IVF Specialist
Medical Director
Akanksha Hospital and Research Institute
Anand, Gujarat, India

Neelam Bhise MS
Scientific Director and IVF Consultant
Acme Fertility
Navi Mumbai, Maharashtra, India

Neharika Malhotra Bora
MD (Obs and Gyn, gold medalist) DRM (Germany) ICOG
Fellowship in Reproductive Medicine and Ultrasound
Infertility Consultant
Rainbow IVF
Agra, Uttar Pradesh, India

Nikita Banerjee
MS DNB OBG Fellowship in Reproductive Medicine
Nova IVI
Mumbai, Maharashtra, India

Nupur Chhabra
Consultant OBG
Jeevan Mala Hospital
New Delhi, India

Parasuram Gopinath MBBS MS (Obs & Gyne)
Senior Consultant and Scientific Director
CIMAR Fertility Center, A Unit of Edappal Hospitals Pvt Ltd
Kochi, Kerala, India

Parikshit Tank
MD DNB FCPS DGO DFP MNAMS MICOG FRCOG
Consultant Obstetrician, Gynecologist, Fertility Care Physician
Ashwini Maternity and Surgical Hospital, Center for Endoscopy
and Assisted Reproduction, Mumbai
Jupiter Hospital
Mumbai, Maharashtra, India

Pinky R Shah DGO DNB FNB
Core Fertility Specialist
Morpheus IVF
Mumbai, Maharashtra, India

Poonam Goyal MDOG
Senior Consultant
Panchsheel Hospital, New Delhi
Max Super Speciality Hospital
Vaishali, Ghaziabad, Uttar Pradesh

Prashanth K Adiga MS
Professor
Department of Obstetrics and Gynecology
Kasturba Medical College, Manipal Academy of Higher Education
Manipal, Karnataka, India

Pratap Kumar
DGO MD FICOG FICS FIMCH
Professor
Department of Obstetrics and Gynecology
Kasturba Medical College
Manipal Academy of Higher Education
Manipal, Karnataka, India

Pratik Tambe
MD FICOG Dip Endoscopic Surgery (France)
Clinical Embryology (UK, Singapore) Assisted Reproduction (Belgium)
ART Consultant and Gyne Endoscopic Surgeon
Chairperson, FOGSI Endocrinology Committee (2017-19)
Managing Council Member, Mumbai (Obs-Gyn Society)
Managing Council Member, AMC, MSR, IAGE (2015-18)
Mentor, MOGS Youth Council

Priyanka Pipara MBBS DGO DNB
Consultant
Gautam Clinic
Kolkata, West Bengal, India

Priyankur Roy
MBBS MS Fellowship in Gyne-Endoscopy
Fellowship in Reproductive Medicine PGDMLS PGDHHM
Senior Consultant
Genome Fertility Centre
Siliguri, West Bengal, India

Priyanka Vora MD DNB FCPS DGO DFP
Consultant Fertility Physician, Scientific Director
Ankoor Fertility Clinic
Mumbai, Maharashtra, India

Rahul Manchanda MD FICOG FACS FICS FICMCH
Head
Gyne Endoscopic Unit
PSRI Multispeciality Hospital
New Delhi, India

Rajeev Agarwal MD (Manipal)
Consultant Gynecologist
Infertility Specialist and Laparoscopic Surgeon
Medical Director
Care IVF
Kolkata, West Bengal, India

Rakhi Singh
MBBS DGO Dip Reproductive Medicine and Embryology
Dip Advance Gynec Laparoscopic Surgery
Consultant
Abalone Clinic and IVF Centre
Noida, Uttar Pradesh, India

Rana Choudhary DNB FCPS DGO DFP MNAMS FICMCH FICOG
Associate Consultant
Ankoor Fertility Clinic, Mumbai
Consultant
Wockhardt Hospital
Mumbai, Maharashtra, India

Richa Sharma MS MNAMS FICOG FICMCH FMAS
Associate Professor
Department of Obstetrics and Gynaecology
UCMS–GTB Hospital
Delhi, India

Rishab Bora MD (Radio)
Head
Department of Radiodiagnosis
Rainbow Hospital
Agra, Uttar Pradesh, India

Ritu Hinduja
MD MRM (UK) DRM (Germany)
Fellowship in Reproductive Medicine (India, Spain, Israel)
Certificate in Genetic Counselling
Consultant Fertility Specialist
Nova IVI Fertility
Mumbai, Maharashtra, India

Rohan Palshetkar MS (Obs & Gyne)
Managing Committee Member of MSR
Mumbai, Maharashtra, India

Ruby Ruprai
MBBS MD (Obs & Gyne) FMAS DMIS
Dip Reproductive Medicine MA-Gyne MBA
Medcare Women and Children Hospital, Dubai
GMC Clinics, Jumeirah, Dubai, UAE

Sandhya Meshram
MS (Obs & Gyne) Fellowship in Reproductive Medicine (ICOG)
Center Head
Morpheus Bliss Fertility Center
Pune, Maharashtra, India

Sankalp Singh MS MRCOG
Director
Reproductive Medicine Unit
CRAFT Hospital
Kodungallur, Kerala, India

Saroj Agarwal MSc (Gold Medalist)
Chief Embryologist
Care IVF
Kolkata, West Bengal, India

Satish Kumar Adiga
MCE PhD Post Doctoral Training (University of Miami, USA)
Professor and Head
Department of Clinical Embryology
Kasturba Hospital
Manipal, Karnataka, India

Sejal Desai MD DNB DHA DGO MICOG DFP
Consultant
Department of Obstetrics and Gynecology
Surya Hospitals
Mumbai, Maharashtra, India

Shaheen Hokabaj MS (Obs & Gyne)
Consultant
Sneh Women's Hospital and IVF Centre
Ahmedabad, Gujarat, India

Contributors

Shally Gupta DGO DNB
Consultant
Rainbow Hospital
Agra, Uttar Pradesh, India

Shaweez Faizi MS
Assistant Professor
Department of Obstetrics and Gynecology
Kasturba Medical College, Manipal Academy of Higher Education
Manipal, Karnataka, India

Sheetal Sawankar
MBBS DNB MNAMS Masters in Reproductive Medicine (UK)
Fellowship in Reproductive Medicine (Germany)
Medical Director
Morpheus Juhu and Mulund Fertility Center, Mumbai
General Manager
Fertility and Gynecology
Morpheus IVF
Mumbai, Maharashtra, India

Shilpa A Reddy MBBS MS (Obs & Gyne) Fellow in Obstetrics and Gynecology Ultrasound Mediscan
Consultant
Lakshmi Kishore Hospital
Proddatur, Andhra Pradesh, India

Shivani Sabharwal MS OBG
Consultant IVF Specialist
Apollo Spectra Hospitals
New Delhi, India

Shubhashree Uppangala PhD
Assistant Professor
Department of Clinical Embryology
Kasturba Medical College
Manipal Academy of Higher Education
Manipal, Karnataka, India

Siddharth MBBS MCE (Australia) Fellowship in Andrology
Andrologist
Manipal Fertility
Bengaluru, Karnataka, India

Simi Fabian MBBS DGO DNB
Consultant
ARMC IVF Fertility Centre
Kozhikode, Kerala, India

Smita Jain MS (Obs & Gyne)
Infertility Specialist and Consultant
Maple Clinic, Uttar Pradesh, India

Sonal Panchal MD
Ultrasound Consultant
Dr Nagori's Institute for infertility and IVF
Ahmedabad, Gujarat, India

Sonia Malik DGO MD FICOG FAMS
Program Director
Southend Fertility and IVF Center
New Delhi, India

Suchetna Sengupta MBBS DRCOG DFFP
Senior Fertility Consultant
Care IVF
Kolkata, West Bengal, India

Sujatha Ramakrishna PhD
Scientific Director
Cloudnine Fertility
Chennai, Tamil Nadu, India

Sunil Jindal MS DNB MNAMS FICMCH
Andrologist and Laparoscopic Surgeon
Scientific Director
Jindal Hospital and Infertility Centre
Meerut, Uttar Pradesh, India

Surbhi Gupta MD OG
Consultant
Urogyn IVF Centre
New Delhi, India

Sushma Mandava MBBS MS DNB FMAS
Consultant
India IVF
Bengaluru, Karnataka, India

Swarnima Das MS
Consultant
Care IVF
Kolkata, West Bengal, India

Vandana Bhatia MD
Senior Consultant
Southend Fertility & IVF Centre, New Delhi
Holy Angels Hospital
New Delhi, India

Vandana Khurd MS OBG
Consultant
Khurd Fertility, Endoscopy and IVF Center
Pune, Maharashtra, India

Vandana Ramanathan MD
Fellow
Reproductive Medicine Unit
CRAFT Hospital
Kodungallur, Kerala, India

Vani Patel MSc (Human Genetics) MSc (Clinical Embryology)
Genetic Counsellors and Embryologist
Vani IVF Centre
Ahmedabad, Gujarat, India

Venu Gopal M MD DNB
Specialist Reproductive Medicine
Asian Reproductive Medicine Centre
Thrissur, Kerala, India

Vijayasarathi Ramanathan
MBBS Mmed Graduate Dip in Health Science
PhD (University of Sydney) FECSM FHEA
Lecturer in Sexual Health and Consultant
Bloom Hospital
Chennai, Tamil Nadu, India

Yasodhara Pallam Reddy MD
Senior Consultant
Sri Durga Hospital and Brain Centre
Nellore, Andhra Pradesh, India

Foreword

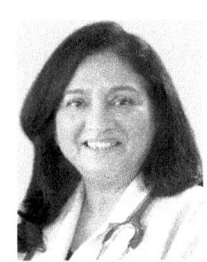

My heartiest congratulations to Dr Apoorva Pallam Reddy and Dr Rajeev Agarwal for coming out with this one of a kind algorithm-based practice-oriented book—*Decision Making in Infertility*. I have complete faith that this will come in handy at all levels of infertility practice. Incredibly, practical topics are presented by the authors who know the pulse of the average Indian practitioner. Largely the book deals with almost every challenge, one can face in managing an infertile couple. The lucid way of writing and the practical tips and tricks make this book a must read for all. I am sure that the readers will be very happy to possess this little endeavor and find it extremely beneficial in their day-to-day practice.

Jaideep Malhotra MD FICOG FMAS FICS FRCOG FRCPI
President ISAR, 2019-2020

Preface

I am still learning
—Michelangelo, at the age of 87

Learning is a never-ending endeavor and even more so for a fertility specialist. The field of infertility is ever changing and the percentage of couples approaching us for fertility management is only increasing with time. Over the past few decades, there has been a tremendous progress in the field of fertility with consistent increase in the pregnancy rates owing to emerging cutting edge technology as well as evidence-based management. Despite there being a surge in the number of books, articles, and literature available over fertility management, long chapters can sometimes be complicated, and very often are not able to provide a step-by-step approach that gives concise and practical perspective to fertility management.

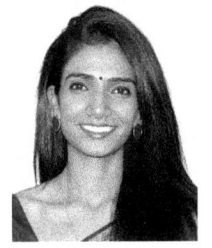

When Shri Jitendar P Vij (Group Chairman) of M/s Jaypee Brothers Medical Publishers (P) Ltd, New Delhi, India approached us for revamping a book on algorithms, which was originally edited by Professor Alan De Churney, it seemed like a herculean task to put forward over one hundred algorithms on infertility. But we realized, that a book like that, is definitely the need of the hour. Thus, began the journey of this baby—*Decision Making in Infertility*. We requested over 70 experts to create a step-by-step approach to fertility management from something as basic as evaluation to something as advanced as genetic evaluation which were subsequently edited into algorithms. All the chapters are written in a format of one page algorithm that catalogs the line of action and one page text, elaborating the algorithm. This simple format makes this book as an excellent choice as a ready reckoner for practicing fertility specialists of all spectrums. The beauty of the book also lies in its crisp, clear cut, and extremely practical approach.

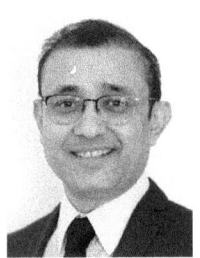

We, along with all the contributors have curated this book with evidence, experience, expertise, and, more importantly, with love. We truly hope you enjoy reading this as much as we enjoyed compiling it.

Happy Learning!!

Apoorva Pallam Reddy
Rajeev Agarwal

Acknowledgments

We sincerely thank Dr Shilpa T, Consultant Radiologist, Prima Diagnostics, Jayanagar, Bengaluru, Karnataka, India for her immense contribution to the radiological images in the book.

We greatly appreciate and thank Ms Jyotirmayi, Ms Jaya, Mr CB Tiwari, Ms Sujatha Manda, Dr Gunjan, Dr Sumera, Ms Shobha, Ms Nandini, Team Care IVF and Team Phoenix Speciality Clinic for their extended support through the entire process of compiling this book.

Lastly, we would like to thank Shri Jitendar P Vij (Group Chairman), Mr Ankit Vij (Managing Director), Ms Chetna Malhotra Vohra (Associate Director—Content Strategy), Dr Savleen Kaur (Development Editor) and the staff of M/s Jaypee Brothers Medical Publishers (P) Ltd, New Delhi, India, for their untiring support.

Contents

SECTION 1: EPIDEMIOLOGY OF INFERTILITY

1. History Taking for an Infertile Couple   3
   Damodar

1B. History Taking for an Infertile Couple- Past Fertility Treatment   6
   Rajeev Agarwal, Apoorva Pallam Reddy

2. Evaluation of Infertility: Female Factors   8
   Ashish Kale, Ashwini Kale

SECTION 2: AMENORRHEA

3. Primary Amenorrhea   10
   Kundan Ingale

4. Secondary Amenorrhea   12
   Kundan Ingale

SECTION 3: OVARIAN FACTORS

5. Ovarian Factor: Evaluation   16
   Kundan Ingale

6. Ovarian Reserve Testing   18
   Apoorva Pallam Reddy, Rajeev Agarwal

SECTION 4: USG IN FERTILITY

7. Role of Ultrasonography in Fertility   22
   Sonal Panchal, Chaitanya Nagori

SECTION 5: ENDOSCOPY IN REPRODUCTIVE SURGERY

8. Laparoscopy: Role in Infertility   26
   Malvika Sabarwal, Shivani Sabharwal, Nupur Chhabra

9. Hysteroscopy: Role in Infertility   28
   Rahul Manchanda, Richa Sharma

SECTION 6: UTERINE FACTORS

10. Uterine Factor Evaluation   33
    Kishore Pandit, Apoorva Pallam Reddy

11. **Endometritis** — 34
    Kishore Pandit

12. **Uterine Anomalies (Müllerian Duct Anomalies)** — 36
    Smita Jain, Meenu Agarwal

13. **Septate Uterus** — 38
    Meenu Agarwal, Sandhya Meshram

14. **Uterine Polyps** — 40
    Sandhya Meshram, Meenu Agarwal

15. **Asherman Syndrome** — 43
    Bimal John

SECTION 7: TUBAL FACTORS

16. **Tubal Evaluation: When and How** — 48
    Ankita Kaushal, Rajeev Agarwal

17. **Role of Tubal Surgery: Tubal Disease** — 50
    Mrugesh Patel

18. **Role of Tubal Surgery: Tubal Re-anastomosis** — 52
    Mrugesh Patel, Apoorva Pallam Reddy

SECTION 8: ENDOCRINE FACTORS

19. **PCOS and Infertility** — 56
    Diksha Goswami

20. **Thyroid Disorders** — 58
    Diksha Goswami

21. **Hirsutism** — 60
    Shally Gupta

22. **Galactorrhea** — 62
    Ruby Ruprai, Chetan Kaur Ruprai

23. **Hyperprolactinemia** — 64
    Ruby Ruprai, Sejal Desai

SECTION 9: CONTROLLED OVARIAN STIMULATION

24. **Ovulation Induction: Oral Ovulogens** — 68
    Yasodhara Pallam Reddy, Apoorva Pallam Reddy

25. **Ovulation Induction: Gonadotropins** — 70
    Hrishikesh Pai, Apoorva Pallam Reddy

26. **Ovulation Induction: Adjuvants in Polycystic Ovarian Syndrome** — 72
    Bhavana Mittal, Poonam Goyal

27. **Ovulation Induction: Adjuvants in Poor Ovarian Reserve** *Rajeev Agarwal, Apoorva Pallam Reddy*	74

SECTION 10: ENDOMETRIOSIS AND FIBROIDS

28. **Endometriosis: Etiology of Infertility in Endometriosis** *Indranil Dutta*	79
29. **Endometriosis: Diagnosis** *Indranil Dutta*	80
30. **Endometriosis: Laparoscopy Staging** *Priyankur Roy, Shaheen Hokabaj*	82
31. **Endometriosis: Fertility Index Staging** *Fessy Louise T, Aparna*	84
32. **Endometriosis and ART** *Shaweez Faizi, Pratap Kumar*	86
33. **Endometriosis: Role of Endoscopy** *Priyanka Pipara, Bhaskar Pal*	88
34. **Endoscopy for Ovarian Endometrioma** *Apoorva Pallam Reddy, Aruna Siddharth*	90
35. **Fibroids in Infertility** *Jiteeka Thakkar, Nandita Palshetkar*	92
36. **Adenomyosis and Infertility** *Basab Mukherjee, Anurag Mallick*	94

SECTION 11: INFECTION IN INFERTILITY

37. **Vaginal Infections** *Shally Gupta*	98
38. **Pelvic Tuberculosis- Diagnosis** *Sonia Malik, Vandana Bhatia*	100
39. **Pelvic Tuberculosis- Management** *Sonia Malik, Vandana Bhatia*	102

SECTION 12: POOR OVARIAN RESPONSE

40. **Poor Ovarian Response: Diagnosis** *Nayana Patel, Molina Patel*	106
41. **Poor Ovarian Response: Medical Management** *Nayana Patel, Molina Patel*	108
42. **Newer Modalities to Improve Poor Ovarian Response** *Nayana Patel, Molina Patel*	110

SECTION 13: ANDROLOGY: A GYNECOLOGIST'S VIEW

43. **Evaluation of the Male Infertility Factors** — 112
    Sunil Jindal, Anshu Jindal

44. **Interpretation of Semen Analysis- Macroscopic Parameters** — 114
    Aditi Kanungo, Rajeev Agarwal, Apoorva Pallam Reddy

45. **Interpretation of Semen Analysis- Microscopic Parameters** — 116
    Aditi Kanungo, Rajeev Agarwal, Siddharth

46. **Male Hypogonadism** — 118
    Sunil Jindal, Anshu Jindal

47. **Azoospermia: Evaluation** — 121
    KK Gopinathan, Parasuram Gopinath

48. **Anejaculation** — 124
    Neharika Malhotra Bora, Chand Mohammad

49. **Genetic Evaluation of the Infertile Male** — 126
    Kamini Patel, Vani Patel

50. **Sperm Deoxyribonucleic Acid Fragmentation** — 128
    Saroj Agarwal, Rajeev Agarwal

51. **Varicocele and Male Infertility** — 130
    Suchetna Sengupta, Rajeev Agarwal

SECTION 14: INTRAUTERINE INSEMINATION

52. **Ovulation Induction in IUI—Oral Ovulogens** — 134
    Bebu Seema Pandey, Apoorva Pallam Reddy

53. **Ovulation Induction in IUI—Gonadotropins** — 136
    Sheetal Sawankar, Pinky R Shah

54. **Follicular Monitoring in IUI** — 140
    Shilpa A Reddy

55. **Doppler in Follicular Monitoring** — 142
    Rishab Bora, Jaideep Malhotra

56. **Doppler in Endometrium Evaluation** — 144
    Rishab Bora, Jaideep Malhotra

57. **Ovulation Trigger in IUI** — 146
    Meenu Handa

58. **10 Steps to Successful IUI** — 148
    Apoorva Pallam Reddy, Rajeev Agarwal

59. **Artificial Insemination: Donor** — 150
    Dorothy P Ghosh, Rakhi Singh

60. **Luteal Phase Support in IUI** — 152
    Apoorva Pallam Reddy, Rajeev Agarwal

SECTION 15: IN VITRO FERTILIZATION

61. **Indications for In Vitro Fertilization-Male Factor** — 157
    Venu Gopal M, Simi Fabian

62. **Indications for In Vitro Fertilization-Female Factor** — 158
    Venu Gopal M, Simi Fabian

63. **Indications for ART—Unexplained and Emerging Factors** — 159
    Venu Gopal M, Simi Fabian

64. **Pre-IVF Evaluation** — 160
    Venu Gopal M, Simi Fabian

65. **Individualized Controlled Ovarian Stimulation** — 162
    Apoorva Pallam Reddy, Nandita Palshetkar

66. **Ovulation Induction in Assisted Reproductive Technique: Agonist Protocols** — 164
    Rohan Palshetkar, Biswanath Ghosh Dastidar, Nandita Palshetkar

67. **Ovulation Induction in Assisted Reproductive Technique: Antagonist Protocols** — 166
    Rohan Palshetkar, Biswanath Ghosh Dastidar

68. **Controlled Ovarian Stimulation in Assisted Reproductive Technique** — 168
    Apoorva Pallam Reddy, Kathyaini VS

69. **Mild Ovarian Stimulation** — 170
    Aswathy Kumaran, Pratap Kumar

70. **Role of LH in Controlled Ovarian Stimulation** — 172
    Sankalp Singh, Vandana Ramanathan

71. **Triggers for Ovarian Stimulation: IVF** — 174
    Meenu Handa

72. **Oocyte Pickup** — 177
    Aditya Khurd, Vandana Khurd

73. **Embryo Transfer** — 181
    Parasuram Gopinath, Kartika D Kumar

74. **Luteal Phase Support in IVF** — 185
    Aarti Deendayal, Hema Desai

75A. **Diagnosis of Ovarian Hyperstimulation Syndrome** — 188
    Kavitha Gautham

75B. **Management of Ovarian Hyperstimulation Syndrome** — 190
    Apoorva Pallam Reddy, Rajeev Agarwal

76A. **Batch In Vitro Fertilization** — 192
    Parikshit Tank, Jaydeep Tank

76B. **Cycle Preparation for Batching Embryo Transfer** — 193
    Apoorva Pallam Reddy, Rajeev Agarwal

77. **Endometrial Preparation for FET: Natural Cycle** — 194
    Apoorva Pallam Reddy, Mithila Mahesh

78. **Endometrial Preparation for FET: Hormonal Replacement Therapy** — 196
Ritu Hinduja, Nikita Banerjee

79. **Oocyte Donor Recruitment Protocol** — 198
Neelam Bhise, Sushma Mandava

80. **Oocyte Donor Controlled Ovarian Stimulation** — 200
Neelam Bhise, Sushma Mandava

SECTION 16: SPERM PREPARATION TECHNIQUES

81. **Sperm Preparation for Assisted Reproduction Techniques** — 202
Saroj Agarwal, Rajeev Agarwal

82. **Advanced Sperm Preparation** — 204
Saroj Agarwal, Rajeev Agarwal

83. **Sperm Retrieval Techniques** — 206
Dorothy P Ghosh, Apoorva Pallam Reddy, Rajeev Agarwal

SECTION 17: ADVANCES IN ART

84. **Assisted Hatching Indications—Technique** — 210
Sujatha Ramakrishna

85. **Endometrial Receptivity Array/Analysis** — 214
Swarnima Das, Rajeev Agarwal

86. **PGT and PGD** — 218
Keshav Malhotra, Neharika Malhotra Bora

87. **Time-lapse Imaging of Preimplantation Embryos** — 222
Shubhashree Uppangala, Pratap Kumar, Satish Kumar Adiga

SECTION 18: DIFFICULT SCENARIOS

88. **Recurrent Implantation Failure** — 227
Divyashree PS, Surbhi Gupta

88A. **Recurrent Implantation Failure: Evaluation** — 228
Divyashree PS, Surbhi Gupta

88B. **Management of Recurrent Implantation Failure** — 230
Divyashree PS, Surbhi Gupta

89. **Recurrent Pregnancy Loss: Management** — 234
Kamini Patel, Vani Patel

90. **Thin Endometrium** — 237
Pratik Tambe, Apoorva Pallam Reddy

91. **Empty Follicular Syndrome** — 240
Kedar Ganla, Priyanka Vora, Rana Choudhary

SECTION 19: PREGNANCY IN ART

92. Ectopic Pregnancy- Diagnosis — 245
Astha Ubeja, Neharika Malhotra Bora

92A. Ectopic Pregnancy: Surgical Management — 248
Narendra Malhotra, Apoorva Pallam Reddy

92B. Ectopic Pregnancy: Medical Management — 250
Apoorva Pallam Reddy, Aruna Siddharth

93. Fetal Reduction — 252
Meenu Batra

SECTION 20: OTHER FACTORS IN ART

94. Unconsummated Marriage — 256
Vijayasarathi Ramanathan

95. Male Sexual Dysfunction — 258
Vijayasarathi Ramanathan

96. Failure to Respond to Gonadotropins — 260
Kedar Ganla, Priyanka Vora, Rana Choudhary

97. Unruptured Follicular Syndrome — 264
Kedar Ganla, Rana Choudhary, Priyanka Vora

98. Diet and Lifestyle in Infertility — 267
Prashanth K Adiga, Anjali M

99. Endometrial Scratching — 270
Kanti Bansal, Meenu Handa

100. Medical Management of Oligoasthenoteratozoospermia — 272
Kedar Ganla, Rana Choudharay, Priyanka Vora

Bibliography — 275

Index — 291

SECTION 1

Epidemiology of Infertility

- History Taking for an Infertile Couple
- History Taking for an Infertile Couple- Past Fertility Treatment
- Evaluation of Infertility: Female Factors

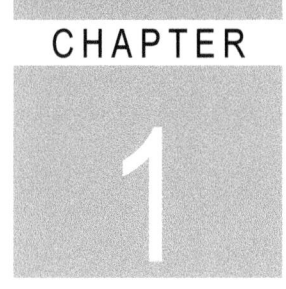

CHAPTER 1

History Taking for an Infertile Couple

Damodar

EPIDEMIOLOGICAL FACTORS

Historical Clues

A detailed history is the first step for evaluation of fertility in a couple. Although it is recommended to investigate, if couples fail to achieve a successful pregnancy after 12 months of regular unprotected intercourse or after 6 months for couples with the female partner age more than 35 years old, with the rise in concept of preconception care, any couple seeking fertility may be evaluated for fertility potential.

The relevant reproductive history should include:

A. *Coital frequency and timing:* Of late, it is not uncommon to see a couple who have not consummated their marriage. Coital frequency and difficulties encountered like dyspareunia, erectile dysfunction, premature ejaculation, inability to ejaculate in the vagina, etc. should be evaluated. In subfertile couples, instructions are usually given for intercourse every other day during the week surrounding ovulation.

B. *Duration of infertility and previous fertility:* Duration of infertility influences the pace and extent of evaluation in infertile couples. Any couple who has not conceived in 1 year of unprotected intercourse requires evaluation or even earlier if either of the couple has a known reproductive cause leading to infertility. Previous fertility does not exclude the possibility of newly acquired secondary male and female infertility factor. The success rate of any fertility treatment is inversely proportional to the duration of infertility.

C. *Impact of age:* Age affects women more harshly than men. The risk of infertility increases with the growing age. Pregnancy before 30 years for women and 35 years for men has more chance of success.

D. *Menstrual history:* Age at menarche, cycle length and characteristics, presence of molimina, and onset/severity of dysmenorrhea give us an insight into conditions like endometriosis, polycystic ovary syndrome (PCOS), luteal phase defect, etc.

E. *Previous methods of contraception:* Conception rates are reduced during the first 2 months after stopping oral contraceptive pills, and the median delay prior to conception is approximately 3 months. This delay is shorter for nulligravid women. Most women (94.3) become pregnant within 2 years of stopping the pill. History of infection post Cu-T use may rise concerns of pelvic inflammatory disease.

F. *Childhood illness and developmental history:* Undescended testicles, varicoceles, mumps hernia, accidental damage, serious illness or surgery may affect male infertility. The reasons for male infertility include unusual characteristics of semen, reproductive infection and disorder, and erectile dysfunction or ejaculation disorder.

G. *Medical and systemic illness:* Systemic illnesses such as diabetes mellitus, thyroid, epilepsy, and systemic lupus erythematosus (SLE) cause infertility and influence reproductive outcome. Testicular function and spermatogenesis especially sperm quality and sperm motility are affected in both type 1 and type 2 diabetic men. SLE affects multiple systems that affect fertility in men and women. Genital tract may be affected by cytotoxic treatment due to the disease activity. Fertility problems such as unsuccessful implantation are encountered.

H. *Previous surgery:* History of pelvic or abdominal surgery, the route of surgery (laparotomy/laparoscopy), and site of surgery (ovary/uterus/vagina) influence current reproductive status. The incidence of injury to vas deferens during inguinal herniorrhaphy has been estimated to be 0.3% in adults, thus may contribute to infertility in some men. Literature shows that bilateral inguinal herniorrhaphies in female children also have had the consequence of accidental tubal ligation that had led to infertility in future.

I. *Medications and allergies:* The patient's medical history can identify risk factors and behaviors of lifestyles that could have significant impact on male infertility. The medical history should include—(1) complete review of systems and (2) family reproductive history. Drugs such as antivertigo agents tend to cause dryness of mouth and therefore are likely to affect cervical mucus also. Drugs affecting male infertility include those used to treat ulcers or gout, which interfere with sperm production; some antidepressants which may cause erection difficulties; beta blockers used to control blood pressure cause impotence and decreased sperm counts and motility.

J. *Exposure to gonad toxins:* Any past or current use of anabolic steroids, recreational drugs, tobacco and alcohol including environmental and chemical toxins and heat. Cocaine and cannabis lower testosterone levels and lead to low sperm count and decrease sperm motility.

K. *Impact of smoking and alcohol consumption:* Meta-analyses have shown that 40% of infertile men are smokers. In men who smoke and drink, the number and motility of sperms decrease; sperm permeability is reduced and the number of sperms with abnormal appearance increases reducing their ability to fertilize eggs. There are no safe levels for smoking and drinking in men planning for fertility.

L. *Impact of cell phone and laptop use:* Mobile and laptop devices emit radiofrequency electromagnetic waves that can reduce sperm quality and disrupt the normal function of the body. Since testicles are shallow organs, these may absorb the radiant energy more than other organs. Oxidative stress (OS) is developed in testicles because cell phones cause free radicals in sperm. OS is a major cause of infertility in men.

M. *Impact of immune responses:* Immunological factors play an important role in sexual problems such as recurrent miscarriage, infertility, and implantation failure. Natural killer (NK) cells play an important role in female sexual function. These cells are correlated with inductive failures such as NK cell cytotoxicity induced abortion or infertility.

N. *Sexual history and sexual violence:* Untreated *sexually transmitted infections (STIs)* are among the factors that cause damage to the reproductive system of men and women. Chlamydia and gonorrhea are the most common STIs that lead to infertility in men and women. As chlamydia is asymptomatic, it is difficult to identify it earlier and treat. Trachoma can affect the sperm function. In vitro experiments show that *Chlamydia trachomatis* tyrosine phosphorylation affects sperm proteins, causes sperm premature death, and develops an apoptosis-like reaction in sperms which increases sperm surface fragmentation levels. Studies show that the *history of sexual violence* is associated with infertility. The psychological trauma caused by sexual violence leads to ovulation infertility or sexual dysfunction.

O. *Obesity:* Researchers have found that obese women with high visceral fat have low chance of successful infertility treatment. In women with body mass index (BMI) more than 25 compared with BMI less than 25, the pregnancy rates were 10.5% and 25.3%, respectively. Some studies show that 30–70% of women with PCOS are obese.

P. *Impact of stress and anxiety:* Stress adversely affects both male and female reproductive abilities. The anxiety may decrease the intimacy between partners and avoid the sexual behavior. Unmatched working schedules might also reduce sexual frequency between couples.

Q. *Effects of nutrition:* A high saturated fat diet is associated with reduced sperm concentration. Severe calorie restriction, malnutrition, and vigorous exercise regimens in women are associated with reduced pregnancy rates.

History Taking for an Infertile Couple

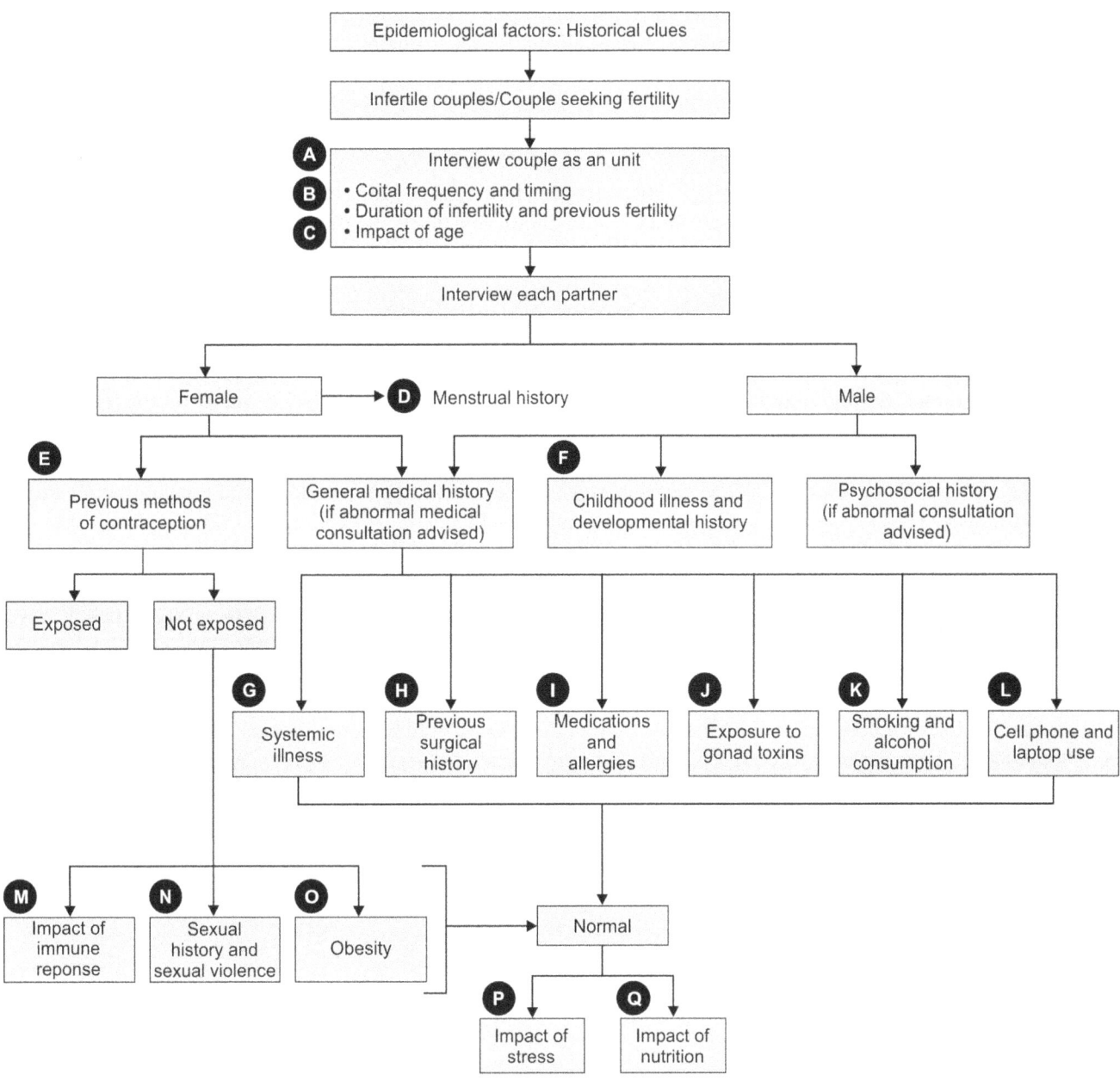

CHAPTER 1B

History Taking for an Infertile Couple- Past Fertility Treatment

Rajeev Agarwal, Apoorva Pallam Reddy

A. Past history of fertility treatment not only acts as source of the patient's response to a particular therapy or medication but also as a valuable information as to how to proceed ahead. The history helps you in planning ahead. In women who have had only ovulation induction, the medication used, patient response for the same, follicular study documenting ovulation, compliance of couple to have intercourse on the fertile days, etc. should be noted.

B. If intrauterine insemination (IUI) was done earlier, then the following details should be the type of ovulogen used, the dose of ovulogen or gonadotropins (GT) used, day of ovulation, tubal patency test, endometrial thickness, single/double IUI, method of preparation, sperm count post-wash, luteal phase support, etc.

C. The total number of IUI done is also important because the success of IUI significantly reduces after 4–6 cycles. The stimulation protocol also influences the pregnancy rate. Hence if only oral ovulogens were used for IUI before, consider GT stimulated IUI subsequently.

D. If in vitro fertilization (IVF) was done, it helps to know in detail regarding the oocyte and embryo quality.

E. The following details should be looked into when analyzing a previous assisted reproductive technique (ART) cycle. Number of attempts has the patient had at an IVF previously, total number of fresh and frozen transfers, type of stimulation protocol used, type and dose of gonadotropin used days of stimulation before oocyte pickup (OPU), peak estrogen and progesterone value on day of human chorionic gonadotropin (hCG), number of oocytes recovered, number of metaphase II (MII) type of sperm used (husband's ejaculated/extracted sperm/donor), fertilization rate, cleavage rate, grades of embryo (D3/D5) cleavage stage or blastocyst, type of endometrial preparation for frozen embryo transfer (FET) cycle and finally outcome of transfer—Biochemical/Clinical/Abortion/live birth/multiple pregnancy.

F. *Improving the uterine factor:* If hysteroscopy was done, review the video if available. Pelvic tuberculosis is very common in our country; see if that was evaluated. Five percent of women may need a personalized day of transfer and endometrial receptivity array can help determine that. Some of the centers routinely performs scratching the endometrial lining in the luteal phase to improve implantation.

G. If the DNA fragmentation is high, then better fertilization is achieved by using testicular sperms. Microfluidics can help sort out highly motile sperms with the assumption that those would be better sperms.

H. Aneuploidy of the embryos can be a reason for failed implantation or biochemical pregnancy. It helps to know if the woman had a PGS or preimplantation genetic screening done before.

I. It helps to know if any established or empirical treatment has been tried for improving implantation.

History Taking for an Infertile Couple- Past Fertility Treatment

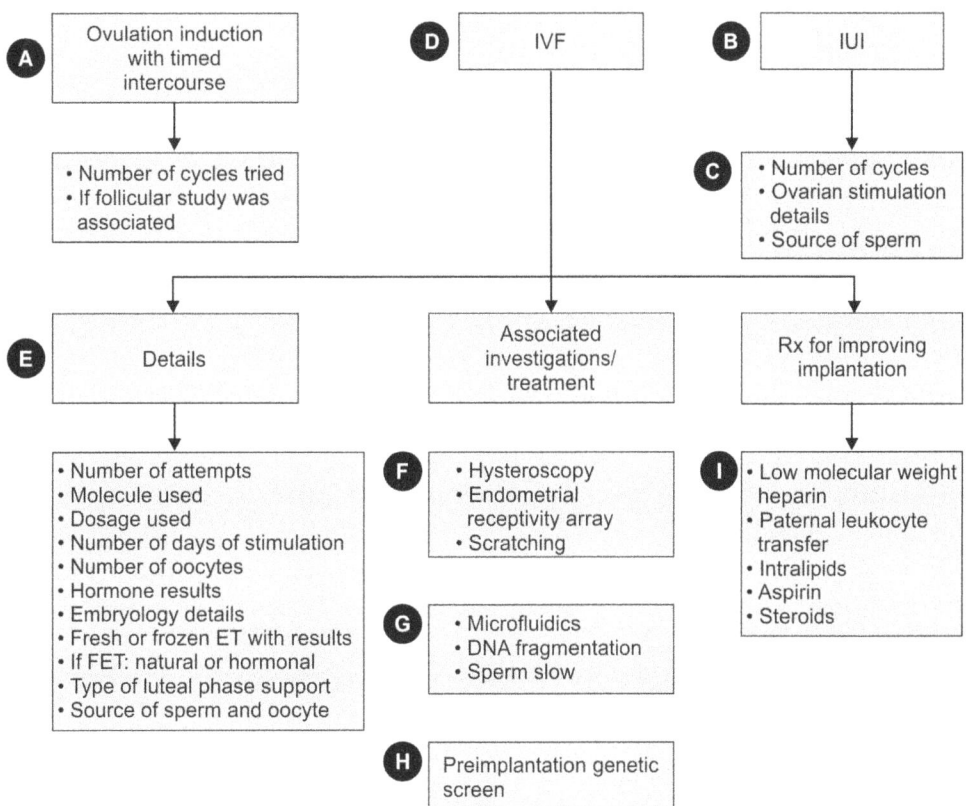

(DNA: deoxyribose nucleic acid; ET: embryo transfer; FET: frozen embryo transfer; IUI: intrauterine insemination; IVF: in vitro fertilization; Rx: treatment)

CHAPTER 2

Evaluation of Infertility: Female Factors

Ashish Kale, Ashwini Kale

The infertility evaluation includes an assessment of both the female and the male partner to discern the factors contributing to their difficulty in conceiving. The basic evaluation of female factor includes a careful history, physical examination of the female partner, investigation of four factors required from the female partner—(1) ovarian factor, (2) uterine factor, (3) tubal factor, and (4) peritoneal factor. As a part of preconception care, women should be offered rubella screening and cervical cytology. Women with polycystic ovary syndrome (PCOS) or/and obesity should be advised for diabetes screening.

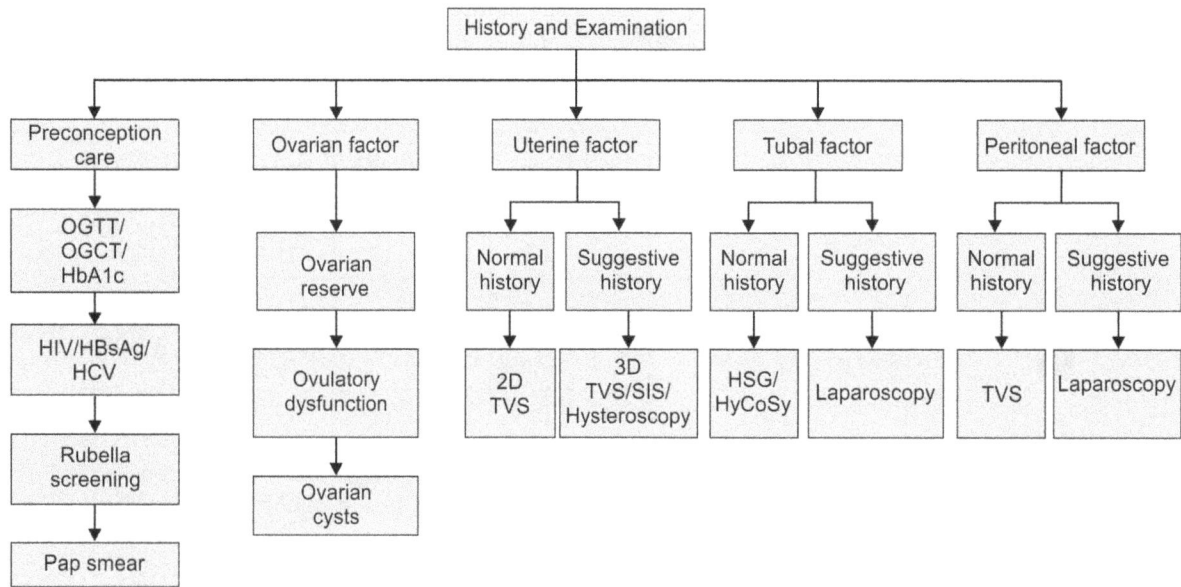

(HbA1c: hemoglobin A1c; HCV: hepatitis C virus; HIV: human immunodeficiency virus; HSG: hysterosalpingography; HyCoSy: hysterosalpingo-contrast sonography; OGCT: oral glucose challenge test; OGTT: oral glucose tolerance test; SIS: saline infusion sonography; TVS: transvaginal sonography; HBsAg: hepatitis B surface antigen)

Suggestive history: Previous surgery, endometriosis, history of pelvic inflammatory disease, k/c/o mullerian abnormality, recurrent miscarriage, dyspareunia, etc.

SECTION 2

Amenorrhea

- Primary Amenorrhea
- Secondary Amenorrhea

CHAPTER 3

Primary Amenorrhea

Kundan Ingale

A. Amenorrhea is defined as the absence of menses in a woman of reproductive age. It is classified as primary and secondary amenorrhea.
B. Primary amenorrhea is defined as an absence of secondary sexual characteristics by age 14 with no menarche or normal secondary sexual characteristics but no menarche by 16 years of age. Secondary amenorrhea is defined as the absence of menses for 3 months in a woman with previously normal menstruation, or 9 months for women with a history of oligomenorrhea.

Primary Amenorrhea

C. The first step of evaluation in primary amenorrhea is physical examination to look for presence of secondary sexual characteristics and pelvic ultrasonography (USG) to look for pelvic organ anatomy.
D. If USG suggest absence of uterus, get karyotype done. If normal karyotype (46XX), diagnosis is Müllerian agenesis. If karyotype report suggests 46XY, cause of amenorrhea is androgen insensitivity. Women with Müllerian agenesis usually have sufficient vaginal length, hence can consummate marriage, yet will not be able to conceive naturally. If the ovarian reserve is normal, self-ART (assisted reproductive technique) with transfer of embryos in a surrogate or considering uterine transplant are options.
E. Androgen insensitivity is seen in 4 per 100,000 live born females. Testes develop in the presence of the Y chromosome, but the lack of androgen receptor activity results in a typical female phenotype. However, anti-Müllerian hormone (AMH) produced by the testes, cause regression of the uterus, cervix, and proximal vagina during fetal development. Prophylactic gonadectomy is done around puberty to reduce the risk of malignancy and women supplemented with hormone replacement therapy. Hormone replacement therapy (HRT) is mainly given in the form of estrogen supplementation—the use of estradiol valerate or alternative esters is preferred over conjugated equine estrogens as the later have an increased risk of thrombosis. Dose depends on the symptomatic improvement and HRT is continued till menopausal. Oocyte donation with surrogacy is an option for women desiring fertility.
F. In the presence of uterus on USG, evaluation of hormonal assays like follicle-stimulating hormone (FSH) and luteinizing hormone (LH) is suggested. If FSH and LH both are low, it is a case of hypogonadotropic hypogonadism. In that case, there is a possibility of either constitutional delay. Sometimes amenorrhea is due to functional delay in conditions like stress, athletes, excessive exercise, etc. If no abnormality is found, give gonadotropin-releasing hormone agonists (GnRHa) challenge test to rule out primary GnRH deficiency. In case of hypogonadotropic hypogonadism, ovarian stimulation can be achieved by using both FSH and LH preparation in combination [either human menopausal gonadotropin (HMG) preparations or rFSH + rLH].
G. If FSH and LH are normal, rule out congenital developmental defects like transverse vaginal septum, imperforate hymen or vaginal agenesis or dysgenesis. In the presence of structural defects corrective surgery is performed at the earliest to prevent back flow of menstrual blood a subsequent deleterious effects. Postsurgery menstruation is established regularly and pregnancy can be tried naturally.
H. If FSH and LH are high, blood karyotype should be done. If karyotype report is 46XO, it is Turner syndrome and if it is 46XX, then it is primary ovarian failure. If diagnosed early, oocyte preservation can be attempted in Turner. Oocyte donation is considered as the final resort.

Primary Amenorrhea

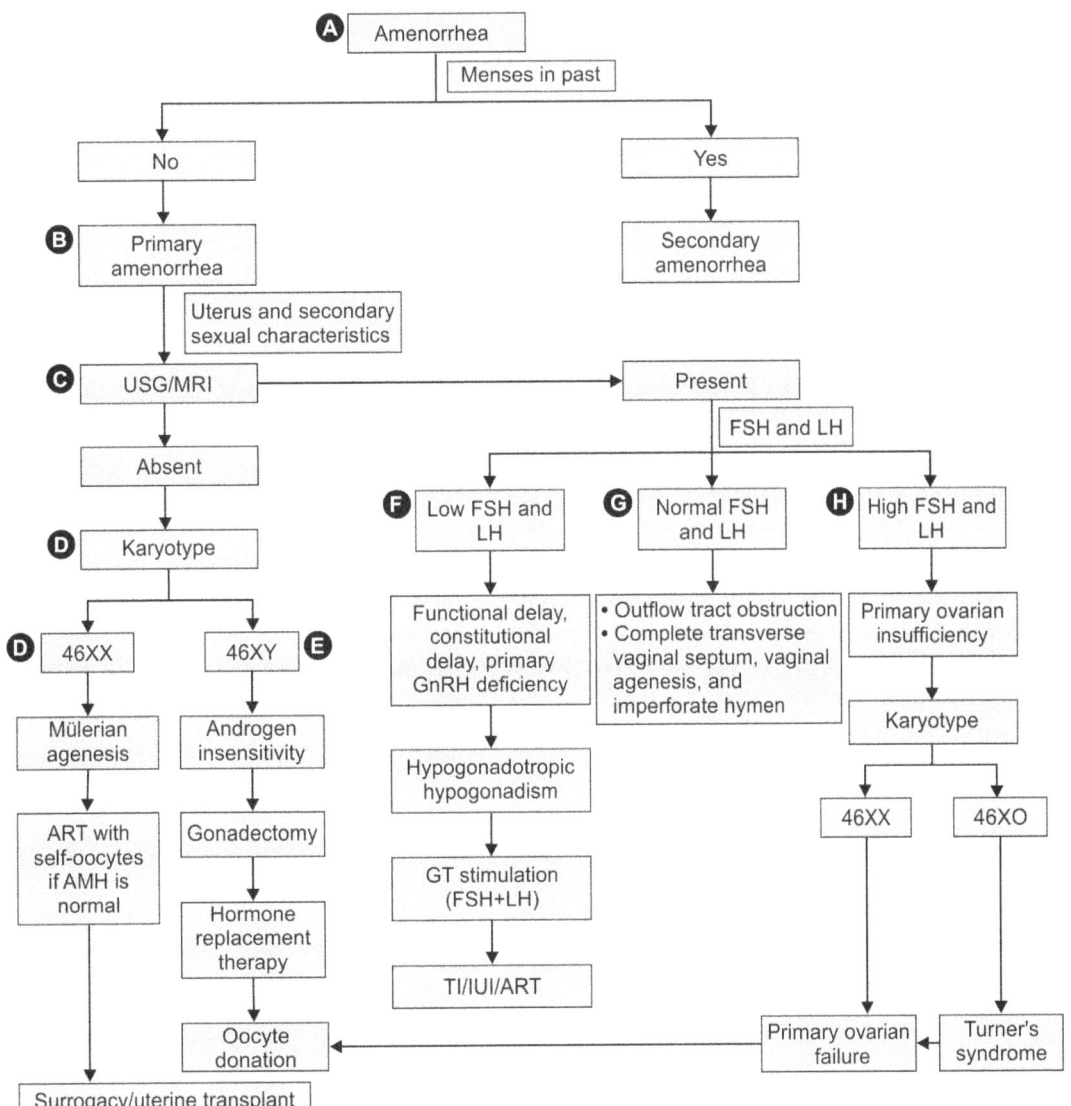

(AMH: anti-Müllerian hormone; ART: assisted reproductive technique; FSH: follicle-stimulating hormone; GnRH: gonadotropin-releasing hormone; IUI: intrauterine insemination; LH: luteinizing hormone; TI: timed intercourse; GT: gonadotropins; USG: ultrasonography; MRI: magnetic resonance imaging)
Note: As the patient is amenorrheic, serum FSH and serum LH can be done randomly at any point.

CHAPTER 4

Secondary Amenorrhea

Kundan Ingale

A. Amenorrhea is defined as the absence of menses in a woman of reproductive age. It is classified as primary and secondary amenorrhea.
B. *Secondary amenorrhea*: Women who have experienced menstruation once or more in their lifetime and are experiencing amenorrhea for more than 3 months. In a patient of secondary amenorrhea, foremost advise her for urine pregnancy rate to rule out pregnancy.
C. If urine pregnancy test (UPT) is negative, she is asked to take progesterone supplement (20 mg of medroxyprogesterone acetate) for 5 days to confirm withdrawal bleeding. If withdrawal bleeding is seen then amenorrhea is due to anovulation.
D. If there is no withdrawal bleeding and endometrial thickness is thin, ask her to take cyclical estrogen and progesterone for 28 days. If there is no menses following hormone replacement therapy, then the cause of amenorrhea is most likely endometrial disease like Asherman syndrome for which hysteroscopy should be done.
E. If there is withdrawal bleeding after either progesterone or estrogen-progesterone, she is advised to undergo hormonal assays like follicle-stimulating hormone (FSH), luteinizing hormone (LH), thyroid-stimulating hormone (TSH) and prolactin (PRL).
F. If FSH and LH are high, (FSH > 25 IU/mL, LH > 25 IU/mL) quiet likely that she has premature ovarian failure.
G. If FSH is normal or low but LH is high and on ultrasonography (USG), there is presence of multiple antral follicles (>12 in each ovary) with she is diagnosed to have anovulation due to polycystic ovarian syndrome. Look for signs of hyperandrogenemia too. If serum TSH is high and serum-free T4 is low, she has most likely amenorrhea due to hypothyroidism. Ovulatory dysfunction is found in both, hypothyroidism as well as hyperthyroidism. Hyperprolactinemia is diagnosed if serum prolactin level is more than 26 ng/mL. High prolactin affects estrogen and testosterone. If prolactin levels are more than 100 ng/mL, rule out pituitary macroadenoma by MRI brain. If there are signs of hyperandrogenemia with normal FSH and LH, check for 17-hydroxyprogesterone, which is elevated in late onset adrenal hyperplasia.

Secondary Amenorrhea

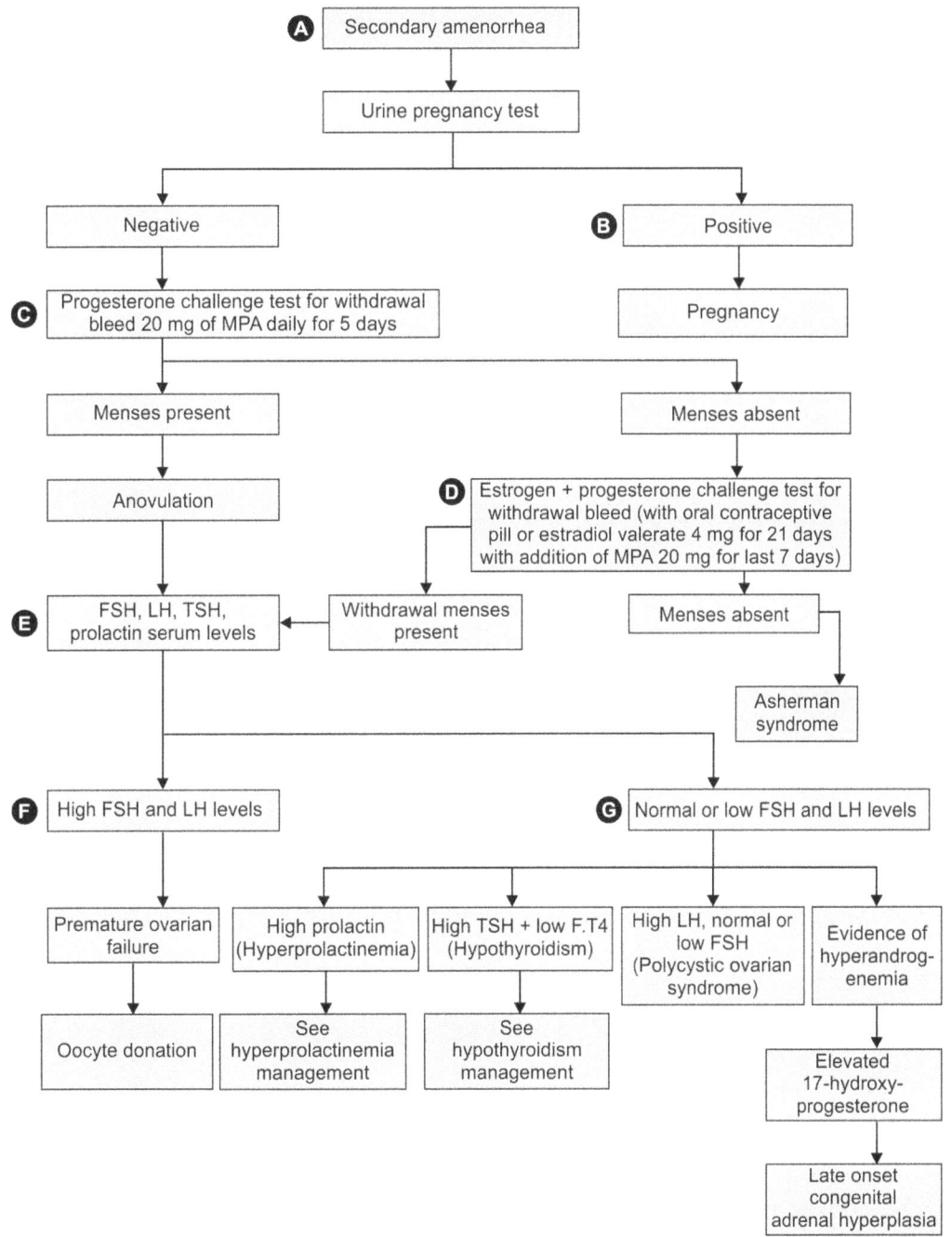

(FSH: follicle-stimulating hormone; LH: luteinizing hormone; TSH: thyroid-stimulating hormone; MPA: medroxyprogesterone acetate)

SECTION 3

Ovarian Factors

- Ovarian Factor: Evaluation
- Ovarian Reserve Testing

CHAPTER 5

Ovarian Factor: Evaluation

Kundan Ingale

A. Of the four factors contributing to conception in the female partner (ovary, tube, uterus and pelvic factors), the female gonad—ovary plays a key role as it stores all the oocytes required for fertility. The ovary can cause infertility in the women on three fronts—(1) Reduction in the number of oogonia and their quality—diminished ovarian reserve, (2) Ovulatory dysfunction—inability of the ovary to respond to hypothalamic-pituitary-ovarian (HPO) axis and failure of ovulation, (3) Ovarian tumors— cysts or masses hampering functionality of the ovary.

B. 25% of the couples experience difficulty in conceiving due to ovulatory dysfunction. The World Health Organization (WHO) categorizes ovulation disorders into three groups. In case of irregular menses or if there is withdrawal bleeding after progesterone, she is advised to undergo hormonal assays like follicle-stimulating hormone (FSH), luteinizing hormone (LH), thyroid-stimulating hormone (TSH), and prolactin (PRL).

C. ***Group I ovulation disorders:*** Hypogonadotropic hypogonadism caused by hypothalamic pituitary failure. This is caused due to failure of the hypothalamus to produce gonadotropin-releasing hormone (GnRH) agonists or failure of pituitary to release FSH and LH resulting in prolonged suppression of the ovary and anovulation. Typically, women present with amenorrhea (primary or secondary) which is characterized by low gonadotropins (FSH < 1 IU/mL LH < 1 IU/mL) and estrogen deficiency (<40 pg/mL). Approximately 10% of women with ovulation disorders have a group I ovulation disorder. Ovulation induction can be achieved by pulsatile gonadotropin-releasing hormone or using both FSH and LH.

D. ***Group II ovulation disorders*** are defined as dysfunctions of the hypothalamic-pituitary-ovarian axis. This constitutes polycystic ovary syndrome majorly and hyperprolactinemic amenorrhea. Around 85% of women with ovulation disorders have a group II ovulation disorder. FSH is normal or low but LH is high and on ultrasonography, there is increase in the number of antral follicles (>12 in each ovary). Look for signs of hyperandrogenemia too. Insulin resistance is present in 20–30% of lean polycystic ovary syndrome (PCOS) patients and 70–80% in obese PCOS patients. Insulin resistance can be detected by standard 75 g 2 hour glucose tolerance test (GTT).

E. ***Group III ovulation disorders*** are caused by ovarian failure. Around 5% of women with ovulation disorders have a group III ovulation disorder. FSH and LH are high. Serum anti-Müllerian hormone (AMH) level is going to help to diagnosis of diminished ovarian reserve. Antral follicle count and AMH levels are the best predictors of ovarian reserve. Ovarian failure can happen prematurely before the age of 40 yrs or perimenopausally at 50 yrs.

F. If serum TSH is high and serum-free T4 is low, she most likely has amenorrhea due to hypothyroidism. Ovulatory dysfunction is found in both, hypothyroidism as well as hyperthyroidism. If TSH is high and free T4 is normal, it is called as subclinical hypothyroidism.

G. Hyperprolactinemia is diagnosed if serum prolactin level is more than 26 ng/mL. High prolactin affects estrogen and testosterone. If prolactin levels are more than 100 ng/mL, rule out pituitary macroadenoma by MRI brain.

H. If there are signs of hyperandrogenemia with normal FSH and LH, check for 17-hydroxyprogesterone which is elevated in late onset adrenal hyperplasia.

Ovarian Factor: Evaluation

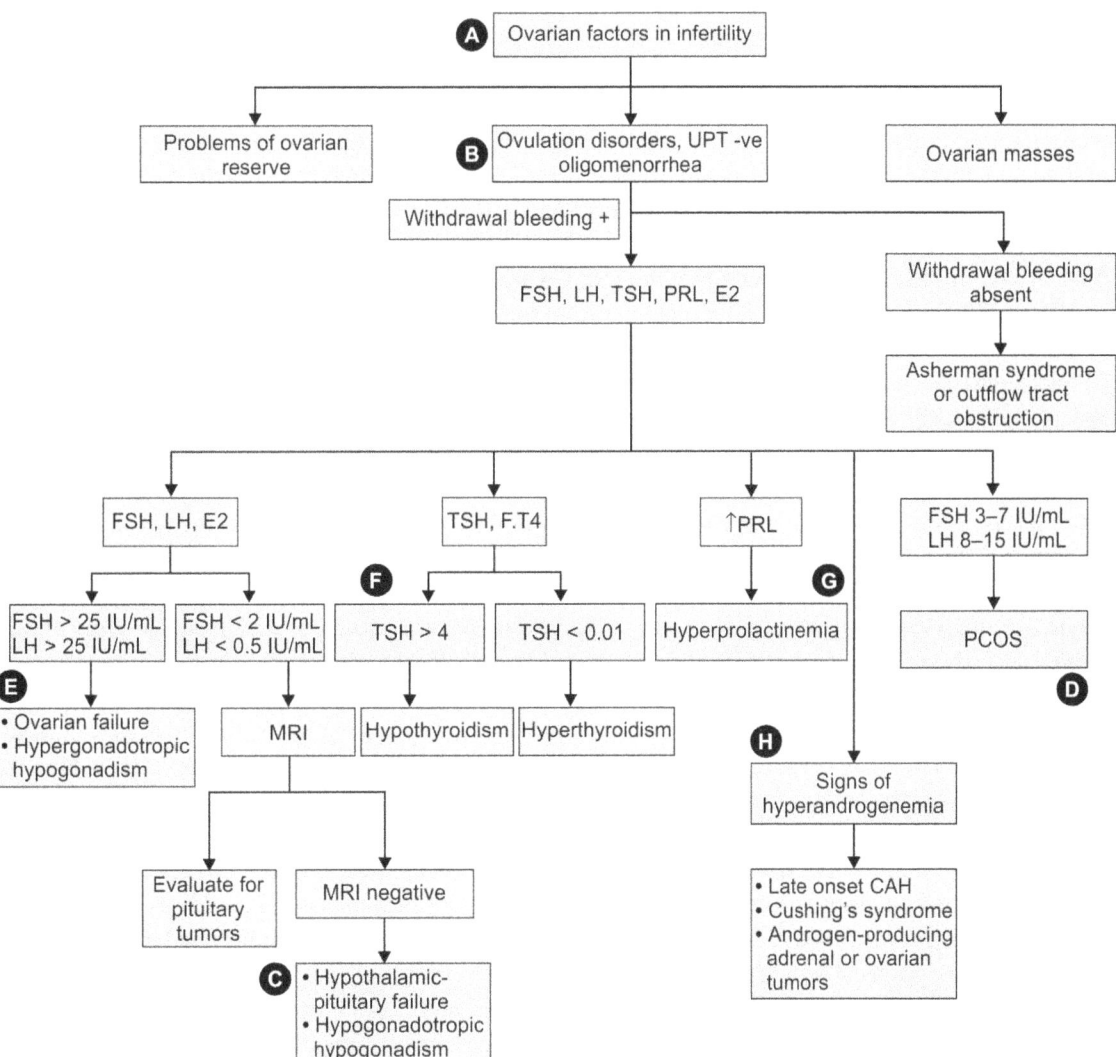

(FSH: follicle-stimulating hormone; LH: luteinizing hormone; PCOS: polycystic ovarian syndrome; TSH: thyroid-stimulating hormone; CAH: congenital adrenal hyperplasia; E2: estradiol; PRL: prolactin level; UPT: urine pregnancy test)

CHAPTER 6

Ovarian Reserve Testing

Apoorva Pallam Reddy, Rajeev Agarwal

Unlike men, women are born with a fixed number of gamets (oocytes) that keep depleting with age. Ovarian reserve is an estimate of the total number oocytes in both the ovaries at the given age. Of the various stages of oocyte development [primordial follicles, primary follicles, secondary follicles, preantral follicles, antral follicles (AFs)], only the secondary follicles, preantral follicles, and AFs are responsive to gonadotropin stimulation. Hence based on their ovarian reserve, women can be classified as normoresponders, hyper-responders, and poor responders. Decline in the number of follicles below a threshold level leads to irregular cycles, poor reproductive outcome, and ultimately menopause. However, it should be emphasized that none of the ovarian reserve tests assist in predicting the probability of ongoing pregnancy and do not shed light on the quality of the oocyte. There is no single test that can be used as the sole criterion for advising assisted reproductive therapy (ART). They probably serve as a surrogate measure to decide the need to speed up the process of conception.

A. *Age:* The fact that there is a progressive reduction in the ovarian reserve with age is well established. This results in a decline of fecundity in natural as well as stimulated ovarian cycles. However, chronological age alone is a poor predictor of individual ovarian responses. The reproductive age (based on ovarian reserve) can be completely different from the biological age (based on their year of birth). This has led to the development and use of various biochemical and biophysical markers of ovarian reserve. Women more than 35 years tend to have reduced fecundity.

B. *AMH or anti-Müllerian hormone:* AMH is a dimeric glycoprotein. As it is exclusively produced by the granulosa cells of preantral (primary and secondary) and the small AFs, it serves as a good means of evaluating the ovarian reserve. The serum levels of AMH positively correlate with basal antral follicle count (AFC) that is measured by transvaginal ultrasonography. The intracycle and intercycle variability of AMH is very less unlike other biochemical markers, making it possible to do the test on any of the cycle. The threshold for normal values is dependent on the method used for evaluation. Although there is no consensus on the cutoff to consider as a poor responder, a threshold of 0.2–1.26 ng/mL is used to classify poor responders with 80–87% sensitivity and 64–93% specificity. There is emerging evidence with the use of AMH in multiple fronts like the diagnosis of polycystic ovary syndrome (PCOS), means to assess reserve in cases with ovarian cyst where AFC cannot be assessed and ability to predict a hyper-response as well. AMH too has its limitations related to assay variability and lack of standardized international assay. The AMH values considered "normal" would also vary from age to age. In addition, there are certain biological, reproductive, and environmental factors that may cause fluctuations in the values. Occasionally, both normal women and those with diminished ovarian reserve have overlapping low to undetectable AMH values. Thus, use of AMH as routine screening tool for diminished ovarian reserve in low-risk population is not recommended. AMH is best measured on day 2–3 of menstrual cycle.

C. *Basal follicle-stimulating hormone (FSH) level on day 2 or 3 of periods:* Most commonly used method to evaluate the ovarian response for decades. Despite the easy availability, use in evaluating ovarian reserve is restricted due to a high inter- and intracycle variability and lack of universally accepted cutoff value to categorize a poor response. Ranges above 25 IU/mL are commonly considered as diagnosis for premature ovarian failure. The assessment of FSH after day 4 of cycle can give false elevations and wrong diagnosis. The usefulness of basal FSH in a general subfertile population or elevated levels in young, regularly cycling women is unclear.

D. *Antral follicle count:* The AFC is assessed by counting the number of AFs seen in both the ovaries by doing a transvaginal ultrasonography in the early follicular phase with a limited intercycle variability. AFs are defined as follicles measuring 2–10 mm on D2–D4 (day 2 to day 4) of cycle. Although both small AF measuring 2–6 mm and large AF measuring 7–10 mm are counted to give AFC, smaller AFs are considered a better predictor for true ovarian reserve. Studies have shown that, AFC of <5 and >14 are good predictors of poor response and hyper-response respectively.

E. *Ovarian volume:* Ovarian volume is calculated with the formula (D1 × D2 × D3 × 0.52 = VOL) where D1, D2, D3 are the measurements of the ovary in three dimensions. Ovarian volume less than 3 cc predicts poor ovarian response with a sensitivity of 80% and specificity of 90% with a poor positive predictive value of only 17%. With the advent of AFC, the use of ovarian volume for predicting ovarian reserve is reduced.

F. It has to be noted that none of the available tests truly determine the primordial oocyte count. When there is discordance between ovarian reserve assessed on AFC and AMH, it is prudent to take an intermediate reference value for prediction. With the use of AMH and AFC, other methods of ovarian reserve testing like dynamic tests, inhibin B, estradiol (E2), clomiphene citrate challenge test (CCCT), exogenous FSH ovarian response test (EFORT), and gonadotropin agonist stimulation test (GAST) have fallen by the wayside.

Ovarian fertility potential	pmol/L	ng/mL
Optimal fertility	28.6–48.5	4.0–68
Satisfactory fertility	15.7–28.6	2.2–4.0
Low fertility	2.2–15.7	0.3–2.2
Very low/undetectable	0.0–2.2	0.0–0.3
High level	>48.5	>6.8

Day 3 FSH level	FSH interpretation
<10	Normal FSH level. Expect a good response to ovarian stimulation.
10–12	Borderline FSH. Response to stimulation is somewhat reduced. Overall, a slightly reduced live birth rate.
13–15	Elevated FSH. Reduced ovarian reserve. Reduced response to stimulation and some reduction in embryo quality with IVF. Reduced live birth rates on the average.
16–20	Markedly elevated FSH. Marked reduction in response to stimulation and usually a further reduction in embryo quality. Low live birth rates.
>20	Very poor (or no) response to stimulation.

Test	Normal responder	High responder	Poor responder
FSH	< 10 IU		> 10 IU
AMH	1.0–3.5 ng/mL	> 3.5 ng/mL	< 1.0 ng/mL
AFC	7–20 AFC	> 20 AFC	< 5–7 AFC

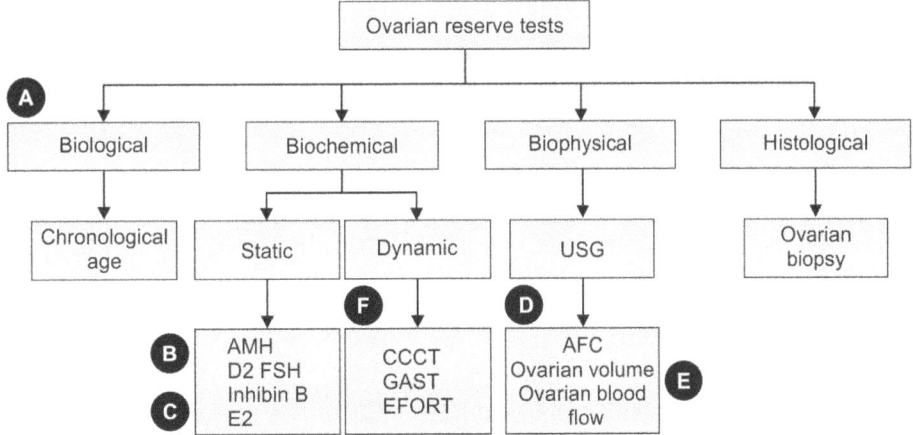

(USG: ultrasonography; AMH: anti-Müllerian hormone; FSH: follicle-stimulating hormone; CCCT: clomiphene citrate challenge test; GAST: gonadotropin agonist stimulation test; E2: estradiol; D2: day 2 of MC; AFC: antral follicle count; EFORT: exogenous FSH ovarian response test).

SECTION 4

USG in Fertility

- Role of Ultrasonography in Fertility

CHAPTER 7
Role of Ultrasonography in Fertility

Sonal Panchal, Chaitanya Nagori

A. Ultrasonography (USG) is the most commonly used instrument useful for both diagnostic and therapeutic purposes in assisted reproductive technique (ART). The use of ultrasonography in reproductive medicine is so common that it is often dubbed as the stethoscope of fertility experts. Apart from the two-dimensional (2D) sonography, addition of latest features like 3D sonography and Doppler has increased the diagnostic value of sonography making this noninvasive tool invaluable in ART.

B. Both the ovaries in the female reproductive system act as the source of oocyte at various stage of development like primordial follicle, primary follicle, secondary follicle, preantral follicle, and antral follicle. Antral follicles (2–10 mm) are responsive to the gonadotropins released by the pituitary [follicle-stimulating hormone (FSH) and luteinizing hormone (LH)] and result in the dominance of follicle before ovulation. Baseline scan on the 2nd day of the menstrual cycle is a good time to assess the antral follicle count that gives an insight into the ovarian reserve of the female partner. Large antral follicles (> 6 mm) on the D2 of the menstrual cycle are considered to result in poor quality oocytes. Any follicle more than 10 mm in size is considered as a cyst. The cyst may be a functional cyst if there is elevation in serum estradiol levels (>60 pg/mL) or a simple cyst if the serum estradiol levels are normal. Presence of a functional cyst hampers the normal development of the follicle. Hence, ovulation induction should be avoided. Small cysts (< 3 cm) that are non-functional, need not be treated as they have a potential to resolve spontaneously in subsequent months. USG is also helpful in the diagnosis of other ovarian cysts like endometriotic cyst, hemorrhagic cyst, dermoid cyst, monitoring of ovarian hyperstimulation syndrome.

C. The main role of USG in ART is monitoring the response to controlled ovarian stimulation, helps in deciding a change of protocol and accurate timing of the procedures like intrauterine insemination (IUI) or occyte pickup (OPU).

D. Ultrasonography is the basic and most preferred method of evaluation of the uterine factor (endometrial/myometrial/serosal). Multiple parameters of the endometrium can be evaluated to assess the probability of pregnancy. Presence of pathologies, like fibroids, adenomyosis, uterine anomalies, can be assessed using a simple 2D sonography. Use of a 3D sonography increases the sensitivity and specificity for detection of anomalies thus reducing the need for invasive testing. Addition of saline in the cavity (saline infusion sonography) helps in better diagnosis of intracavitary lesions polyps, adhesions, submucosal myoma, etc.

E. Healthy fallopian tubes are not visualized on USG. Infusion of saline or sono-opaque dye (Echovist) helps in establishment of tubal patency. Pathologically enlarged tubes (hydrosalpinx-fluid filled fallopian tubes or pyosalpinx-infective or pus-filled tubes or hematosalpinx-blood filled fallopian tubes can be visualized on USG and should mandatorily be followed-up with laparoscopy.

F. Introduction of transvaginal USG has been revolutionary for OPU in the field of ART prior to which OPU was done laparoscopically. Incorporating sonography guided embryo transfer (ET) has shown to significantly improve the pregnancy rate compared to blind transfer. With the onset of ART, the incidence of multiple pregnancy is rising. Use of sonography for fetal selective fetal reduction decreases the adverse effects of higher order pregnancies. For more details, see in respective chapters on OPU, ET, and fetal reduction.

Role of Ultrasonography in Fertility

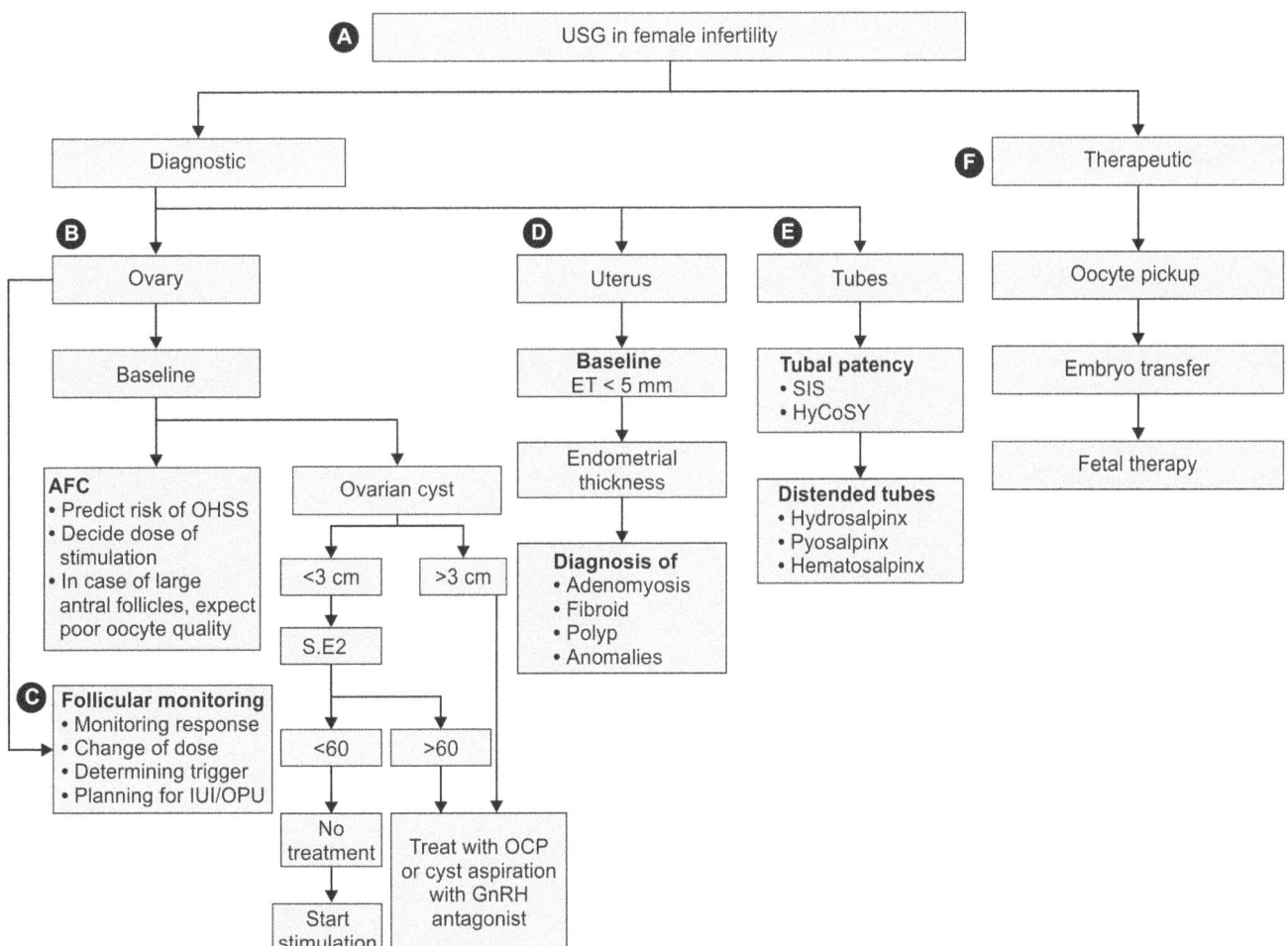

(AFC: antral follicle count; ET: embryo transfer; GnRH: gonadotropin-releasing hormone; HyCoSY: hysterosalpingo-contrast sonography; IUI: intrauterine insemination; OCP: oral contraceptive pill; OHSS: ovarian hyperstimulation syndrome; OPU: oocyte pickup; SIS: saline infusion sonography; USG: ultrasonography)

Section 4: USG in Fertility

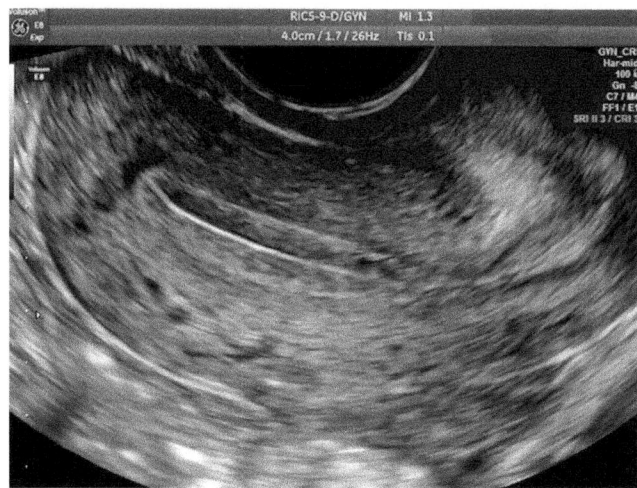
Normal uterus with trilaminar endometrium on 2D

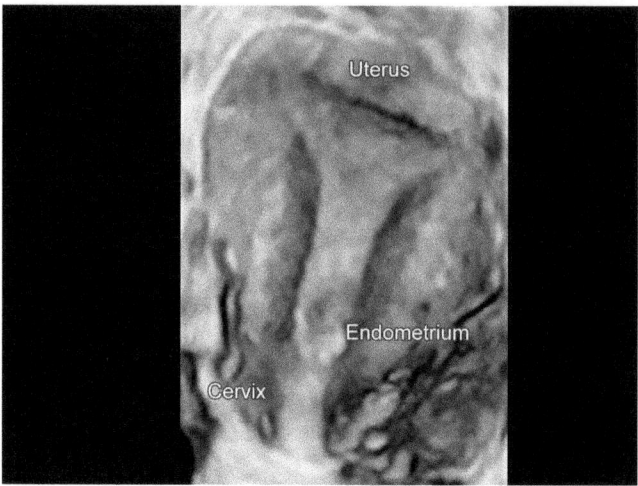
Normal uterus on 3D

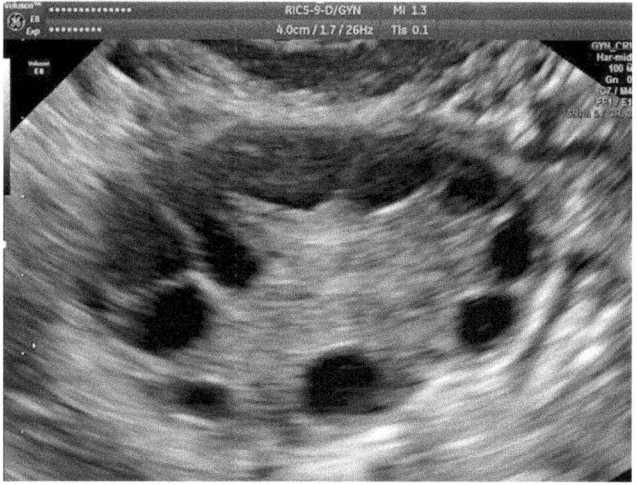
Polycystic ovary on 2D

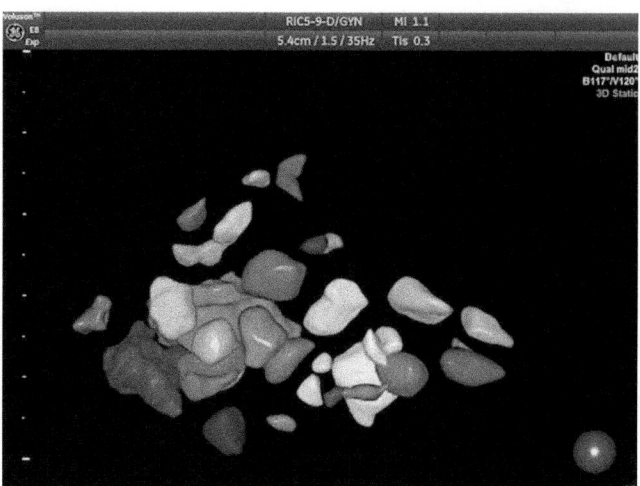
Polycystic ovary on sonovac

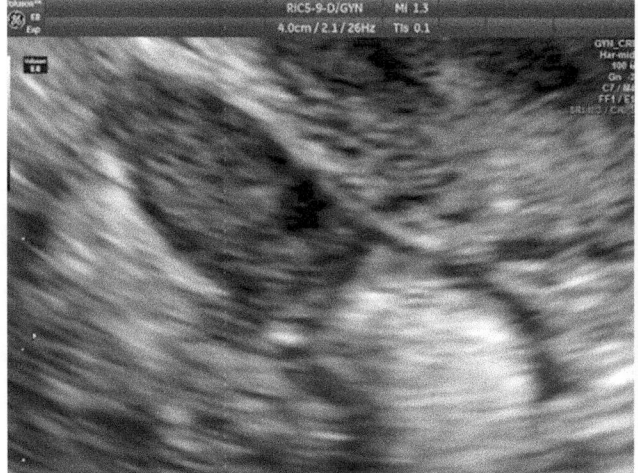
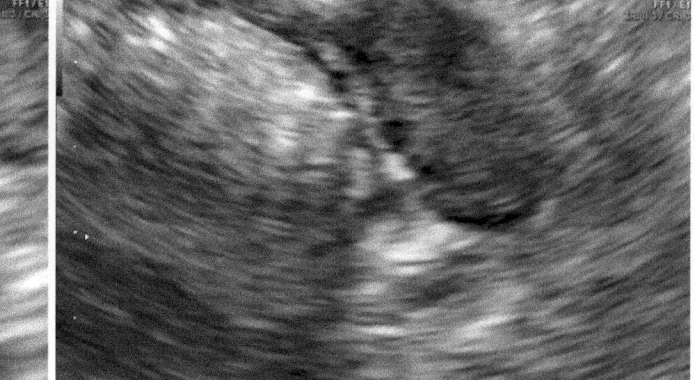
Ovary with poor ovarian reserve

SECTION 5

Endoscopy in Reproductive Surgery

- Laparoscopy: Role in Infertility
- Hysteroscopy: Role in Infertility

CHAPTER 8

Laparoscopy: Role in Infertility

Malvika Sabarwal, Shivani Sabharwal, Nupur Chhabra

A. Laparoscopy offers the unique opportunity to diagnose and treat in the same sitting. It is considered the gold standard for evaluation of tubal and pelvic factor. This algorithm highlights the role of laparoscopy in evaluating and managing female infertility.

B. Laparoscopic ovarian drilling is considered the second-line treatment for polycystic ovary syndrome (PCOS) women not responding to maximum dose of ovulation inducing agents. Gonadotropins and laparoscopic ovarian drilling (LOD) are both equally effective second-line agents. However, LOD has the advantage of generating unifolliculogenesis, reducing the risk of multiple pregnancy, does not require intensive follicular monitoring, lesser incidence of ovarian hyperstimulation syndrome (OHSS), and higher chances of spontaneous pregnancy within the first 6 months of therapy.

There are various hypotheses regarding the mechanism of action, such as nonspecific stromal destruction or the opening of follicular capsules that release follicular fluid, which contains androgens, thereby removing the ovulation block. A significant reduction in serum androgen levels, an increase in follicle-stimulating hormone (FSH) levels, and a decrease in luteinizing hormone (LH) pulse amplitude have been observed, independent of the mechanism. However, LOD is associated with permanent reduction in the ovarian reserve if used over zealously. Four punctures with monopolar current at 40 watts for 4 seconds each are recommended to prevent excessive ovarian damage. Also, there is risk of adhesion formation. Therefore, LOD may be an option in highly resistant cases of PCOS with large bulky ovaries after thorough counseling of patient.

C. If there is strong suspicion of pelvic factor or tubal pathology, laparoscopy may be suggested as the first-line of investigation to evaluate tubal function.

D. In patients with unexplained infertility, the best line of action is ovulation induction (OI) with or without intrauterine insemination (IUI) for 3–6 cycles. No randomized controlled trials (RCTs) have evaluated the effects of diagnostic laparoscopy in unexplained infertility after failed ovarian stimulation with or without IUI; however, at least 50% of patient pathologies, such as endometriosis or adhesions, can be detected if laparoscopy is performed. In addition, no evidence suggests that laparoscopy with adhesiolysis before assisted reproductive technique (ART) increases the pregnancy rate in ART cycles.

E. Laparoscopy can be postponed after a normal patency or if unilateral obstruction is revealed by hysterosalpingogram (HSG), particularly in females less than 36 years of age with normal ovarian reserves. However, in patients with a history of endometriosis, pelvic infections, or ectopic pregnancy, evaluation with hysteroscopy and laparoscopy is recommended.

F. Hydrosalpinx has deleterious effects on fertility even after ART. Clipping of the hydrosalpinx increases pregnancy rates.

G. If ultrasound reveals any abnormality, then management is individualized as per case scenario. Laparoscopy has a crucial role both in the diagnosis and management of endometriosis. Refer to Chapter Role of Endoscopy in endometriosis for more details.

H. In patients with infertility and fibroids, an effort should be made to adequately evaluate and classify fibroids, particularly those impinging on the endometrial cavity, using transvaginal ultrasound, hysteroscopy, saline sonography, or magnetic resonance imaging. Role of laparoscopy in managing fibroids is dealt in Fibroid Management.

I. In suspected cases of uterine malformations, it is highly recommended to perform both hysteroscopy and laparoscopy to increase the diagnostic accuracy and enhance safety threshold.

Laparoscopy: Role in Infertility

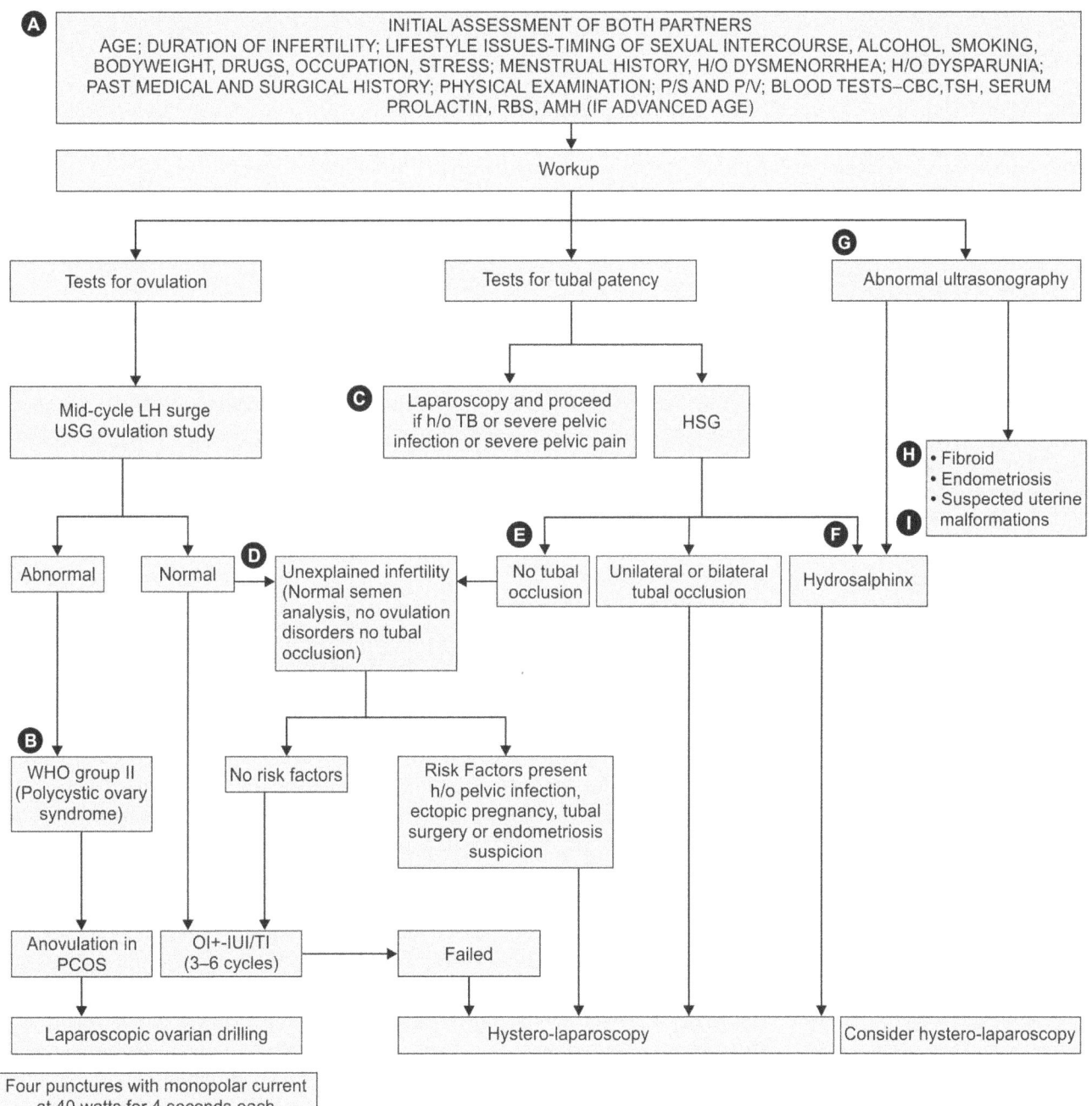

(AMH: anti-Müllerian hormone; CBC: complete blood count; h/o: history of; HSG: hysterosalpingogram; IUI: intrauterine insemination; LH: luteinizing hormone; OI: ovulation induction; PCOS: polycystic ovary syndrome; P/S: per speculum; P/V: per vaginal; RBS: random blood sugar; TB: tuberculosis; TI: timed intercourse; TSH: thyroid-stimulating hormone; USG: ultrasonography)

Hysteroscopy: Role in Infertility

Rahul Manchanda, Richa Sharma

INTRODUCTION

Structural defects in the endometrial cavity of the uterus can affect the reproductive outcome negatively, by interfering with the implantation potential of the embryo or increase the possibility of spontaneous pregnancy losses. Hence, evaluation of the endocervical canal and endometrial cavity is an important step in the infertility workup.

A. *Indications of hysteroscopy*: Endometrial cavity may be evaluated using noninvasive modalities like hysterosalpingography (HSG), two-dimensional (2D) or three-dimensional (3D) transvaginal sonography (TVS), sonohysterography (SHG), minimally invasive techniques like office hysteroscopy and invasive techniques like hysteroscopy. Although HSG is very sensitive (98%), it is limited by low specificity (34.9%). TVS has the benefit of being both specific (96.3%) and sensitive (100%) in detected uterine abnormalities. Use of SHG along with 3D increases the detection rate of intrauterine anomalies. Hysteroscopy is considered the "gold standard" in the diagnosis of intrauterine abnormalities. Similar to laparoscopy, hysteroscopy also offers the benefit of concurrent treatment option. Abnormal hysterogram, diagnosis and treatment of suspected intrauterine pathology, unexplained infertility, recurrent pregnancy loss, persistent thin endometrium suggesting intrauterine adhesions (IUAs), misplaced or embedded foreign bodies, and proximal tubal cannulation are all indications to prompt an hysteroscopic evaluation of the uterus.

B. *Proximal or distal tubal block*: Hysteroscopic insertion of soft 3-F catheter with wireguide of less than 0.5 mm diameter into the tubal lumen, bypassing the intramural portion. Doing a hysteroscopic cannulation with concurrent laparoscopy prevents inadvertent tubal injury and confirms tubal patency postcannulation, failing which microsurgical tubal reconstructions is considered. Success is 72–92%.

C. *Submucous myomas*: Small submucous myomas, (4–5 cm diameter) of types 0, 1, and 2 can be effectively treated with hysteroscopic transcervical resectoscopic myomectomy (TCRM), with high success rates. However, type 2 myomas may require a multistage procedure. Women with enlarged uterus and more than three myomas are at a risk of repeat surgery of 9.7% and 35%, respectively at 5 years compared to women with a normal size uterus or less than two submucous myomas. Patient satisfaction symptomatically is in the range of 70–80%.

D. *Endometrial polyps* can be effectively and safely treated with hysteroscopic polypectomy, with reduced recurrence rate. Symptom resolution occurs in 75–100% of the women and risk of recurrence is hardly 2.5–3.7% in 9 years.

E. *Uterine synechiae*: The hydrodistension of the uterus during hysteroscopy may itself lyse mild adhesions, and blunt dissection using only the tip of the hysteroscope may further lyse adhesions. Controlled division of adhesions by scissors and needle has best results. Monopolar and bipolar electrosurgical instruments and the neodymium-doped yttrium aluminum garnet (Nd:YAG) laser can be used in a resectoscope for dense adhesiolysis. Use of electrical source increases the risk of perforation and inadvertent visceral damage. Myometrial scaring is another method to create a uterine cavity in women with severe IUAs where six to eight incisions of 4-mm depth are made in the myometrium using a Collins knife electrode. Anatomic success has been reported to 50–71%.

F. *Septate uterus*: Hysteroscopic metroplasty or hysteroscopic transcervical division or incision of the uterine septum using cold scissors, unipolar or bipolar cautery, laser, bipolar electrosurgical needle, or resectoscope with an operating loop. Moving the hysteroscope from side-to-side and visualization of both the ostia on a panoramic view from the level of internal os verifies completion of resection. Concurrent laparoscopy or transabdominal ultrasound decreases the risk of uterine perforation. Reduction in the dimpling and blanched appearance of the uterine fundus on laparoscopy are considered reassuring for the complete removal of the septum.

G. *Unicornuate uterus*: Transcervical uterine incision (TCUI) procedure using hysteroscopic bipolar electroresectoscope is effective means to create new uterine fundus with a width of more than or equal to 2 cm. TCUI involves shallow transverse incision over the narrowed fundal part with a loop or needle electrode, followed by 4 cm long and 1 cm deep vertical incision over the lateral walls starting at fundus tapering to stop at the level of the isthmus. An inverted triangular-shaped uterine cavity is created at the end of surgery.

H. In patients with recurrent pregnancy loss, hysteroscopy aids as an important tool in the diagnosis of aforementioned uterine pathologies and their respective management. This eventually improves significantly the reproductive outcome.
I. Presence of any foreign body like fetal bones or tissue from previous miscarriages, lost intrauterine devices, etc. can be visualized and removed under hysteroscopic guidance.

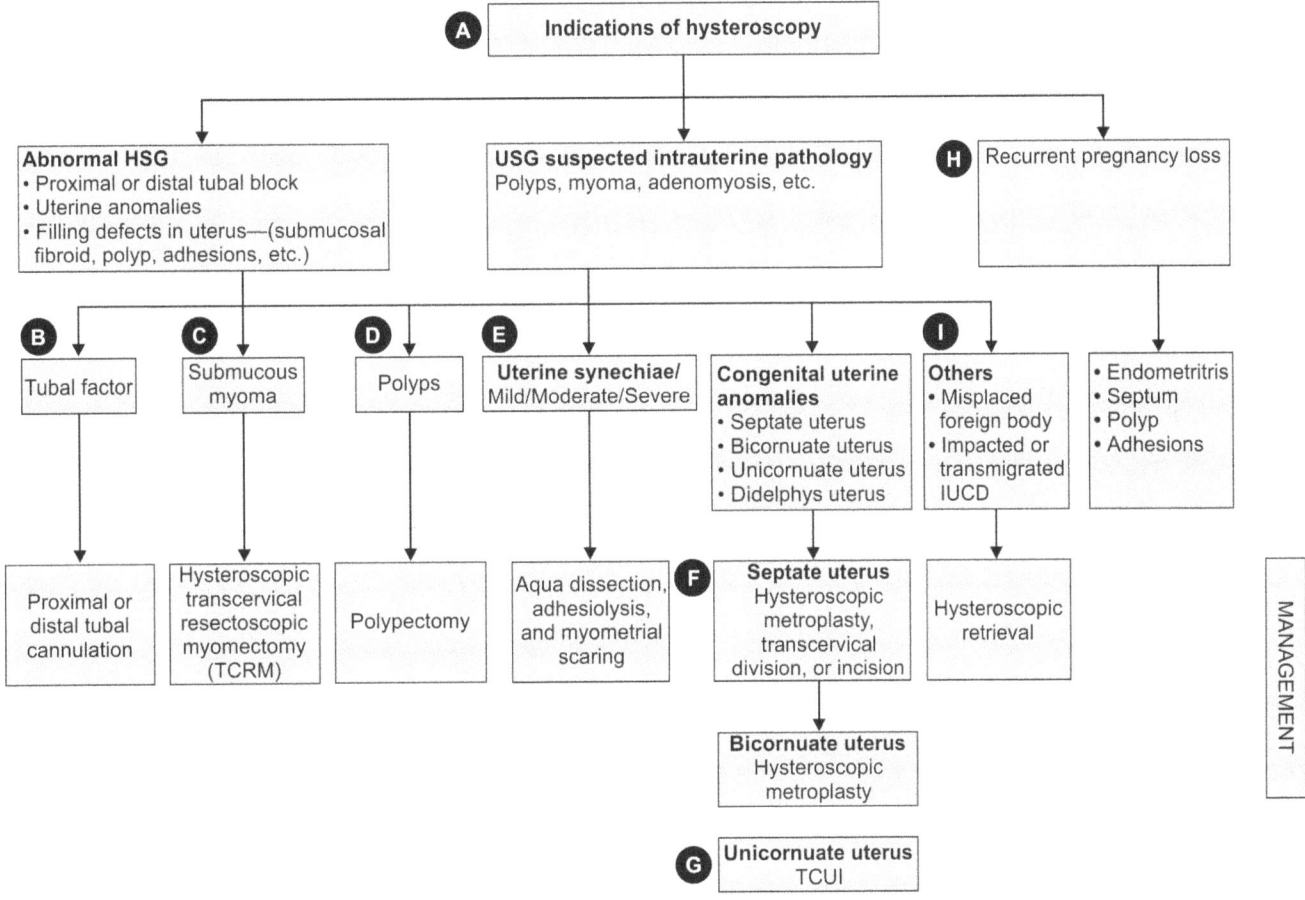

(HSG: hysterosalpingography; IUCD: intrauterine contraceptive device; TCUI: transcervical uterine incision; USG: ultrasonography)

SECTION 6

Uterine Factors

- Uterine Factor Evaluation
- Endometritis
- Uterine Anomalies (Müllerian Duct Anomalies)
- Septate Uterus
- Uterine Polyps
- Asherman Syndrome

Section 6: Uterine Factors

3D imaging of the uetrus

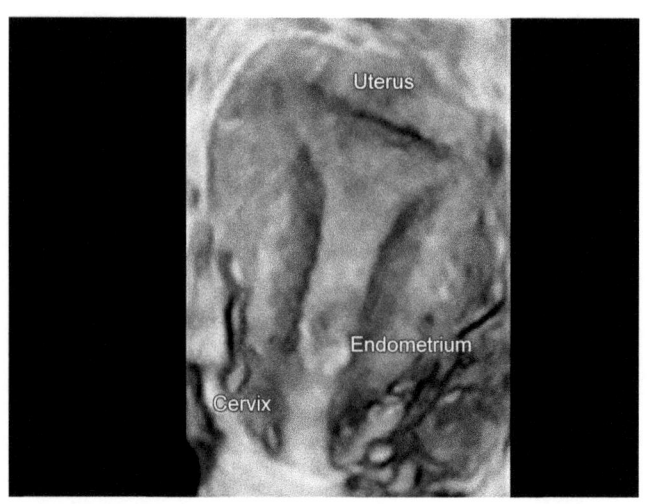

Normal uterus

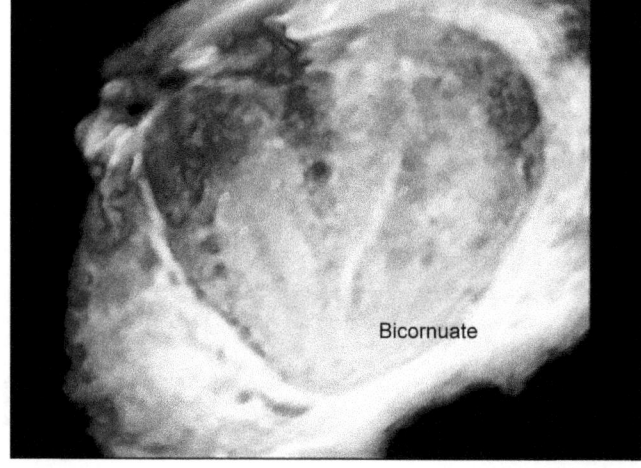

Bicornuate uterus

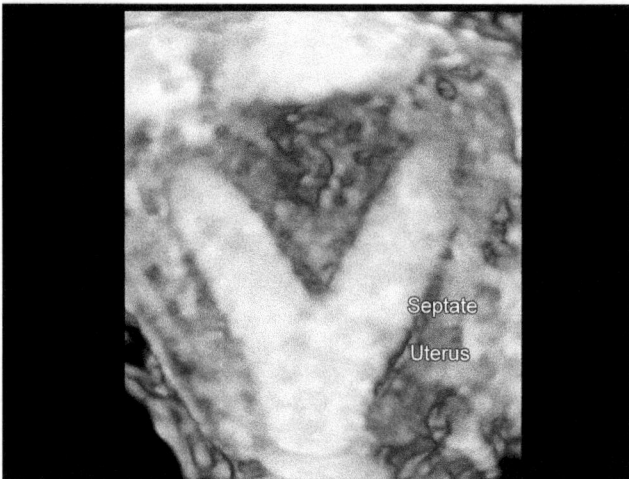
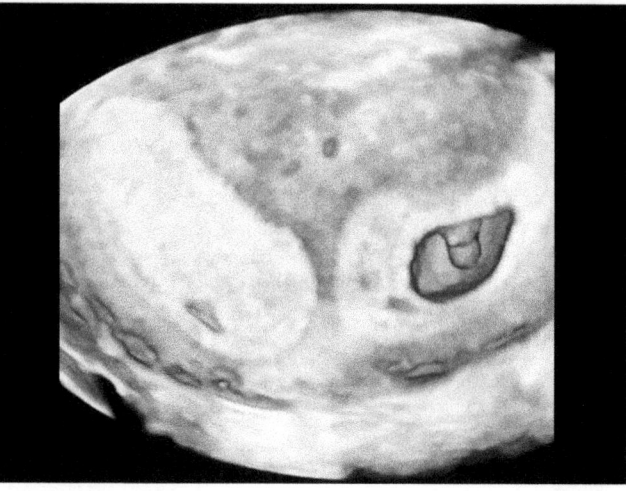

Sepatate uterus

CHAPTER 10

Uterine Factor Evaluation

Kishore Pandit, Apoorva Pallam Reddy

A. Assessment of uterine abnormalities is a core part in infertility evaluation. Uterine irregularities can be one of the causes of infertility by interfering with implantation.

B. A variety of investigations can be used to evaluate the uterine factor. The structural defects are usually evaluated using modalities like hysterosalpingography (HSG), transvaginal sonography (TVS), diagnostic hysteroscopy, saline infusion sonography (SIS), three-dimensional hysterosonography (3-DHS). However, diagnostic hysteroscopy has remained the gold standard in infertility investigation.

C. The functional ability of the uterus can be tested by endometrial biopsy for assessing endometritis especially tuberculosis. Analysis of Infectious Chronic Endometritis (ALICE)™ is a newer molecular diagnostic tool that can detect pathogens even at nonculturable levels and detects the nine pathogens responsible for chronic endometritis, including Enterobacteriaceae, *Enterococcus, Streptococcus, Staphylococcus, Mycoplasma*, and *Ureaplasma*.

D. Studies show that endometrium that is not dominated by *Lactobacillus* (NDL) has a lower implantation rate and a higher miscarriage rate (60%). Endometrial Microbiome Metagenomic Analysis (EMMA)™ test allows us to determine the complete profile of bacteria in the patient's endometrium—the endometrial microbiome.

E. Endometrial receptivity is the ability of the endometrium to interact with the inbound embryo and result in a successful Implantation. The only test available so far to predict this is the endometrial receptivity array (ERA).

It is to be noted that the efficacy of newer investigations like EMMA, ALICE, and ERA are yet to be established by stronger research.

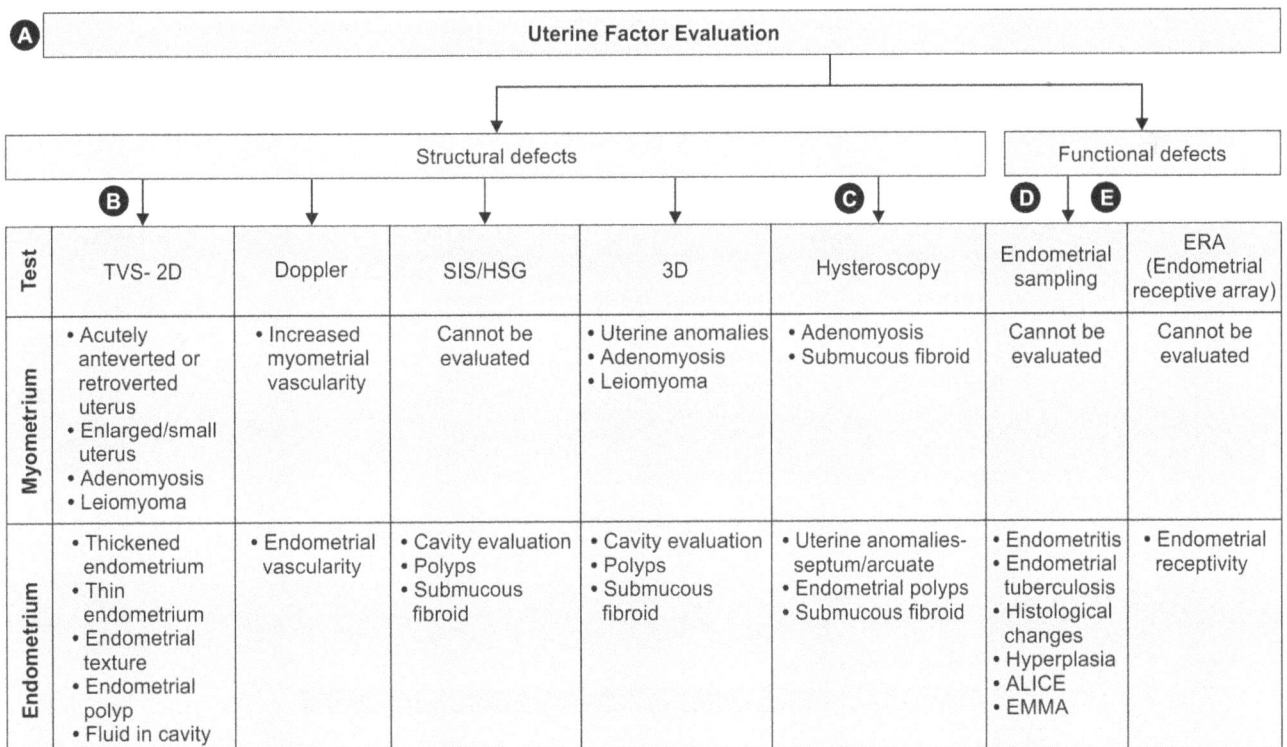

CHAPTER 11

Endometritis

Kishore Pandit

A. *Acute endometritis* is puerperal in nature is most often limited to the endometrium. It is most commonly seen following cesarean section, in prolonged labor with rupture of membranes and following multiple pelvic examinations. This infection is common in the lower socioeconomic status, and is effectively treated with antibiotics. It rarely progresses to chronic endometritis. It is not a common cause of infertility.

B. *Chronic endometritis* is generally asymptomatic or vague symptoms like abnormal uterine bleeding, pelvic pain, and white discharge. Incidence is about 10% in fertile women but reported as high as 40% in infertile women and 42–58% in those with recurrent implantation failure or recurrent pregnancy losses. More prominent TH1 (T-helper 1) response, increased IGFBP1 (insulin-like growth factor-binding protein 1) and decreased IGF1 (insulin-like growth factor 1) and IL II (interleukin-II) downregulation is observed in women with chronic endometritis.

C. Plasma cell identification in the endometrial stroma (on histology) is the ideal way of diagnosing chronic endometritis but it is quite nonspecific and is also dependent on the date of the menstrual cycle when sampling is done. Unfortunately, histology is still the current gold standard for diagnosis.

D. Infection forms the basis of chronic endometritis. The most common infectious agents responsible for chronic endometritis are *Streptococcus* species, *Enterococcus faecalis*, *Staphylococcus* species, Enterobacteriaceae, *Mycoplasma*, *Gardnerella vaginalis*, *Chlamydia trachomatis*, *Neisseria gonorrhoeae*, *Ureaplasma urealyticum*, and *Mycobacterium tuberculosis*. The other problem is that not all microorganisms responsible for chronic endometritis can be cultured and even if culture does happen, the turnaround time is very long.

E. On hysteroscopy the following features of chronic endometritis can be seen: focal or diffuse periglandular hyperemia, stromal edema and polyps of less than 1 mm size. Hysteroscopies should be done in the follicular phase (cycle day 6–12).

F. Molecular testing uses real-time polymerase chain reaction (RT-PCR) and next-generation sequencing (NGS) for detecting bacterial DNA from the sample. It has the advantage of identifying and quantifying presence of small quantities of bacterial DNA. Results are similar to all other three methods together in 76.9% of cases.

G. Appropriate treatment of women with chronic endometritis significantly improves reproductive outcome.

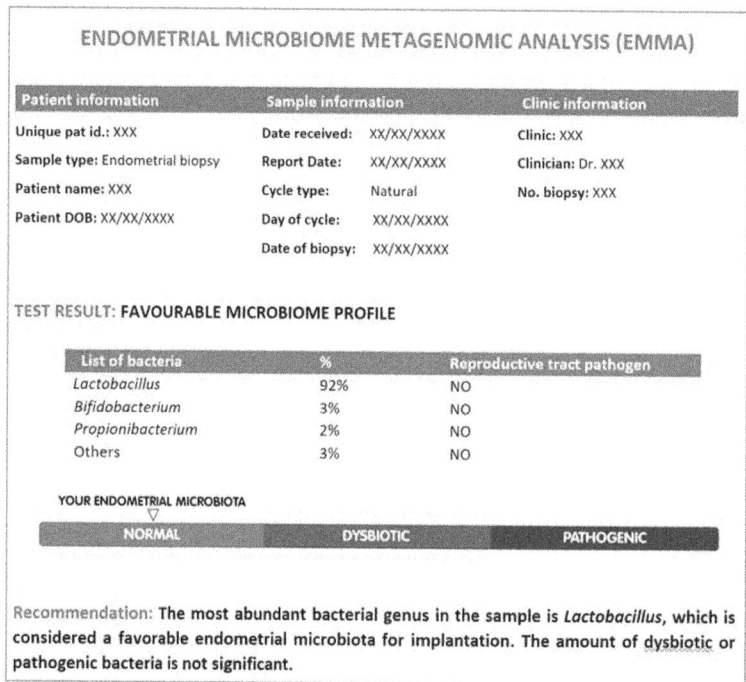

Sample EMMA report

Endometritis

Endometritis

- **A** Acute endometritis
  - ↓ Unresolved/persistent
- **B** Chronic endometritis
  - ↓
- Methods of diagnosis
  - **C** Histology
    - Evidence of plasma cells (bacterial infection)
    - Intranuclear inclusions (viral infection)
    - Noncaseating granulomatous lesions (tuberculosis)
  - **D** Culture
    - Culture of offending microorganisms
  - **E** Hysteroscopy
    - Hyperemia
    - Edema
    - Micropolyps
  - **F** Molecular testing
    - Highly sensitive
    - Quantifies bacterial DNA instead of live bacteria thus samples can be frozen/fixed and easily transported
    - Detects both culturable and nonculturable bacteria

Treatment

- **G**
  - Doxycycline 100 mg twice daily for 14 days (First line)
  - Ofloxacin 400 mg twice daily + Metronidazole 500 mg twice daily for 14 days
  - Anti-tubercular therapy where indicated

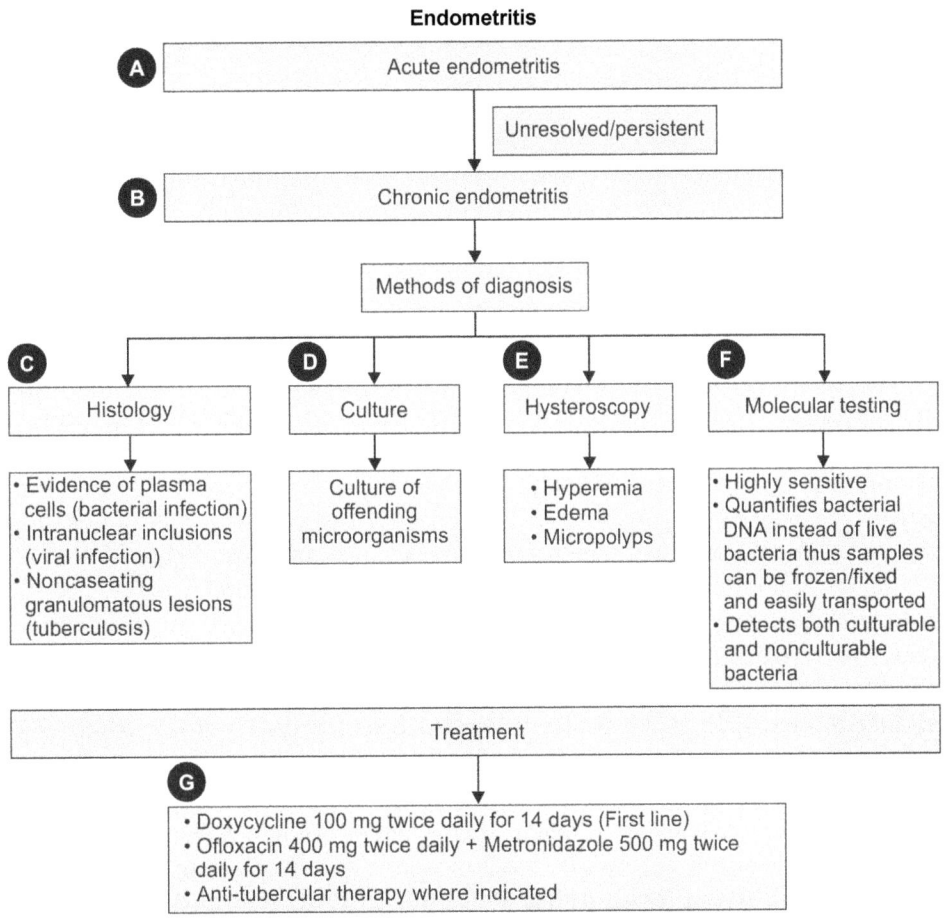

Sample report of ALICE

CHAPTER 12

Uterine Anomalies (Müllerian Duct Anomalies)

Smita Jain, Meenu Agarwal

A. *Uterine anomalies:* The uterus, cervix, vagina, and the fallopian tubes are formed due to the transformation of Müllerian ducts (fusion and reabsorption) in a female fetus between 7 weeks and 12 weeks of gestation. Any defects in this transformation results in anatomical and functional deficiencies. Interruption of Müllerian duct development during organogenesis will result in aplasia or hypoplasia of uterus, cervix, and vagina. Fusion defects result in anomalies like uterine didelphys and bicornuate uterus variants. Reabsorption defects result in septate and arcuate uterus effects. Müllerian duct *anomalies* (MDAs) are not associated with ovarian anomalies. Most anomalies are diagnosed accidentally as a part of routine investigation or after reproductive mishap or menstrual disturbance like primary amenorrhea. As the functionality of the uterus and prognosis of reproductive outcome depends on the type of anomaly, it is extremely important to determine the type of defect. Although most anomalies do not require any attention, managing others become imperative.

B. *Diagnosis:* Despite the limited role of two-dimensional (2D) sonography in the diagnosis of Müllerian defects, the emergence of 3D has revolutionized the diagnostic value of sonography and diminished the need to perform invasive tests. It helps in evaluating not only the cavity but also differentiates septate from bicornuate uterus. When the apex of the fundal contour is more than 5 mm *above* a line drawn between the tubal ostia, the uterus is septate. When the apex of the fundal contour is *below* or less than 5 mm above a line drawn between the tubal ostia, the uterus is bicornuate. When Müllerian defects are suspected, it is always prudent to look for presence of any associated renal anomalies. Hysterosalpingography (HSG), which is routinely performed to evaluate female infertility, can bring to light any defects in the uterine cavity. As a key component of MDA characterization is the external uterine fundal contour, HSG is not an optimal test to differentiate between septate uterus and bicornuate. A diagnostic hystero-laparoscopy not only serves as an excellent diagnostic test, but also has the singular benefit of management in the same sitting. It also helps in the analysis of pelvic and tubal factor. Magnetic resonance (MR) imaging is typically not done on a routine basis and is reserved only for complex and indeterminate cases. Use of MR imaging for evaluation of MDAs reduces the number of invasive procedures and related costs by guiding management decisions.

C. *Treatment:* Most women with uterine anomalies do not require treatment and the cases that require, can be corrected through minimally invasive techniques, such as laparoscopy or hysteroscopy. In the case of a unicornuate uterus, an obstructed hemiuterus can be removed if the other side of the uterus is intact and functional.

Uterine Anomalies (Müllerian Duct Anomalies)

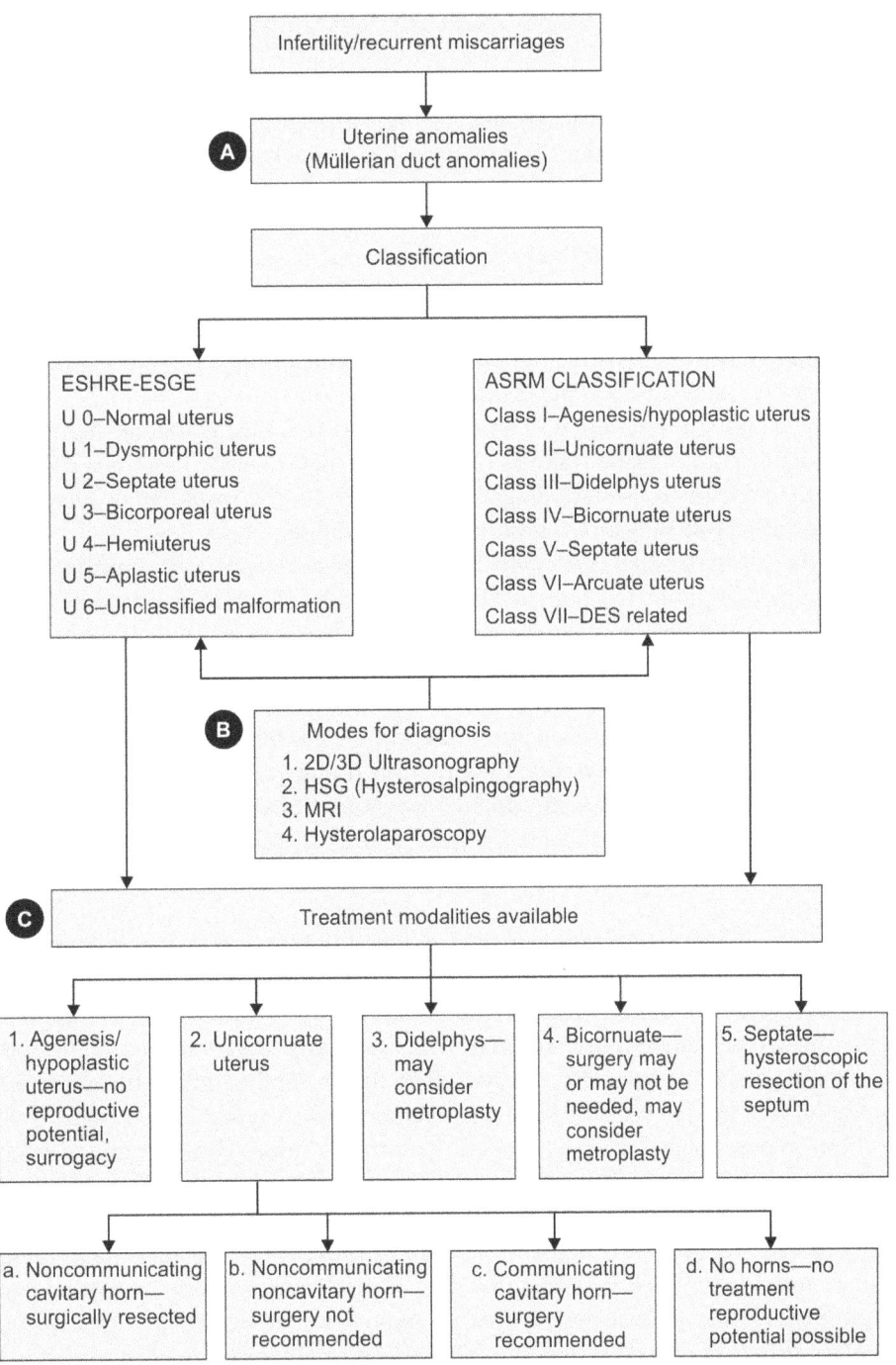

(ASRM: American Society for Reproductive Medicine; DES: diethylstilbestrol; ESHRE-ESGE: European Society of Human Reproduction and Embryology-European Society for Gynaecological Endoscopy; HSG: hysterosalpingography; MRI: magnetic resonance imaging)

CHAPTER 13

Septate Uterus

Meenu Agarwal, Sandhya Meshram

A. Uterine anomalies are commonly found in infertile women with a prevalence of 7.3% and it rises up to 16% in women with recurrent pregnancy losses. Uterine anomalies may be suspected in the presence of features like recurrent pregnancy loss, splitting of cavity on 2D scan, abnormal cavity on hysterosalpingography (HSG) done to assess tubal patency.
B. A 3D ultrasonography (USG) along with saline infusion sonography is as effective as hystero-lap in diagnosis of septum. A line is traced joining both horns of the uterine cavity at the level of ostia. If this line crosses the fundus or is less than 5 mm, it is bicornuate uterus. If this line is more than 5 mm it is septate uterus.
C. The American Society for Reproductive Medicine (ASRM) guidelines diagnose septum on the basis of internal and external fundal indentation. The internal indentation should be more than 1.5 cm and external indentation less than 1 cm for the diagnosis of a septate uterus as per ASRM.
D. The European Society of Human Reproduction and Embryology (ESHRE) guideline states that if internal fundal indentation is more than 50% of uterine wall thickness, it is septate uterus. There is a risk of overdiagnosis and overtreatment if ESHRE guideline is used for diagnosing septum. Thus, it would be prudent to subject a female to hysteroscopic resection of septum only on the basis of ASRM guideline.
E. There is fair evidence that all uterine septa are associated with increased reproductive mishaps and resecting all septa longer than 1.5 cm improves reproductive outcome (Grade C evidence). Before the surgical treatment of septum, all other endocrinological, autoimmune, and chromosomal causes for recurrent pregnancy loss should be ruled out. There is insufficient evidence for or against recommending danazol or gonadotropin-release hormone agonists to reduce endometrial vascularity prior to septal resection.
F. Hysteroscopic resection can be done as an office procedure without anesthesia using office hysteroscope with scissors in case of thin septum. It can be done with regular hysteroscope under anesthesia, also using scissors. The distension media used is normal saline in such cases. The main advantages of using scissors are less thermal damage, less scarring, lesser chances of perforation, lesser postoperative complications like fluid overload and pulmonary edema. The resectoscope and the microscissors are equally valid instruments to correct a septate uterus, with an optimal feasibility rate.
G. Hysteroscopic resection with resectoscope can be done using bipolar resectoscope or monopolar needle or resectoscope. The advantage of bipolar resectoscope is the use of normal saline as distending media while glycine has to be used for use of monopolar current. But the disadvantage is the need for cervical dilatation with resectoscope, while in monopolar needle, dilatation is not required. While resecting, always stay in midline, and progress toward the base, observing and preserving symmetry of cavity at all times. Till the pinkish myometrial fibers are seen, the procedure is continued. The septum is cut till both the tubal ostia are seen in the same plane in a panoramic view.
H. One of the late complications of septal resection is uterine rupture in subsequent pregnancy, either following uterine contractions or spontaneous. In a study by Sentilhes et al. reported that using modalities like hysterosalpingography or ultrasonography scan for prediction of rupture or increased interval between resection and the subsequent pregnancy, and performing elective cesarean sections are not effective to prevent and to detect the impeding ruptures in the subsequent pregnancies. It is worth noting that there is moderate evidence suggesting that use of scissors for hysteroscopic metroplasty has lesser chances of ruptured compared to resectoscope. The clinicians should keep the procedure in mind while deciding mode of delivery and use labor augmenting medications judiciously.
I. Postoperatively antibiotics according to hospital policy must be given. Hormone replacement is not routinely required. Only in cases of large septal resection, estradiol valerate 2 mg thrice a day to be given for 21 days with progesterone in last 10 days for endometrial regeneration. Postoperative intrauterine device (IUD) or balloon not recommended. Pregnancy can be planned 2 months postsurgery. Unless resecting a complete septum, there is no role of second look hysteroscopy to assess cavity.

Septate Uterus

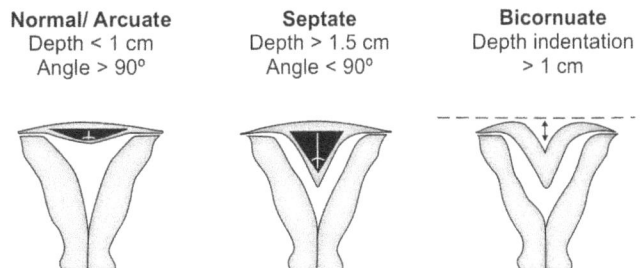

Diagrams of the ASRM definitions of normal/arcuate, septate, and bicornuate uterus based on assessment of available literature, understanding that these anomalies reflect points on a spectrum of development normal/arcuate: depth from the interstitial line to the apex of the indentation <1 cm and angle of the indentation >90°. Septate: depth from the interstitial line to the apex of the indentation >1.5 cm and angle of the indentation <90°. Bicornuate: external fundal indentation >1 cm. Internal endometrial cavity is similar to a partial septate uterus.
(ASRM: American Society for Reproductive Medicine)

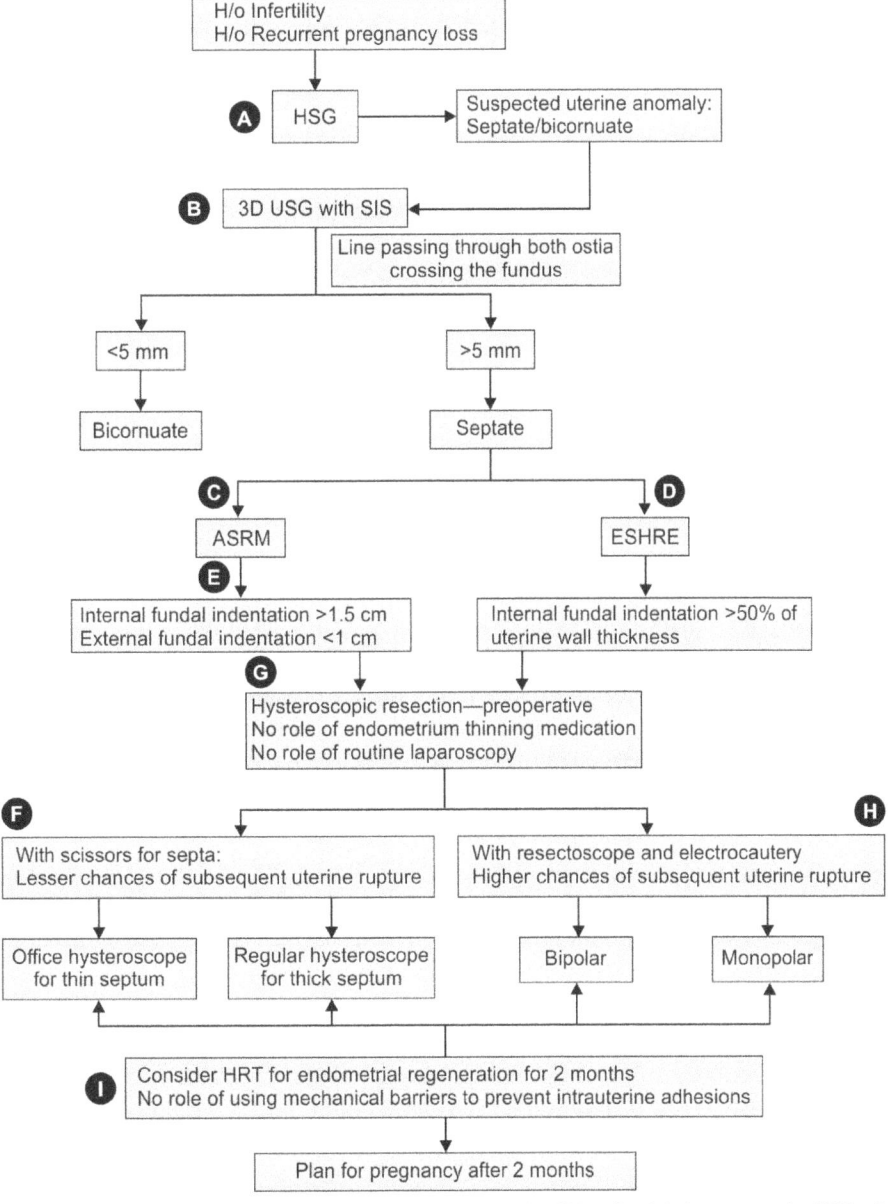

(H/o: history of; HRT: hormone replacement therapy; HSG: hysterosalpingography; SIS: saline infusion sonography; USG: ultrasonography; ASRM: American Society for Reproductive Medicine; ESHRE: European Society of Human Reproduction and Embryology)

CHAPTER 14

Uterine Polyps

Sandhya Meshram, Meenu Agarwal

A. Endometrial polyps are the most common uterine anomaly, seen in 15% of infertile females. The mechanism by which the polyp causes infertility is still not clearly understood but the most possible explanation is decreased endometrial receptivity preventing embryo implantation. Age, hypertension, obesity, use of tamoxifen and diabetes are well known risk factors for the development of endometrial polyps. SuprQphysiological estrogen levels or unopposed estrogen action like in assisted reproductive technique (ART) cycles also increases incidence of polyps.

B. Mostly seen as an incidental finding on a transvaginal 2D ultrasound done in the proliferative phase of the menstrual cycle more common in women with H/o infertility or recurrent pregnancy loss. The sensitivity of 2D ultrasonography (USG) alone is 19–96% and specificity is 53–100% in diagnosing a polyp.

C. A polyp can be confused with a polypoidal endometrium, but on Doppler flow, a feeding vessel can be clearly seen in a polyp, which cannot be seen in a polypoidal endometrium. The use of color Doppler increases the sensitivity of detection of polyp to 99%.

D. The most accurate diagnosis of polyp is with transvaginal sonography (TVS) with saline infusion sonography with both sensitivity and specificity almost 100%. It not only helps in diagnosing a polyp but also gives a clear perspective for management as it tells about the number, size, and location of polyp, which indeed is the most decisive factor.

E. In non in vitro fertilization (IVF) cycles, a polyp that is less than 15 mm, can await spontaneous regression. Most studies suggest that 27% of polyps show spontaneous regression over an average period of 8 weeks. If there is no spontaneous regression, if there are uterotubal polyps or multiple polyps, performing hysteroscopic polypectomy increases the spontaneous pregnancy rates. (6 months postsurgery is 57% for uterotubal polyps and 40% for multiple polyp removal).

F. If the size of polyp is more than 15 mm, hysteroscopic polypectomy followed by timed intercourse or intrauterine insemination (IUI) is advisable. Removal of endometrial disease by blind curettage is successful less than 50% of the time, and in many cases, removal is incomplete. Blind dilation and curettage or biopsy should not be used for diagnosis or management of endometrial polyps (level B).

G. If the patient is for IVF and a polyp of less than 15 mm (G1) is seen before ovarian stimulation, it is resected only if there are multiple polyps, or there is h/o recurrent implantation failure or h/o recurrent pregnancy loss. If the size is more than *15 mm (G2)*, hysteroscopic polypectomy is done and IVF-ET is done in immediate next cycle.

H. If a polyp of more than *15 mm (H1)* is seen during ovarian stimulation, the decision of performing a hysteroscopic polypectomy on the day of oocyte pickup (OPU) or opting for a freeze all is taken after discussing the options and prognosis with the patient. If the size is less than *15 mm (H2)*, a decision to do the transfer or not can be taken after discussing the pros and cons with the patient with due consideration to patient's previous reproductive history. If the controlled ovarian stimulation (COS) is continued, a freeze all option can be considered depending on the number of embryos formed, previous history of patient and the frozen transfer success rate of the clinic. Embryo transfer (ER) in the same cycle can be done for patients if the number of embryos is very less or the embryos are not good enough to be frozen.

I. Hysteroscopic polypectomy can be done with scissors or with resectoscope. It can be done as an outpatient procedure with scissors and office hysteroscope where cervical dilatation is not required.

J. Undergoing ovarian stimulation or planning for pregnancy in the immediate next cycle after resection of the polyp is not associated with decrease in pregnancy rates.

K. There is higher chance of recurrence in patients with multiple polyps. If more than 6 months has elapsed from the corrective surgery, it is advised to re-evaluate the cavity with saline infusion sonography (SIS) before performing embryo transfer.

Uterine Polyps

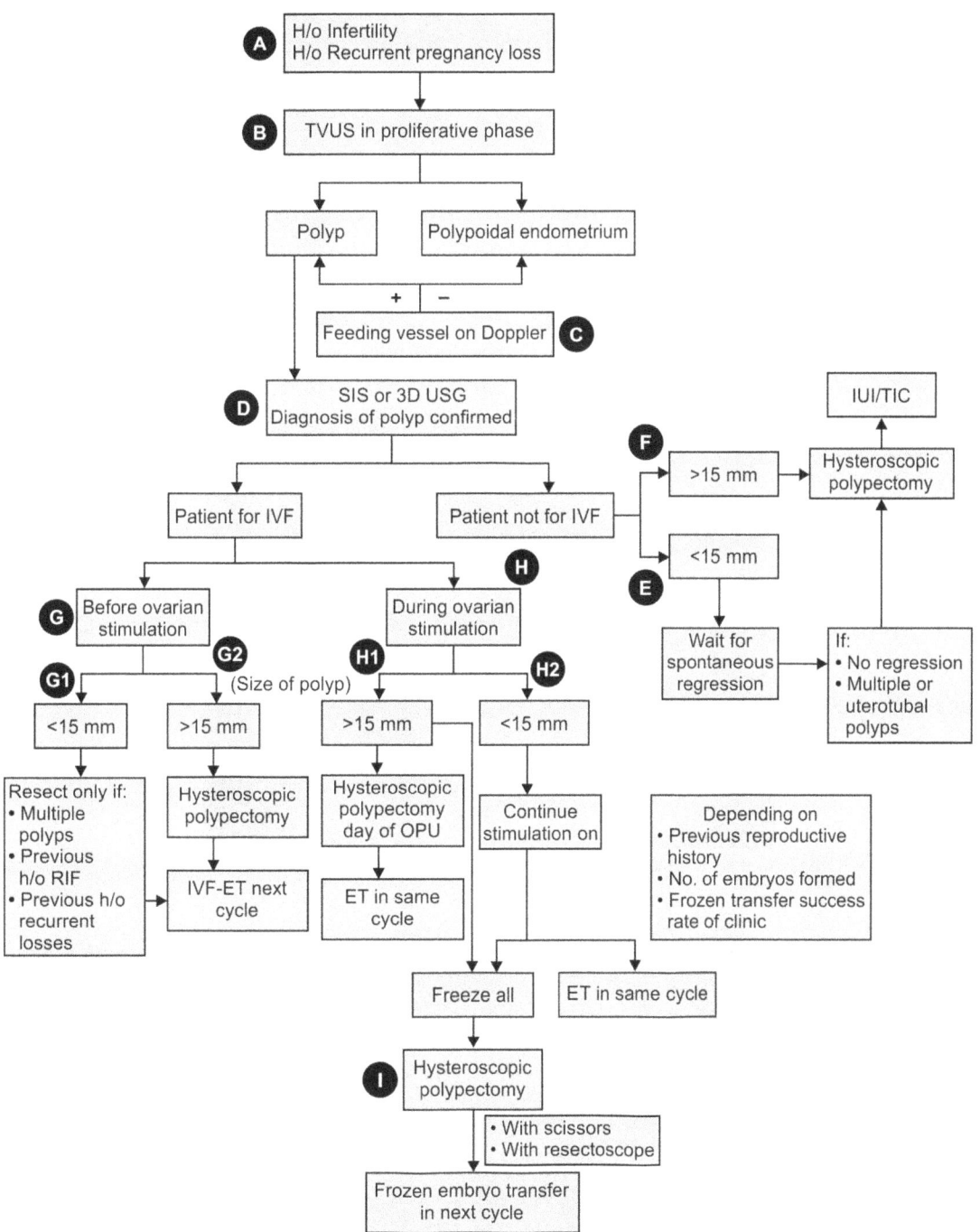

(H/o: history of; IUI: intrauterine insemination; IVF: in vitro fertilization; SIS: saline infusion sonography; TVUS: transvaginal ultrasound; ET: embryo transfer; TIC: timed intercourse; OPU: oocyte pickup; USG: ultrasonography; RIF: recurrent implantation failure)

Section 6: Uterine Factors

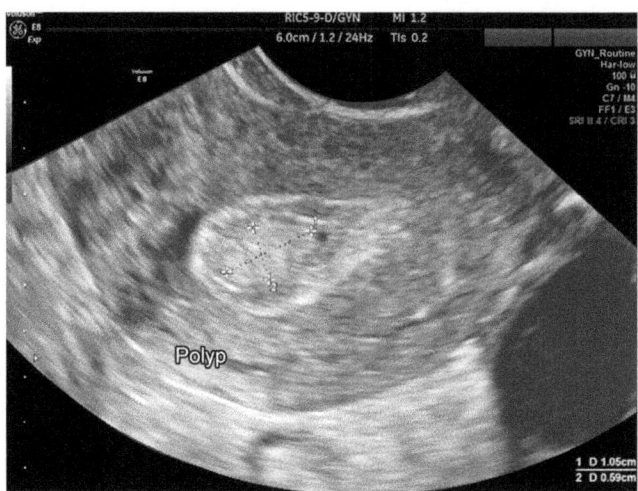
Fundal polyp seen on 2D scan

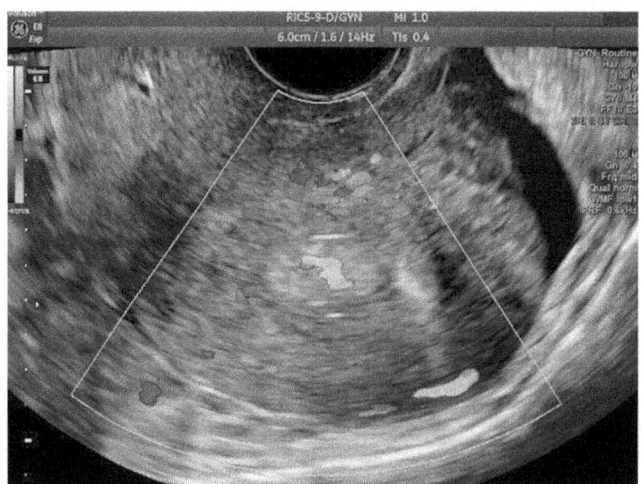
Feeding vessels of polyp seen of color Doppler

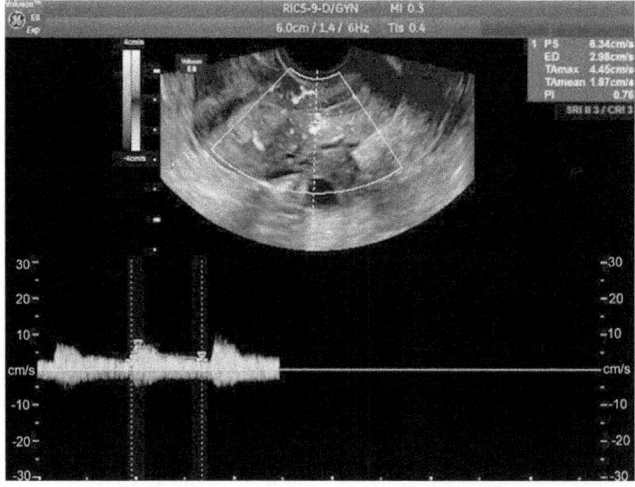
Feeding vessels of polyp seen of color Doppler

CHAPTER 15

Asherman Syndrome

Bimal John

A. Asherman syndrome, which is also referred to as intrauterine adhesions (IUAs) or intrauterine synechiae, occurs when scar tissue (adhesions) forms inside the uterus and/or the cervix.
B. Asherman syndrome should be suspected when the female partner gives history of menstrual disturbances oligomenorrhea or amenorrhea, immediately after an intrauterine procedure, infertility, cyclic pelvic pain, recurrent pregnancy loss, etc. history of procedures on a gravid uterus [missed/incomplete abortion, postpartum hemorrhage (PPH), etc.], repeat procedures 2 × fold risk, history of submucous/intramural myomectomy; infection, especially tuberculosis, intrauterine contraceptive device (IUCD) placement, etc.
C. Two-dimensional and 3D transvaginal ultrasonography have a sensitivity of 52% and specificity of 11% compared with hysteroscopy. 3D ultrasonography (USG) may be more helpful in the evaluation of IUAs, with sensitivity reported to be 87% and specificity of 45% compared to hysteroscopy. Thin endometrium in peri/postovulatory period; less than 4 mm is highly suggestive. Transvaginal USG does not offer any extra advantage over transabdominal USG.
D. Hysterosalpingography (HSG) has a sensitivity of 75–81%, specificity of 80%, and positive predictive value of 50% compared with hysteroscopy for diagnosis of IUAs. Findings can be in the form of filling defects—homogeneous opacity surrounded by sharp edges. Completely distorted and narrow cavity in severe cases. Ostial occlusion may be evident in some cases.
E. Saline infusion sonography or SIS also called SHG or sonohysterography was found to be as effective as HSG, with both reported to have a sensitivity of 75% and positive predictive value of 43% for SHG or SIS/gel infusion sonography (GIS) and 50% for HSG, compared with hysteroscopy. Findings can be in the form of:
    – *Mild*: Narrow, echogenic, and mobile bands in distended cavity.
    – *Moderate*: Thick, broad-based bridging bands.
    – *Severe*: Difficult distension during saline injection.
F. Hysteroscopy is the gold standard investigation of choice as well as the most accurate method of diagnosis of IUAs. If hysteroscopy is not available, HSG and SHG are reasonable alternatives. Magnetic resonance imaging should not be used for diagnosis of IUAs outside of clinical research studies.
G. Intrauterine adhesions should be classified as prognosis is correlated with severity of adhesions. The American Fertility Society classifies the severity of IUAs as follow:
    – *Mild disease*: Few filmy adhesions involving less than third of the uterine cavity with normal menses or hypomenorrhea.
    – *Moderate disease*: Filmy and dense adhesions, the involvement of one-third to two-thirds of cavity and hypomenorrhea.
    – *Severe Disease*: Dense adhesions involving more than two-thirds of the cavity with amenorrhea.
    Prognosis decreases with increase in severity of disease.
H. Hysteroscopic lysis of adhesions is the recommended approach for symptomatic IUAs. Mere distension separates mild adhesion. Tip of the scope can be used to tackle flimsy adhesions. Adhesiolysis should begin from the lower part of the cavity and progress upward. Central and filmy adhesions should be released first—this will allow better distension of cavity. Dense and lateral adhesions should be treated last. Serial hysteroscopy (second hysteroscopy after 7–14 days of first adhesiolysis to tackle severe adhesions) and repeat hysteroscopy (hysteroscopy to ensure no adhesion reformation, usually done after 3 months) may be done in severe cases of IUA. Dilation and curettage done blindly should be avoided as there is no evidence to support it. There is always a risk of perforations when adhesiolysis is performed. The procedure can be aided by ultrasound, fluoroscopy or laparoscopy but there is no evidence to suggest that these can prevent a perforation but may minimize the complications, if perforation does happen.
I. The use of solid barriers like an intrauterine device (IUD), stent, or catheter (Foleys—No 10–12 with 3.5–5 mL bulb, balloon uterine stent inflated with 1 mL saline, etc. for 7–10 days) appears to reduce the chances of adhesions

reforming postoperatively. Although the risk of infection is minimal when solid barriers are used as compared to no treatment at all, there is not much data on whether these will favor future fertility outcomes. Grade A. Similarly, there is no evidence to support or challenge the use of preoperative, intraoperative, or postoperative antibiotic therapy in surgical treatment of IUAs. If an IUD is used postoperatively, it is preferred to use something like a Lippes Loop, which is inert and has a large surface area as compared to an IUD which contains progestin or copper (should not be used). Semisolid barriers such as hyaluronic acid and auto-cross-linked hyaluronic acid gel increase pregnancy rates as compared to solid barriers by reducing adhesion reformation.

J. Hormone treatment using conjugated estrogen, with or without progesterone stimulates regeneration and re-epithelialization of scarred tissue. Estrogen for 4 weeks ± progesterone in last 2 weeks—usually 2-3 months course.

Severity of adhesions	Conjugated estrogen (21 days)	Medroxyprogesterone acetate (7 days)
Mild adhesions	0.625 mg BD	10 mg BD
Moderate adhesions	1.25 mg BD	10 mg BD
Severe adhesions	1.25 mg QID	10 mg BD

K. Stem cell treatment/platelet rich plasma may in future provide an effective additional treatment (along with surgical) to the management of Asherman syndrome; however, current evidence is very limited and thus this treatment should not be offered outside of research settings. The role of medications like sildenafil citrate, aspirin, and nitroglycerin, which are used as adjuncts to improve vascular flow to the endometrium, has not been proven.

Asherman Syndrome

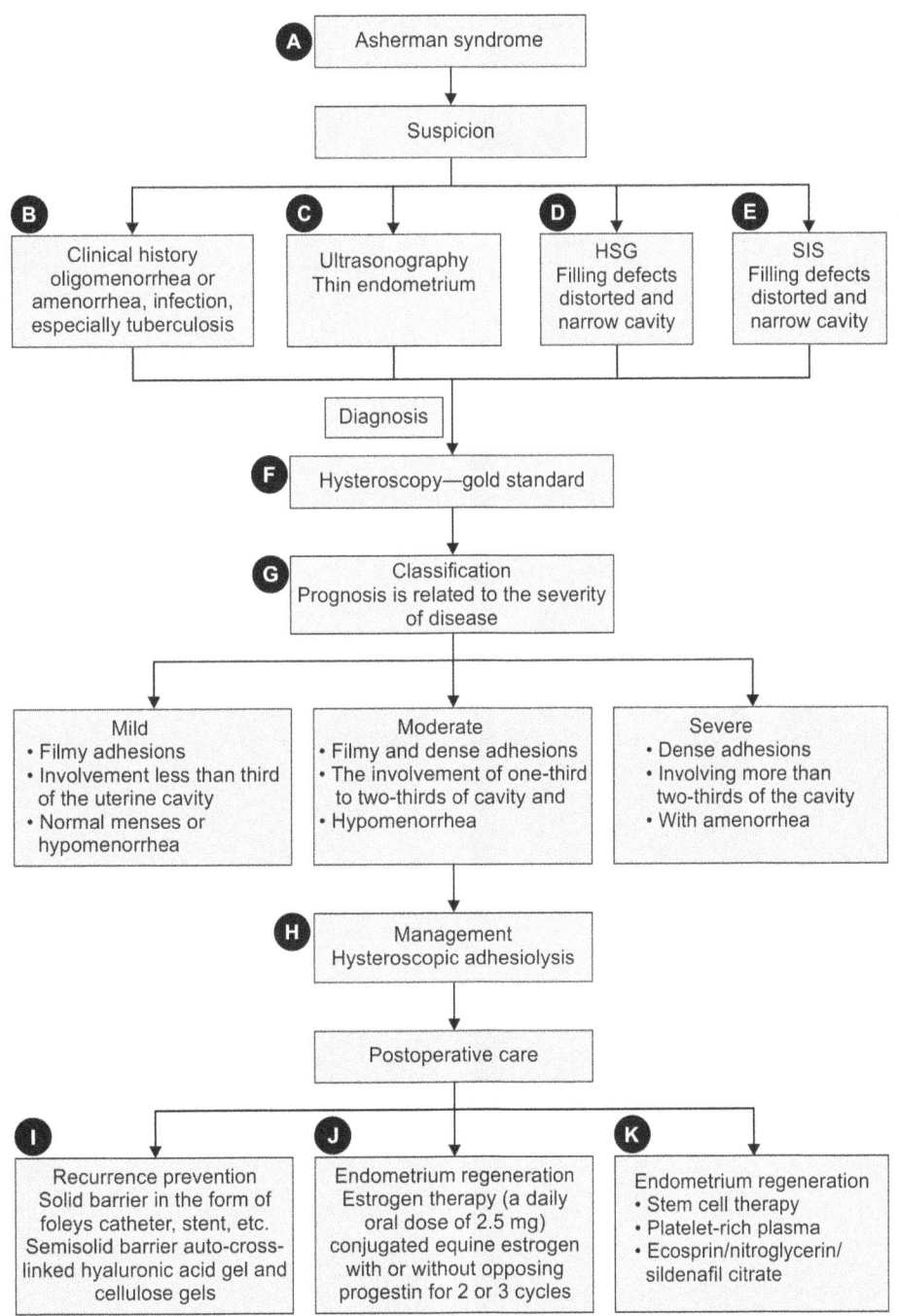

(HSG: hysterosalpingography; SIS: saline infusion sonography)

Section 6: Uterine Factors

Hysterosapingography images of various uterine and tubal anomalies

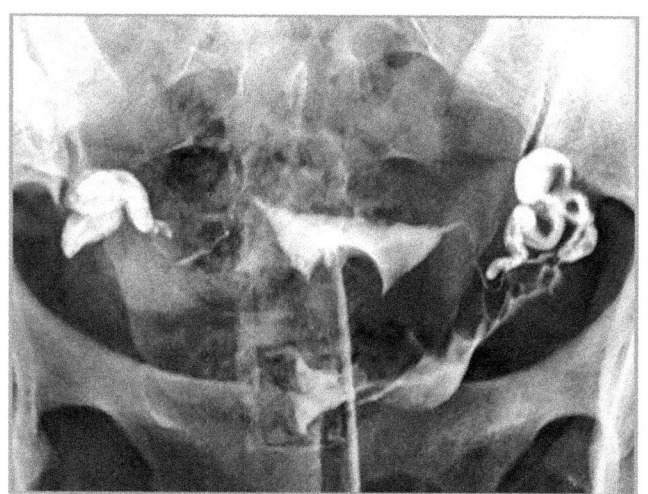
Distal hydrosalphinx and block

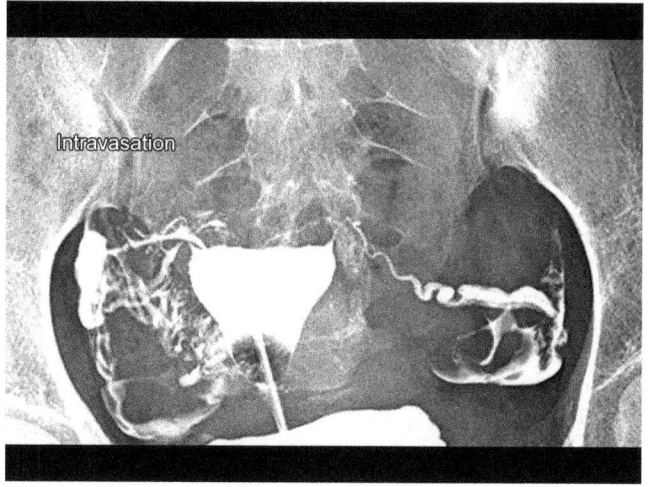
Intravasation of the dye

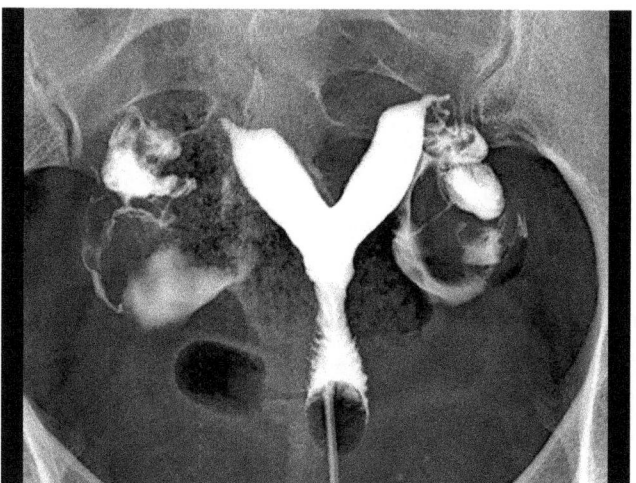
Septate uterus

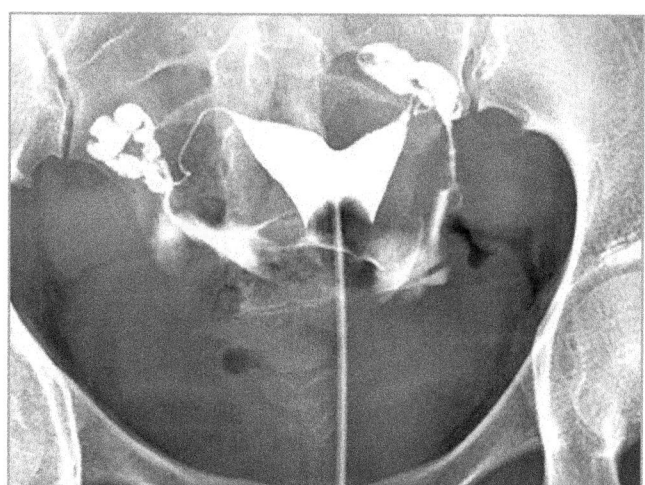
Arcuate uterus

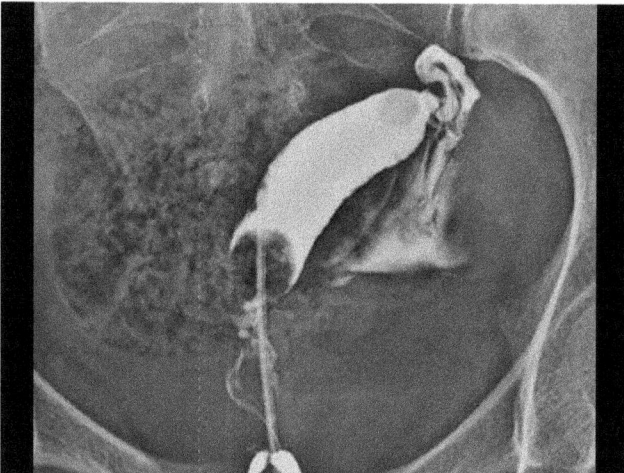
Unicornuate uterus

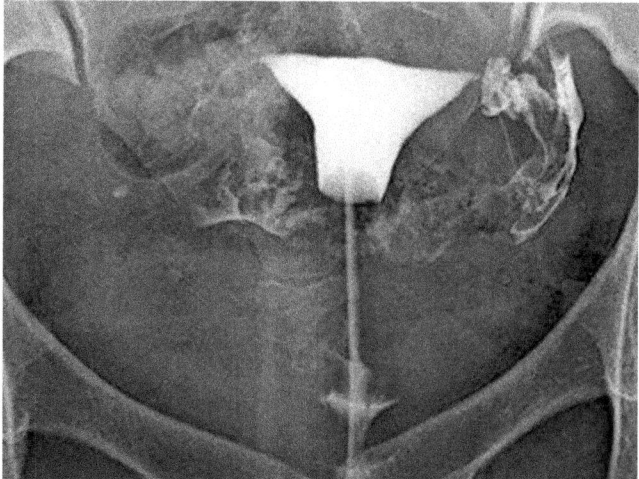
Unilateral tubal block

SECTION 7

Tubal Factors

- Tubal Evaluation: When and How
- Role of Tubal Surgery: Tubal Disease
- Role of Tubal Surgery: Tubal Re-anastomosis

CHAPTER 16

Tubal Evaluation: When and How

Ankita Kaushal, Rajeev Agarwal

INTRODUCTION

In a female undergoing evaluation for subfertility, tubal factors account for 25–35% of cases. For proper tubal functioning, a coordination of hormone secretion, ciliary action, and neuromuscular activity is required. The role of the fallopian tube is to aid in sperm transport and capacitation, retrieving the ova, facilitating the meeting of ova and sperm, fertilization, storing the formed embryo, nourishing it and finally transporting it to the uterine cavity for implantation. Normal tubal function can be compromised by any external or internal injury.

A. A female should be subjected to tubal evaluation after one year of unprotected intercourse if she is less than 35 years of age and has no other associated pathology with no or mild male factor infertility. However, if she is more than 35 years of age or has associated moderate to severe male infertility or any other risk factors that increase the risk for tubal pathology then early evaluation (i.e. after 6 months of unprotected intercourse) is recommended. The risk factors for tubal damage are history of ectopic pregnancy/pregnancies, pelvic inflammatory disease (PID), endometriosis, previous pelvic surgery, and tuberculosis (with pre-existing pathology preconceptional evaluation is recommended). Prior abortions and myomectomy may also predispose to subclinical inflammation or infection ultimately leading to tubal damage. Chlamydia antibody test is not a reliable test for tubal pathology; with negative Chlamydia antibody test, chances of tubal pathology are less than 15%.

B. Tubal disease includes both anatomical pathology and any factors that hamper normal functions of the tube. Anatomical factors such as obstruction, narrowing, and dilatation. Tubal function is also affected by factors external to the tube, changes in the muscular wall or to the tubal mucosa. Tubal block might involve the distal part, middle part or the proximal part.

C. Proximal tubal obstruction comprises of 10–25% of all tubal disease. It is most commonly due to muscular spasm and PID. Tubercular infection when involving the tube can be a mild one with damage to mucosa of the tube or it can be severe with peritubal scarring, kinking, rigidity of the tube, steno-occlusions, dilatation, formation of hydrosalpinx, and pelvic adhesions. Commonly used tests are hysterosalpingogram (HSG), laparoscopy, hystero-contrast sonography, and saline infusion sonography (SIS) or sonosalpingography (SSG).

D. Hysterosalpingogram is the most commonly used test for evaluation of patency of tubes. If it states patent tubes, tubal blockage is very unlikely (of those who have a normal HSG, 5% will get detected with tubal occlusion on laparoscopy). Normal HSG reduces the risk tubal factor might play a role in future infertility of that particular couple. Around 60% of patients with blocked tubes on first HSG, when repeated after a month, show bilateral patent tubes. Patients with subfertility should undergo repeat HSG after 1 month, if first report suggests proximal bilateral tubal block.

E. Other imaging modalities commonly employed for tubal patency tests include hystero contrast sonography (HyCoSy) and SSG/SIS. Results of SSG correlate positively with laparoscopy in 97% and SSG and HSG showed 93% correlation. The shortcoming of the procedure is that even when patency of tube can be confirmed, it does not give any information about the site of the block, condition of the lumen and tubo-ovarian relationship. Modifications such as use of pulse Doppler, color Doppler, combining air and saline, use of three-dimensional (3D) saline sonosalpingography were applied for better results. HyCoSy is a safe, low-cost, and high accuracy outpatient procedure. A meta-analysis, which compared the results of HyCoSy and laparoscopy and dye tests in 428 infertile women, showed that the sensitivity was 93.3% and specificity was 89.7%.

F. Laparoscopy is the "gold standard" for assessment of tubal pathology. It is an operative procedure and is associated with anesthesia risks. Experience and training is required with proper operation theater (OT) set up and operating team.

G. Not so commonly used tests, salpingoscopy (used to inspect the tubal mucosa), falloposcopy (endoscopy of lumen of the fallopian tube), transvaginal hydrolaparoscopy or fertiloscopy (done under local anesthesia or sedation) still need more research work in terms of diagnostic evaluation of tubes.

H. Royal College of Obstetricians and Gynaecologists (RCOG) recommendations for tubal assessment:
   - *HSG*: Recommended for women with no comorbidities [pelvic inflammatory disease (PID), previous ectopic pregnancies, and endometriosis].
   - *HyCoSy*: In women without comorbidities, where appropriate expertise is available.
   - *Laparoscopy with dye test*: In women with associated comorbidities, where assessment of other pelvic structures is also important along with tubal assessment.

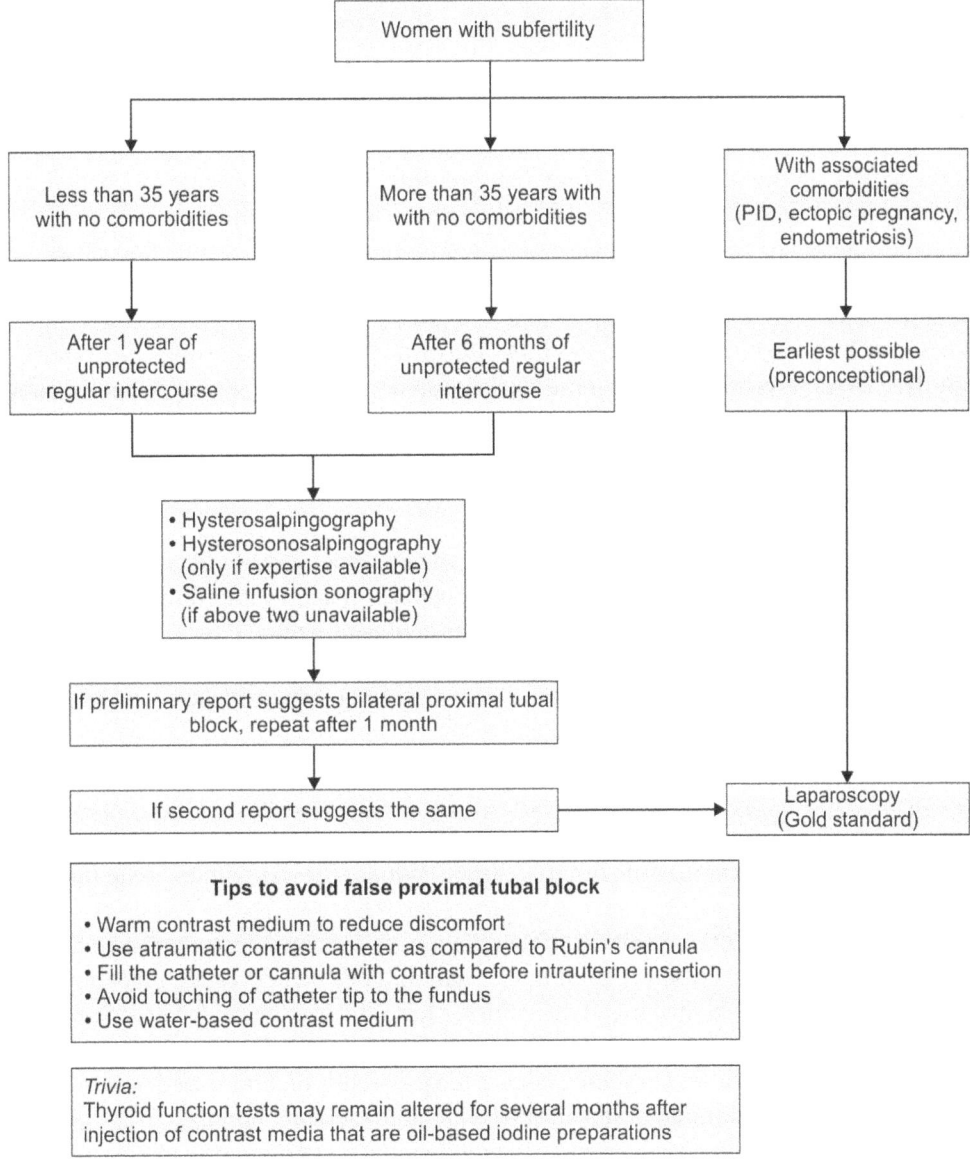

(PID: pelvic inflammatory disease)

CHAPTER 17

Role of Tubal Surgery: Tubal Disease

Mrugesh Patel

A. Laparoscopy is the gold standard for diagnosing tubal as well as pelvic factor.
B. If tubal patency test is confirmed on laparoscopy, the couple may be advised to proceed with intrauterine insemination (IUI) or try naturally based on the other factors. The decision to perform a laparoscopy in the presence of single patent tube should be taken after measuring the advantages and disadvantages of the same. Presence of a single patent tube is good enough to plan for pregnancy either naturally or through IUI. Even if the dominant follicle releases on from the contralateral ovary of patent tube, pregnancy can still be achieved due to transperitoneal migration. Older women with long standing infertility, other subfertility factors and unilateral tubal block should be considered for laparoscopic evaluation, on the other hand younger and recently married women with normal fertility evaluation apart from unilateral block should be considered for conservative management.
C. If a proximal tubal block is seen, a coaxial catheter system is introduced for tubal cannulation either under fluoroscopic guidance or with the help of a hysteroscope (confirmation by laparoscope). An outer catheter is introduced into the uterotubal ostium and a selective salpingogram is done. If tubal blockage is indeed seen, then an inner catheter with a flexible guidewire is advanced through the outer tube. The distal part of the tube must be of course normal as seen on laparoscopy. If gentle pressure does not clear the blockage then true occlusion is conformed. In about 85% of cases, this procedure clears the blockage. Ongoing pregnancy rates are higher with hysteroscopic cannulation.
D. Distal tubal disease can be fimbrial adhesions or hydrosalpinges. Both occur due to pelvic inflammatory disease but may also occur due to some prior tubal surgery or due to peritonitis. Mildly dilated tubes or flimsy adnexal adhesions have good prognosis.
E. E1. Yonger women with milder forms of tubal disease and no other associated subfertility factors have the best prognosis and benefit the most from tubal surgery. Older women with associated subfertility factors should be counseled for assisted reproductive technique (ART) to increase the conception rate.
   E2. Women with massively dilated tubes, extensive peritubal adhesions or damaged luminal mucosa have poor prognosis at establishing tubal functionality postsurgery. These women benefit from either tubal occlusion or complete salpingectomy.
F. Proximal tubal occlusion (mechanical clipping preferred over salpingectomy since it preserves ovarian reserve) has been shown to increase the pregnancy rates in women with hydrosalpinx visible on ultrasonography (USG) undergo in ART.
G. Incising the hydrosalpinges at the time of proximal occlusion reduces the risk of increase in the size of hydrosalpinx postsurgery.
H. Laparoscopic salpingectomy is indicated when the fallopian tube is damaged beyond repair. Numerous studies have shown that hydrosalpinges negatively affect in vitro fertilization (IVF) success rates. This may be due to decreased endometrial receptivity, mechanical flushing of the embryos from the uterine cavity, or a direct embryotoxic effect. Those hydrosalpinges, which are visible on ultrasound, may be more significantly affected. Staying closer to the fallopian tube while coagulating the mesosalpinx reduces the possibility of diminished ovarian reserve postsurgery. Presence of unilateral hydrosalphinx diagnosed on USG is an indication for clipping.
I. Patient should be evaluated and counseled based on their individual merit of success of tubal surgery against the risk of failure and ectopic pregnancy. IVF should be given as the choice of management for all women with severe tubal disease or failed tubal surgery.

Role of Tubal Surgery: Tubal Disease

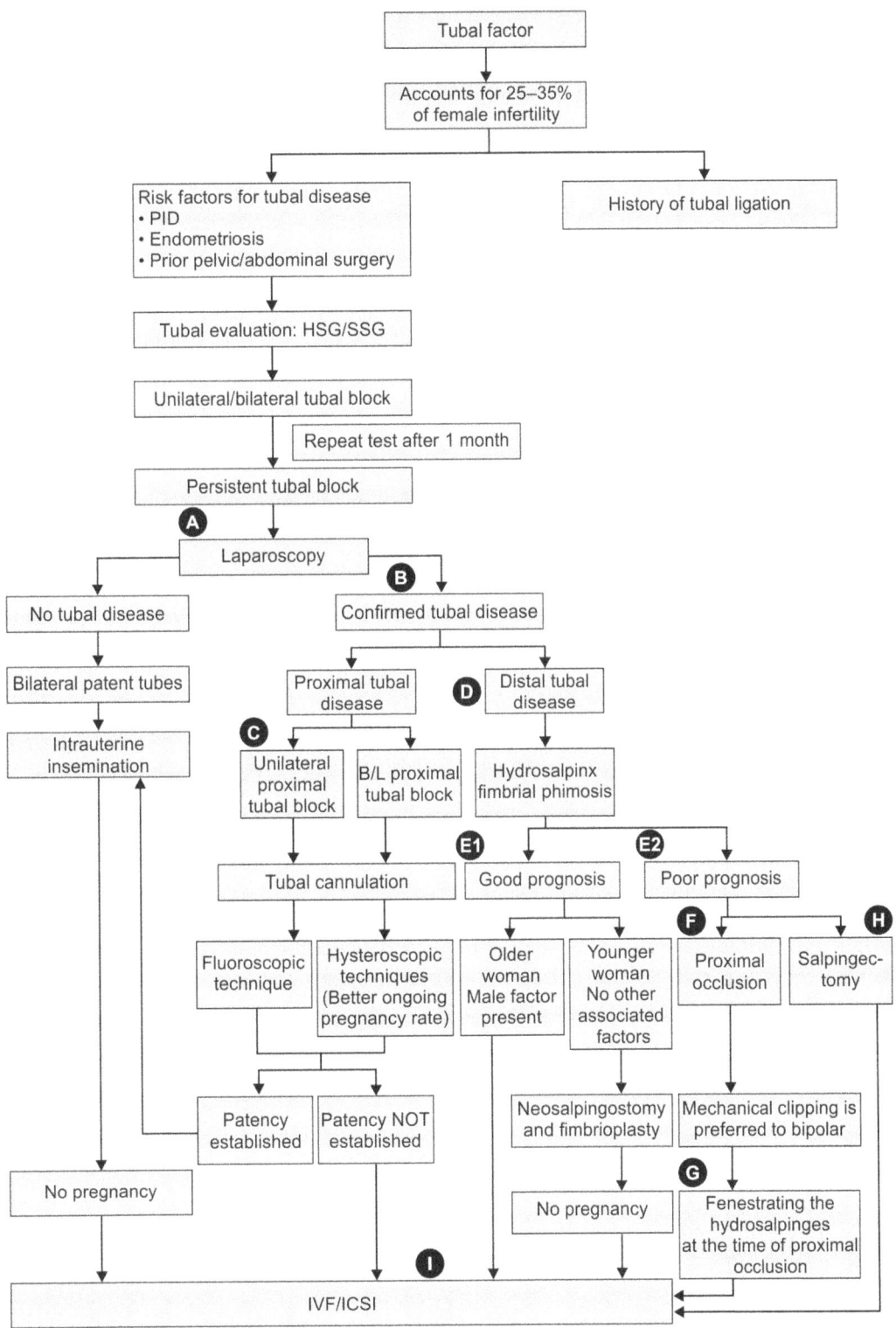

(HSG: hysterosalpingography; ICSI: intracytoplasmic sperm injection; IVF: in vitro fertilization; SSG: sonosalpingography; PID: pelvic inflammatory disease; B/L: bilateral)

CHAPTER 18

Role of Tubal Surgery: Tubal Re-anastomosis

Mrugesh Patel, Apoorva Pallam Reddy

A. Tubal reanastomosis or tubal reversal, a surgical method used to reverse tubal ligation (an operation to prevent pregnancy by the surgical tying, or coagulation of the fallopian tubes or application of fallope rings to prevent fertilization of the oocyte) may be an option for women who wish to re-establish their fertility. Pregnancy and birth rates vary widely depending on age and prior sterilization method. Since microsurgical principles have been applied to tubal anastomosis surgery, studies consistently have reported success, whether performed by laparotomy or by laparoscopy with or without a surgical robot. Definitions of success have varied. The definitions include: tubal patency, pregnancy, uterine pregnancy, ongoing pregnancy, viable pregnancy, term pregnancy, delivery and birth. Various factors need to be taken into account before an apt choice of management is considered for women seeking tubal re-anastomosis.

B. The fallopian tube assessment is basically divided into two parts:
   1. Assessment of the proximal part of fallopian tube
   2. Assessment of the distal part of fallopian tube.

   The proximal part of fallopian tube is accessed by hysterosalpingography. If the proximal tubal length is less than 2 cm, the couple should be counseled for in vitro fertilization as tubal anastomosis is highly likely to fail.
   If the proximal fallopian tube is ≥ 2 cm, a laparoscopy is recommended to assess the distal tube segment.

C. If the fimbria are absent, she is not a good candidate for tubal anastomosis; and in vitro fertilization (IVF) should be considered. In women with intact fimbria and good effective length of the fallopian tube, reanastomosis may be considred.

D. Intraoperatively, if abnormal/obliterated endosalpinx is detected, the patient has a higher probability of ending up with an ectopic pregnancy—tubal implantation even if tubal patency is established. Hence, they are advised to opt for assisted reproductive technique (ART).

E. Both laparotomy and laparoscopy are equally effective in establishing tubal anastamosis based on the type of setting, expertise of the surgeon and condition of the patient.

F. In cases with a healthy normal endosalpinx, a tubo-tubal anastomosis is carried out after both proximal and distal tubal segments are pepared and anastamosed. Patency is checked post procedure on the table by injceting methylene blue into the cavity.

G. The couple is counseled extensively regarding prognosis for pregnancy and complications. In younger women, with no other associtaed infertility factors in either of the couple and longer proximal segment with normal endosalpinx, tubal anastomosis offeres an effective and cheaper alternative to achieving pregnancy compared to ART.

Role of Tubal Surgery: Tubal Re-anastomosis

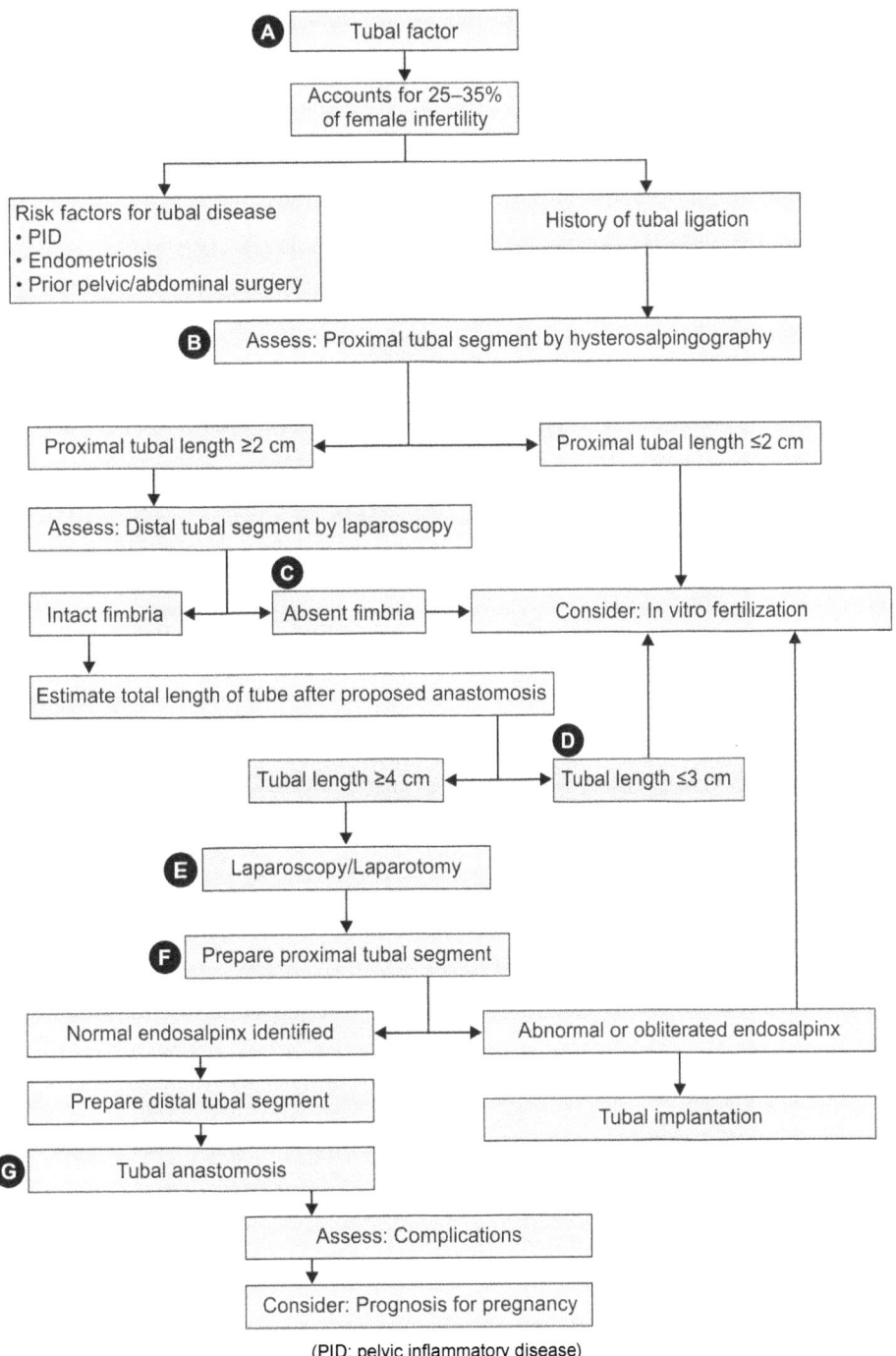

(PID: pelvic inflammatory disease)

Hydrosalpinx on 2D-USG

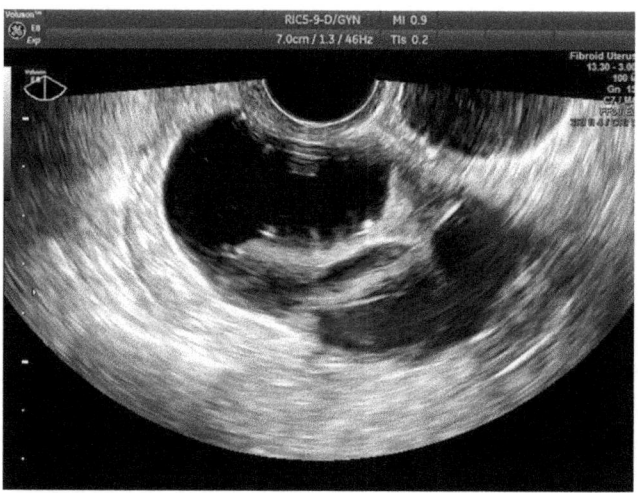

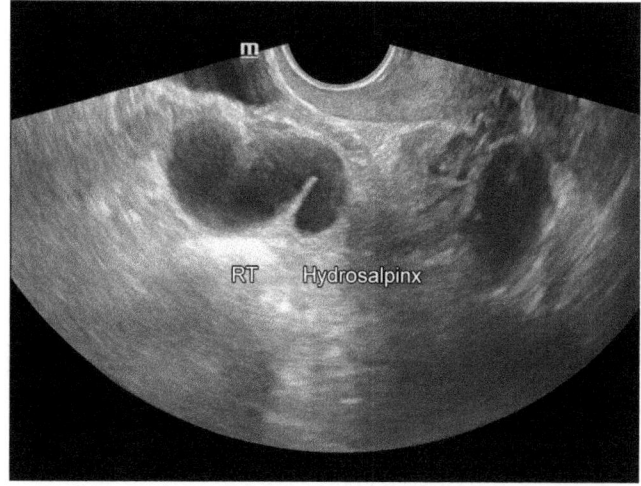

SECTION 8

Endocrine Factors

- PCOS and Infertility
- Thyroid Disorders
- Hirsutism
- Galactorrhea
- Hyperprolactinemia

CHAPTER 19

PCOS and Infertility

Diksha Goswami

PCOS WITH INFERTILITY

A. Polycystic ovarian syndrome (PCOS) is the most common endocrinopathy amongst subfertile women. It accounts to as high as 80% of the women with ovulatory dysfunction (WHO Type II). About 40% of the women diagnosed with PCOS have associated metabolic syndrome, which has severe implications for maternal and fetal health. Hence all PCOS women should be evaluated for metabolic syndrome and specially obese PCOS should have a lipid profile, oral glucose tolerance test, and waist circumference and blood pressure measurement to rule out metabolic syndrome. They should be counseled regarding long-term health implications of the same.

B. Lifestyle interventions, which include diet and physical activity, should be recommended for all women with PCOS to optimize the health. Weight loss of 5–10% yields significant clinical improvements and this can be achieved by consuming hypocaloric diet hypocaloric diet (500 kcal deficit) with reduced glycemic load. Regular moderate intensity physical activity, no less than 150 minute/week is an important component of weight loss programs and enhances the overall health benefit. Bariatric surgery should be offered to morbidly obese women or in presence of comorbidities.

C. At present, international consensus of all major societies endorses that letrozole should be considered first-line pharmacological treatment for ovulation induction (OI) in women with PCOS with anovulatory infertility and no other infertility factors to improve ovulation, pregnancy, and live birth rates, Dose: 2.5–7.5 mg/day for 5–10 days. Where letrozole is not available or use is not permitted or cost is prohibitive, health professionals can use other ovulation induction agents. Clomiphene citrate (CC) alone can also be used for OI in these women (Dose: 50–150 mg/day for 5–10 days). Male factor and tubal infertility should be ruled out before OI especially in patients with risk factors. Choice of drug for OI should be decided after considering previous response, anticipated response, availability of drug and local guidelines. Patients who do not respond to maximal possible dosage (Resistance) can shift to second-line agents. In women with adequate response and ovulatory cycles, same drug and dosage can be continued for 3–6 cycles.

D. Metformin 1,500–2,000 mg/day in divided doses can be added to women who are CC resistant especially if body mass index is more than 30 kg/m^2 after explaining the gastrointestinal side effects.

E. Gonadotropins (GT) are the second-line drugs indicated in women with PCOS who have not conceived on first-line agents (CC or letrozole) or have resistance to CC after ruling out other infertility factors. Chronic low-dose protocol is preferred in these women in order to reduce the side effects of multiple pregnancy and ovarian hyperstimulation. The principle is to use the least possible dosage for response with strict ultrasonography (USG) monitoring and cancellation criteria. Adding metformin to these patients not only increases the ovulation rates, but also reduces the chance of hyperstimulation.

F. Laparoscopic ovarian surgery (LOS) is the second line modality for OI in resistant or failed cases. Choice between LOS and gonadotropins depends on surgical expertise, cost, monitoring, and potential side effects. LOS is preferred over GT in the presence of other indications for laparoscopy. LOS has better results in lean women with high luteinizing hormone (LH) more than 10 and high free androgen index values.

G. In vitro fertilization (IVF) is usually the third-line treatment in women with PCOS where first-line or second-line therapies have failed unless there are other absolute indications for IVF. Problems faced in these women include risk of hyperstimulation and subsequent ovarian hyperstimulation syndrome (OHSS), poor oocyte quality, and altered endometrial receptivity. Due to increased incidence of fertilization failure in these women, some advocate intracytoplasmic sperm injection (ICSI) to improve the fertilization rates. In vitro maturation (IVM) of oocytes has also been advocated though largely experimental at present to reduce incidence of OHSS.

H. Strategies to optimize the IVF outcome in women with PCOS include using an antagonist protocol with agonist protocol in women at risk of OHSS. Elective cryopreservation can be done in these women to reduce chances of early OHSS and if agonist trigger has been used.

PCOS and Infertility

TRIVIA ABOUT PCOS

- There is 40% chance of affliction with PCOS if sister is affected and 10% if mother has PCOS.
- Polycystic ovary syndrome is also known as Stein-Leventhal syndrome, names of the two scientists who first described this syndrome.
- It is the most common endocrinological disorder affecting 5–10% women in reproductive age group.

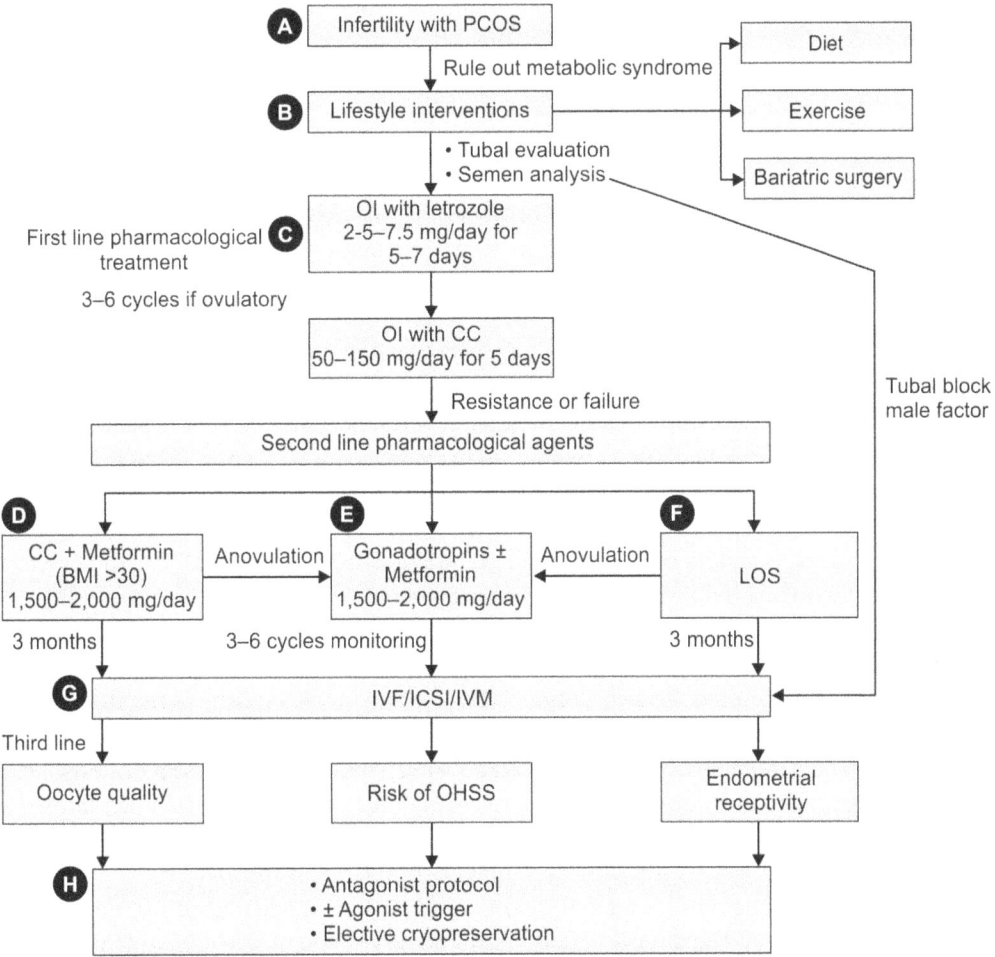

(BMI: body mass index; CC: clomiphene citrate; ICSI: intracytoplasmic sperm injection; IVF: in vitro fertilization; IVM: In vitro maturation; LOS: laparoscopic ovarian surgery; PCOS: polycystic ovary syndrome; OHSS: ovarian hyperstimulation syndrome; OI: ovulation induction)

CHAPTER 20

Thyroid Disorders

Diksha Goswami

THYROID DISORDERS IN INFERTILITY

A. The National Institute for Health and Care Excellence (NICE) and American Association of Clinical Endocrinologists (AACE) all recommend against universal screening for thyroid in infertile women. It is recommended that aggressive case finding should instead be the norm. Serum thyroid-stimulating hormone (TSH) should be used to screen all women presenting with signs or symptoms suggestive of thyroid disease, undergoing assisted reproductive technique (ART) procedures or history of diabetes/autoimmune disorders.

B. Women with high TSH levels more than 4.2–4.5 mIU/L despite normal free T3 and free T4 levels are defined as having subclinical hypothyroidism. Anti-peroxidase antibodies (Anti-TPO) should be checked if repeated TSH levels more than 2.5 mIU/L or recurrent miscarriages or other risk factors for thyroid disease are present. Treatment with levothyroxine is started if TSH levels are more than 4 mIU/L or if more than 2.5 mIU/L and anti-TPO antibodies are positive. There is limited evidence to support treatment with levothyroxine in asymptomatic women with TSH more than 2.5. If these women are not treated, they should be monitored every 4 weeks when pregnant.

C. Women with overt hypothyroidism have high TSH levels and low free triiodothyronine (FT3) and free thyroxine (FT4) levels. Treatment with levothyroxine improves the pregnancy rates, decreases risk of miscarriage, and improves the pregnancy outcomes in these women. Dose of levothyroxine is between 25 µg and 75 µg if TSH is less than 10 and 1.6 µg/kg/day if TSH levels are ≥ 10.

D. Women on thyroxine replacement should be monitored every 4–8 weeks after initiating therapy or any change in dose. Once pregnant TSH levels should be checked and maintained to below 2.5 mIU/L in the first trimester. Usually 30–50% increase in levothyroxine requirement is there in pregnancy.

E. Subclinical hyperthyroidism is diagnosed if TSH level is low in presence of normal FT3 and FT4 levels. Treatment with antithyroid drugs can be considered if TSH is persistently below <0.1 mIU/L or if symptomatic. Women with levels between 0.1 and 0.4 can be monitored. Propylthiouracil (PTU) is the preferred drug in first trimester.

F. Women with Grave's disease demonstrate positive TSH receptor stimulating antibodies and diffuse uptake of radioactive iodine (RAI). These women should be treated along with an endocrinologist. Treatment options include radioactive iodine/antithyroid drugs or thyroidectomy. In women receiving RAI, pregnancy should be planned after 6 months. Doses of carbimazole are 10–30 mg once daily and for PTU—50–150 mg three times. Minimal dose of drugs should be given to normalize thyroid function until which pregnancy should be postponed.

G. Total T3 and FT4 levels should be monitored 2–6 weeks after starting antithyroid drugs. Baseline complete blood count and liver function test should be done and patient should be warned of side effects. Once woman is euthyroid, dose of drugs can be reduced. Consider switching over to PTU or withdrawal of drugs or definitive treatment like RAI/surgery in these women before planning conception.

Thyroid Disorders

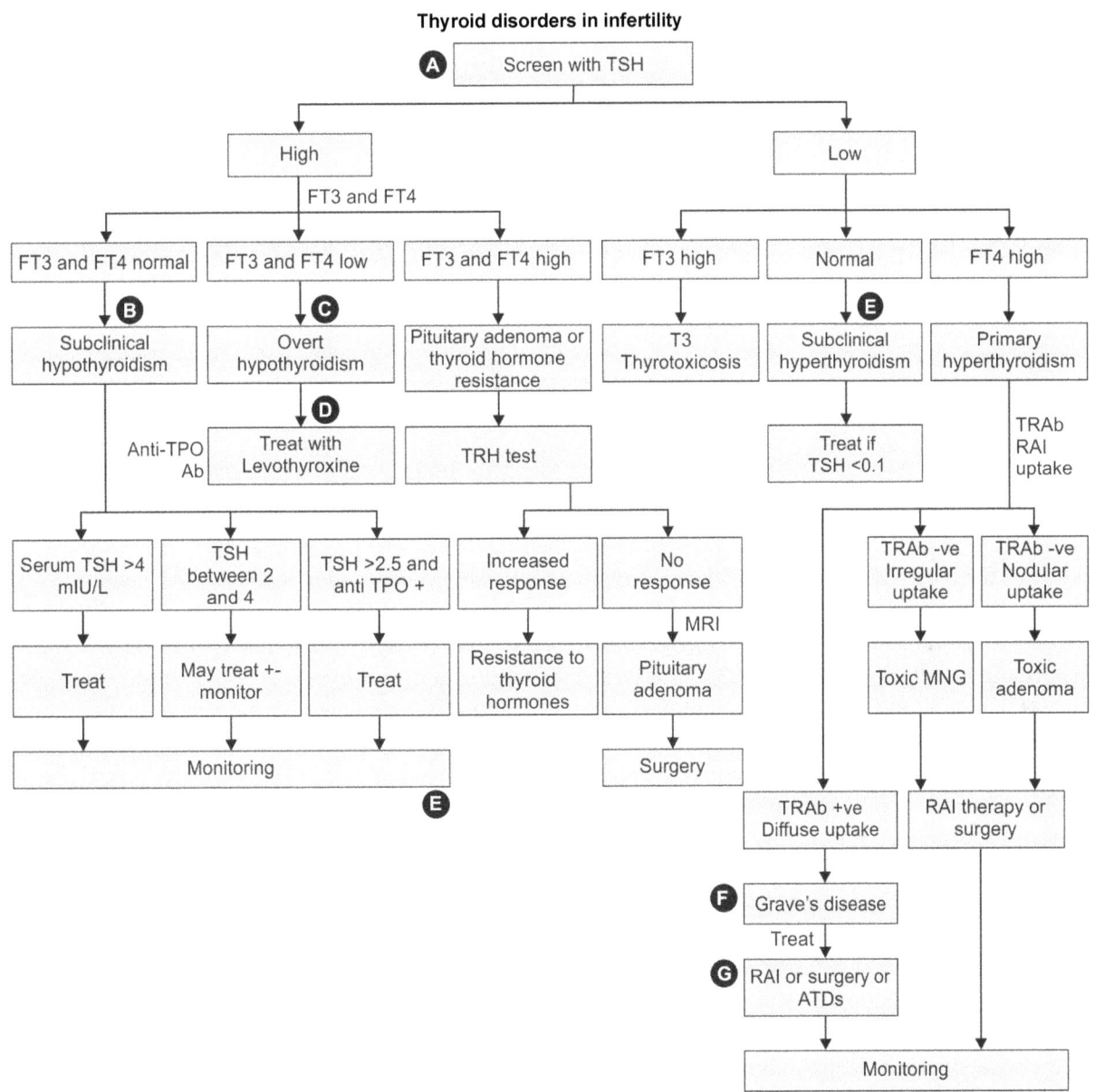

(TSH: thyroid-stimulating hormone; FT3: free triiodothyronine; FT4: free thyroxine; TPO: thyroid peroxidase; TRH: thyrotropin releasing hormone; TRAb: thyrotropin receptor antibody; MNG: multinodular goiter; RAI: radioactive iodine; ATDs: antithyroid drugs)

CHAPTER 21

Hirsutism

Shally Gupta

INTRODUCTION

Hirsutism is a hormonal disorder in which there is excess growth of terminal hair in androgen-dependent areas in women such as abdomen, upper back, breasts, upper lip and chin. About 5–10% of women of reproductive age are affected. Hirsutism is confused with hypertrichosis sometimes. However, hypertrichosis is defined as excessive hair growth, in non-androgen-dependent areas of the body and can be terminal or villus in nature. It can be acquired or congenital.

A. Evaluation involves a detailed history, physical examination, and blood tests to find out the cause and rule out idiopathic hirsutism. A simple way to quantify hair growth is the Ferriman–Gallwey (FG) score.

B. The Endocrine Society guidelines discourage routine evaluation of androgen levels when women have mild hirsutism. Biochemical testing is recommended in women with sudden onset, moderate to severe, rapidly progressive hirsutism, and when associated with acanthosis nigricans, irregular menses, central obesity, and fertility.

C. Total testosterone is initial investigation of choice in hirsute women and signifies androgen production. Further evaluation of free testosterone can be done if total testosterone is significantly elevated.

D. If the total testosterone level is more than 150 ng/dL further investigation is required as it could be because of ovarian hyperthecosis or ovarian or adrenal testosterone-secreting tumor. If dehydroepiandrosterone sulfate (DHEA-S) levels are more than 700 µg/dL it could be because of hormone secreting adrenocortical carcinoma. Elevated 17-hydroxy-progesterone levels with severe hirsutism is strongly suggestive of congenital adrenal hyperplasia (CAH). Prolactin needs to be evaluated in women with menstrual abnormalities. In those with signs of cortisol excess a 24-hour urine free-cortisol examination is needed. To rule out any ovarian or adrenal tumor, a pelvic ultrasound and CT scan respectively is needed.

E. Estrogen-progestin combinations are usually first-line treatment options in mild to moderate hirsutism. The level of sex hormone-binding globulin (SHBG) is increased with estrogen thus decreasing the levels of free testosterone and other SHBG-bound androgens. Adrenal androgens are also inhibited by interfering with their synthesis. Combination of low-dose ethinyl estradiol (0.03–0.035 mg) in combination with a progestin that has low androgenic or antiandrogenic properties is usually started as first line. It has been seen oral contraceptive pills (OCPs) with cyproterone acetate (CPA) is more effective than drospirenone, for the treatment of hirsutism in polycystic ovarian syndrome (PCOS).

F. Antiandrogens are second-line drug therapy for hirsutism. Spironolactone is an aldosterone antagonist. Various enzymes involved in androgen biosynthesis are inhibited. Finasteride is a type-2, 5-α reductase inhibitor. As it does not affect type-1, 5-α reductase inhibitors a partial inhibitory effect is anticipated. It should always be used with a contraceptive since it can cause feminization of a male fetus because dihydrotestosterone (DHT) is involved in the development of male external genitalia. Flutamide is a nonsteroidal antiandrogen, which works by blocking androgen receptors thus preventing the binding of DHT. Flutamide is associated, with liver toxicity. Other treatment options include down regulation with GnRH agonists and insulin sensitizing agents like metformin. Topical creams containing eflornithine hydrochloride 13.9% (Vaniqa) inhibit the enzyme ornithine decarboxylase and stop hair growth. Combination with laser and photoepilation gives best results. Nonpharmacological permanent or temporary hair removal methods can also be used.

CAUSES OF HIRSUTISM

- Hirsutism is most commonly caused by PCOS. It develops at puberty and presents with other complaints of PCOS such as menstrual irregularities, infertility, weight gain, anovulation, and insulin resistance. Idiopathic hirsutism is responsible for approximately half the patients.

Hirsutism

- Congenital adrenal hyperplasia has three forms: 3-β hydroxysteroid dehydrogenase deficiency, 21-hydroxylase deficiency, and 11-hydroxylase deficiency. 21-hydroxylase deficiency is the most common. They present at birth or in early infancy, with sign and symptoms of androgen excess, genital ambiguity, hirsutism, and cortisol deficiency.
- 5% of all ovarian tumors are androgen secreting tumors. They cause hirsutism that presents later in life and has rapid progress and very high testosterone levels.
- Adrenal tumors are mostly adrenal carcinoma that secretes DHEA and DHEA-S. Cushing's disease is usually due to ACTH-secreting adenoma that causes increased cortisol and adrenal androgens.
- Drug-induced hirsutism can be due to phenytoin, danazol, glucocorticoids, cyclosporine, and progesterone.

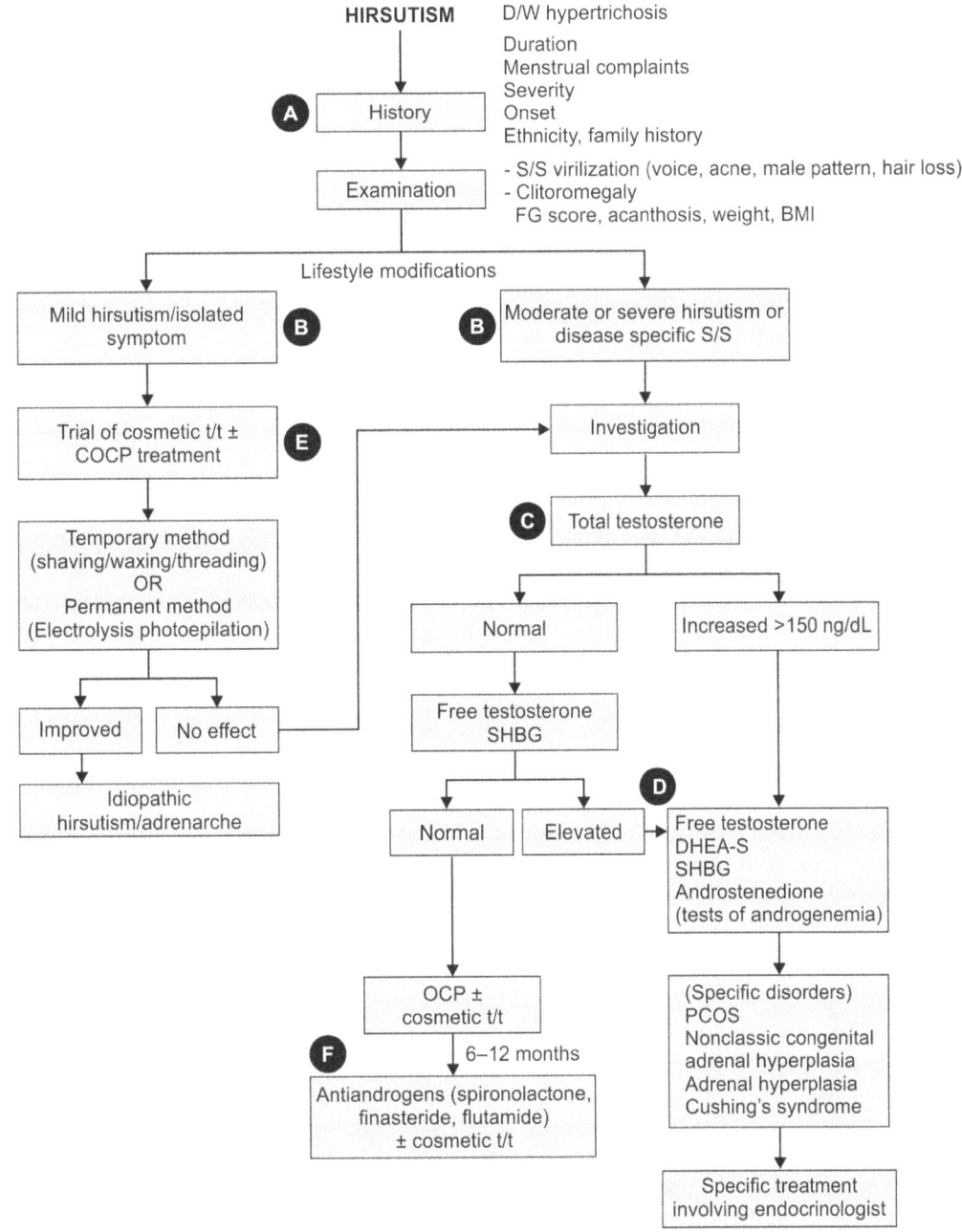

(COCP: combined oral contraceptive pill; DHEA-S: dehydroepiandrosterone sulfate; FG: Ferriman–Gallwey. OCP: oral contraceptive pill; PCOS: polycystic ovarian syndrome; SHBG: sex hormone-binding globulin; BMI: body mass index; S/S: signs and symptoms; D/W: differentiate with)

CHAPTER 22

Galactorrhea

Ruby Ruprai, Chetan Kaur Ruprai

INTRODUCTION

Galactorrhea is the secretion of breast milk at a time remote from nursing and is usually due to hyperprolactinemia or excessive sensitivity of the breast to normal circulating levels of prolactin. Galactorrhea warrants an evaluation regardless of the patients' menstrual status.

Isolated galactorrhea, with normal menses and normal serum prolactin levels, occurs in up to 20% of women at some point in their lives.

A. True galactorrhea may be *caused by* a variety of disorders, including pituitary tumors, primary hypothyroidism, chronic renal failure or hepatic disease, and neurogenic stimulation from breast manipulation, infectious and traumatic lesions of the chest wall (herpes zoster, rib fracture, and chest wall scar). Several classes of drugs may cause hyperprolactinemia and galactorrhea. The *most common causes* of hyperprolactinemia include prolactin-secreting pituitary tumor, use of dopamine antagonist (metoclopramide, phenothiazines, and risperidone), use of neuroactive medications (selective serotonin reuptake inhibitors), pregnancy, renal disease, and primary hypothyroidism.
   - *When associated with normal ovulatory menses*, the most likely cause is excessive sensitivity of the breast to normal circulating levels of prolactin.
   - *When associated with amenorrhea*, the circulating prolactin level (PRL) is likely elevated. The clinical picture of *hyperprolactinemia* mimics the puerperal period, characterized by irregular menses or amenorrhea, galactorrhea, infertility, and a decreased libido. Patients can also exhibit hypopituitarism, visual impairment, and headache due to an expanding mass.

B. Whenever galactorrhea is identified, *serum prolactin* should be measured, preferably in morning fasting sample. Because the secretion of prolactin is labile and episodic, an elevated prolactin level should be confirmed on at least two occasions when the patient is in a fasting, nonexercised state, with no breast stimulation (nipple stimulation/breast examination should be avoided for at least 30 minutes before checking PRL levels). *Stress* can increase PRL secretion; therefore, levels just outside the normal range should be repeated. Nearly 30% of hyperprolactinemia can be stress related.

C. If *PRL level is not elevated, then no further evaluation* is needed. Observation or treatment with a dopamine receptor agonist is an option, since galactorrhea may occur in the presence of normoprolactinemia. In *women with galactorrhea, normal ovulatory menses, and normal prolactin concentration*, low doses of dopamine agonists, bromocriptine (1.25–2.5 mg) or cabergoline (0.25 mg once or twice weekly) are often effective.

D. *If level is greater than 30 ng/mL*, serum thyroid-stimulating hormone (TSH) and *creatinine* levels should be measured to rule out secondary causes of hyperprolactinemia and prolactin determination repeated. Because about *5% of primary hypothyroidism patients also have hyperprolactinemia*, it is important to exclude thyroid disease. If TSH is high, complete thyroid evaluation should be performed. With thyroid replacement, TSH and PRLs should return to normal.

E. If no cause for the hyperprolactinemia is found by history, examination, and routine testing, *MRI of the pituitary fossa*, with gadolinium enhancement should be performed to rule out intracranial lesion. *CT is inferior to MRI and* may not be sensitive enough to identify small lesions or large lesions that are isodense with surrounding structures. Serum prolactin greater than 200 ng/mL virtually assures the presence of a prolactinoma. About 40% of microadenomas are prolactin secreting. *Pituitary adenoma should be suspected in every patient who has hyperprolactinemia*, even in those with relatively minor elevations, since a microadenoma has been reported in a patient with a prolactin level of only 23 ng/mL. Suprasellar lesions (craniopharyngioma) frequently cause only marginal hyperprolactinemia. Incidental pituitary adenomas are found by MRI scanning in 10% of normal population. An elevated prolactin level coincident with a pituitary lesion does not always imply a prolactinoma is present.

Galactorrhea

TREATMENT OF GALACTORRHEA WHEN PROLACTIN LEVELS ARE HIGH

Since most galactorrhea is associated with hyperprolactinemia, treatment is classified based on the underlying causes or effects of hyperprolactinemia. Treatment is not recommended for patients with asymptomatic microprolactinoma.

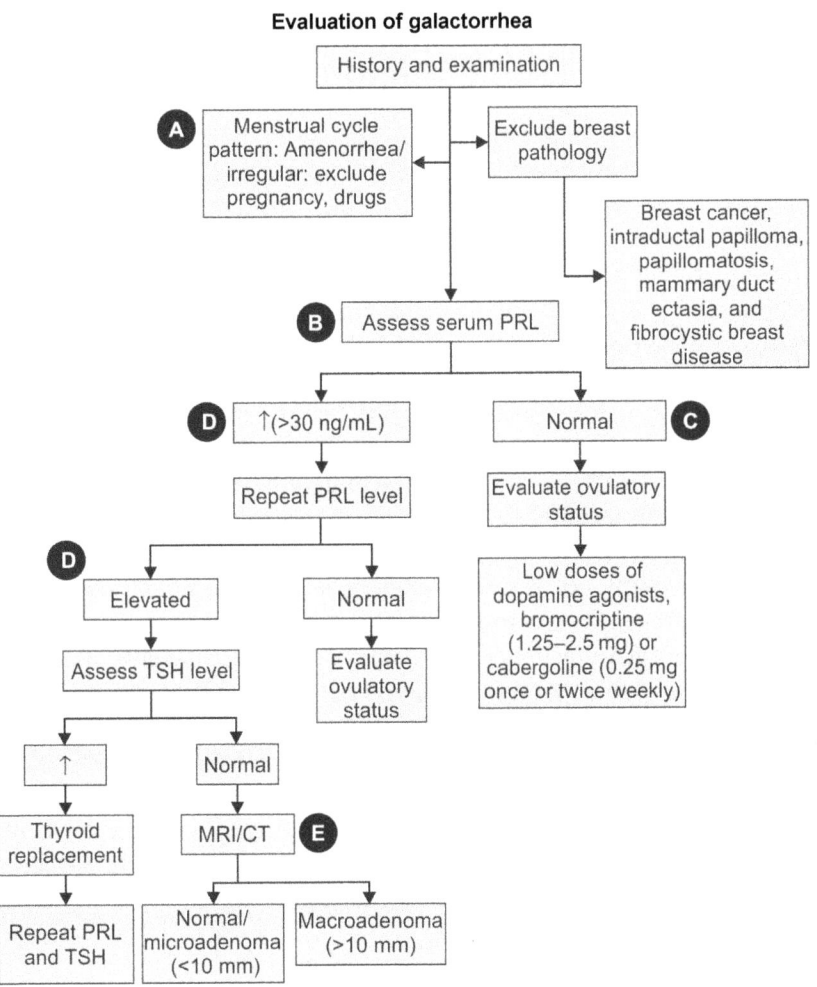

(TSH: thyroid-stimulating hormone; PRL: prolactin)

CHAPTER 23

Hyperprolactinemia

Ruby Ruprai, Sejal Desai

A. For patients with symptomatic prolactinomas (both macroadenomas and microadenomas), medical therapy with dopamine agonists is the treatment of choice. Prolonged suppression may be required to prevent tumor growth and the return of hyperprolactinemia, galactorrhea, and ovulatory dysfunction. Because of the inherent risks of surgery and the efficacy of dopamine agonists, surgery or radiation therapy is rarely needed for prolactinomas. Surgery should be considered only in cases of resistance or intolerance to optimal medical therapy, when there clearly are neurologic or other problems caused by direct expansion of the tumor. Trans-sphenoidal surgery is the conventional procedure. Stereotactic radiosurgery is more popular as MRI allows more accurate dose planning.
B. Pituitary gland secretes prolactin (PRL), follicle-stimulating hormone (FSH), luteinizing hormone (LH), adrenocorticotropic hormone (ACTH), and thyroid-stimulating hormone (TSH). PRL-secreting pituitary adenomas can reduce the secretion of FSH and LH and cause amenorrhea. Estrogen replacement is considered safe for the patient with a microadenoma or idiopathic hyperprolactinemia. However, its use should be individualized in macroadenomas because estrogen has the potential to increase tumor growth. Because estrogen replacement does not correct the LH and FSH deficiencies, women should be counseled that such replacement does not restore ovulation.
C. In patients with hyperprolactinemia, PRL levels should be monitored, and MRI should be performed every 2 years (more often if pituitary tumor is suspected).
D. Dopamine agonists have been shown to be effective in normalizing PRL, restoring hypothalamus-pituitary-gonadal axis function and reproductive hormones, shrinking adenomas and abrogating galactorrhea, and increasing bone density via normalization of estrogen/testosterone levels.
E. Serum PRL levels may remain normal after drug withdrawal in one-third of patients. Therefore, in patients who attain normoprolactinemia, treatment with dopamine should be periodically discontinued according to the Endocrine Society's clinical guidelines for diagnosis and treatment of hyperprolactinemia.
F. Compared with bromocriptine, cabergoline is more effective at normalizing PRL (52% taking bromocriptine vs 92% taking cabergoline), at restoring menstrual function (68% taking bromocriptine vs 82% taking cabergoline), and better tolerated (patient compliance: 3% vs 12%, $P < 0.001$). Both drugs are safe for the facilitation of ovulation and pregnancy. Although no detrimental effects on fetal outcomes have been reported, the current recommendation is to discontinue cabergoline 1 month before conception is attempted.

FOLLOW-UP

Approximately 16% of patients with "idiopathic" hyperprolactinemia (negative imaging and no other apparent cause) will develop evidence of microadenomas in follow-up.

Once the therapy is initiated, fasting PRL levels should be monitored monthly and later every 3–6 months. Shrinkage of the tumor should be followed by formal visual-field testing and MRI.

PROGNOSIS

- When monitored for longer than 7 years, 90–95% of microadenomas remains stable or gradually decreases PRL secretion.
- One-third of patients with idiopathic hyperprolactinemia may experience resolution without treatment. This increases to two-thirds if the patient's basal PRL level is less than 40 ng/mL.
- Recurrence rates of hyperprolactinemia are as high as 80%, and, subsequently, patients require long-term medical therapy.
- Surgery is often not curative for macroprolactinomas, with a recurrence rate of as high as 40% within 5 years.

Hyperprolactinemia

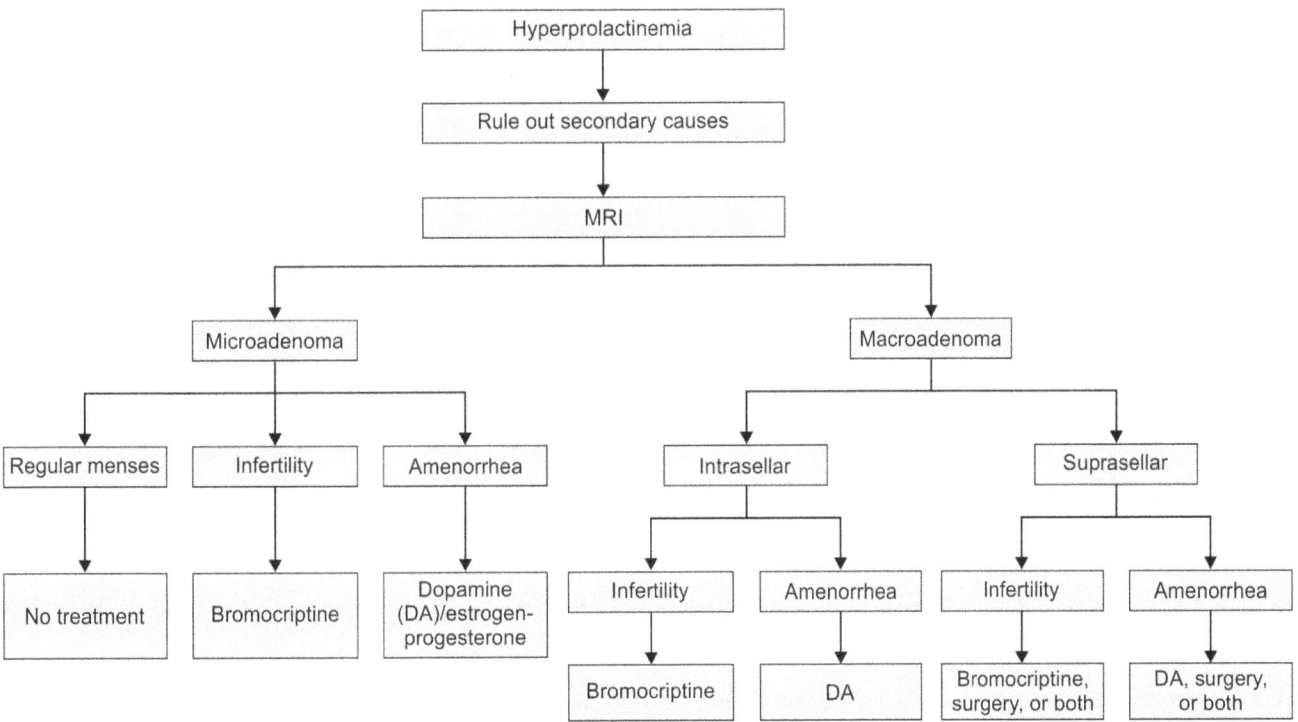

SECTION 9

Controlled Ovarian Stimulation

- Ovulation Induction: Oral Ovulogens
- Ovulation Induction: Gonadotropins
- Ovulation Induction: Adjuvants in Polycystic Ovarian Syndrome
- Ovulation Induction: Adjuvants in Poor Ovarian Reserve

CHAPTER 24

Ovulation Induction: Oral Ovulogens

Yasodhara Pallam Reddy, Apoorva Pallam Reddy

A. About 10–25% of all cases of infertility are caused by ovulatory dysfunction. The oral ovulogens act by inhibiting the negative feedback mechanism of estrogen on the hypothalamus thus increasing the endogenous follicle-stimulating hormone (FSH) levels and increasing the FSH window.

B. *Clomiphene citrate (CC)* is a selective estrogen receptor modulator that has both agonistic and antagonist effects on the receptors at various levels. It blocks the estrogen receptors at the hypothalamus and pituitary, thus eliminating the negative feedback of ovarian estrogens and increasing the pulse frequency of FSH and luteinizing hormone (LH). This raise in FSH is observed only for 5 days and does not increase even after continuing the medication beyond 5 days. Despite having an ovulatory rate of 70–92%, the low pregnancy rate is due to negative impact on endometrium, cervical mucus, tubal transport, oocytes, uterine blood flow, and placental protein synthesis.

Starting dose is 50 mg/day from day 2 of periods for 5 days. The dose is body mass index (BMI)-dependent. In case, the patient remains anovulatory to this dose; it may be increased to a maximum of 200–250/day keeping in mind that higher doses have lesser pregnancy chances despite achieving ovulation. 51% of the drug is excreted within 5 days. Thus, repeated dosage has cumulative effect. It can appear in feces up to 6 weeks. A check of liver function is necessary. Use for more than six cycles consecutively or more than 12 cycles in total is not recommended in view of slight increase in future risk of ovarian cancer.

Clomiphene resistance defined as failure to ovulate after receiving 150 mg of CC daily for 5 days per cycle, for at least three cycles, is common and occurs in approximately 15–40% in women with polycystic ovarian syndrome (PCOS). Management options for CC resistance include weight loss, addition of dexamethasone, bromocriptine, metformin, pretreatment suppression with oral contraceptive pills, laparoscopic ovarian drilling or gonadotropin usage.

C. *Tamoxifen* is also a selective estrogen receptor modulator (SERM) and has a similar mechanism of action as CC. It is started with a dose of 20 mg daily and increased by 10 mg daily in the subsequent cycle till ovulation is achieved or a maximum of 40 mg/day. Tamoxifen has been found to be as effective as CC and also effective in CC-resistant cases. It has a better endometrial morphology and cervical score than CC. The incidence of ovarian carcinoma is also lower than CC. Has higher incidence of developing endometrial polyps.

D. *Letrozole* belongs to the third-generation nonsteroidal inhibitory (type II) group of aromatase inhibitors. It has a central and peripheral mechanism of action. Letrozole inhibits the rate limiting step (aromatization) of conversion of androstenedione and testosterone to estrone and estradiol. This result in two things: (1) fall in circulating and local estrogens and (2) rise in intraovarian androgens. Thus, in the central action there is fall in estrogen levels, releasing the hypothalamo-pituitary axis from the negative feedback of estrogens. Thus, there is a surge in FSH release, which results in follicular growth. Since, the feedback mechanism is intact; normal follicular growth, selection of dominant follicle, and atresia of smaller growing follicle occurs; and thereby facilitating monofollicular growth and ovulation. Peripherally the increased intraovarian androgens increase the sensitivity of the FSH receptors. It also causes upregulation of the estrogen receptors in the endometrium, thus causing rapid growth of it upon replacement of estrogen.

Letrozole is more potent than the other aromatase inhibitors. It is 99.9% absorbed orally. Its half-life is 42 hours. A dose of 2.5 mg daily from day 2 to day 6 is used. It has been shown that a 5 mg daily dosage has better clinical pregnancy rate than 2.5 mg and 7.5 mg daily. Unlike CC, letrozole dosage is independent of BMI. Letrozole has no increased risk of congenital abnormalities as compared to CC (Badawy et al.).

E. All cycles stimulated with oral ovulogens should be monitored for ovulation preferably with ultrasonography. This helps in assessing the response to medication as well as assesses factors like endometrial thickness.

Ovulation Induction: Oral Ovulogens

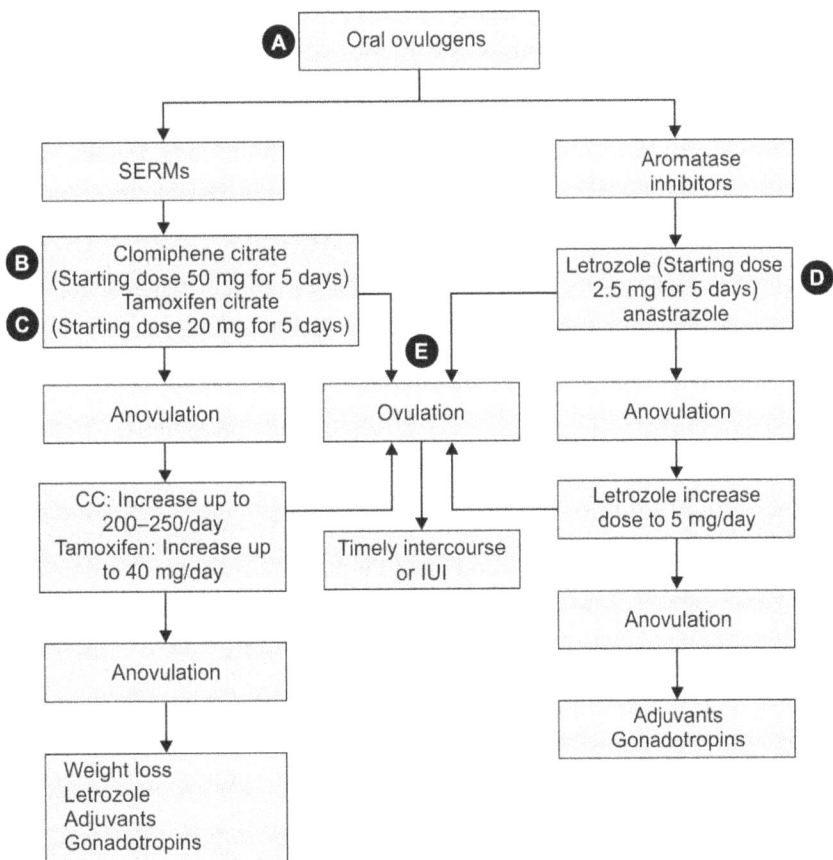

(IUI: intrauterine insemination; SERMs: selective estrogen receptor modulators; CC: clomiphene citrate)

CHAPTER 25

Ovulation Induction: Gonadotropins

Hrishikesh Pai, Apoorva Pallam Reddy

GONADOTROPINS

A. External supplementation of gonadotropins (GT) is indicated in cases of clomiphene citrate (CC) resistance, failure of ovulation with use of oral ovulogens, for inducing ovulation in hypogonadotropic hypogonadism, to improve the pregnancy rates in intrauterine insemination, mild/minimal endometriosis, and for controlled ovarian stimulation in assisted reproductive technique (ART). This significantly increases the follicle-stimulating hormone (FSH) window, thereby causing multi-follicular genesis. The pregnancy rates in GT-stimulated intrauterine insemination (IUI) are significantly higher than the oral ovulogens stimulated cycles.

B. Gonadotropins were first extracted from the urine of menopausal women that contained both FSH and luteinizing hormone (LH) in equal components—human menopausal gonadotropin (HMG). But there were other protein impurities like Tamm Horsfall protein, urokinase, tumor necrotic factor binding protein, etc. which resulted in local side effects like pain, allergic reactions, etc. Hence, these preparations resulted in inconsistent responses and could be given only as deep intramuscular preparations.

C. With the improvement of technology, these impurities were removed from the HMG preparations resulting in highly purified HMG (HP-HMG). However, the bioassay of 75 IU of HMG can range between 60 IU and 90 IU. Thus, varied response is observed. The half-life after intramuscular injection is about 35 hours.

D. Urinary FSH is prepared by separating the LH component using LH monoclonal antibodies from the original HMG preparation.

E. If the monoclonal antibodies of FSH were used to extract the FSH component of HMG, the resultant GT was highly purified FSH (HP-FSH).

F. Both human chorionic gonadotropin (HCG) and LH have same alpha unit and similar beta unit, HCG beta subunit contains an additional 23 amino acids apart from the ones present in LH. These additional amino acids increase the half-life of HCG to 24 hours compared to the 20 minutes half-life of LH. The similarities in structure make HCG an ideal component for creating a surrogate LH surge and cause the final ovulation trigger. The prolonged $t_{1/2}$ of HCG results in unwanted effects like prolonged luteotropic effect, supraphysiological levels of estrogen and progesterone, and higher chances of ovarian hyperstimulation syndrome (OHSS). Residual HCG may be mistaken for early pregnancy. Both 5,000 IU and 10,000 IU of HCG are equally effective in inducing ovulatory changes.

G. Due to the presence of human prion proteins in the commercially available preparation, the urinary preparations always carry a theoretical risk of transmission of the prion disease. This prompted the development of recombinant preparations.

H. With the development of recombinant technology, it was possible to insert the genes encoding for the alpha and beta subunits of FSH into expression vectors that are transfected into Chinese hamster ovary cell lines and produce recombinant FSH. Both follitropin alpha (rFSHα) and follitropin beta (rFSHβ) are structurally identical to native FSH and have both alpha and beta units of FSH. The alpha and beta in their names refer to the post-translational glycosylation process and purification procedures of the two recombinant FSH preparations. Most recombinant preparation use an analytic technique called size exclusion high performance liquid chromatography (SE-HPLC), a physicochemical robust technique, that results in a batch to batch variation less than 2%. This is as high as 20% when techniques like Steelma-Pohley in vivo assay are used that quantify the FSH activity by rat ovarian weight gain. Recently, a newer recombinant preparation called follitropin delta derived from the human fetal retinal origin has been introduced. Follitropin delta constitutes the first prospectively evaluated and validated biomarker-driven FSH dosing regimen. It uses serum anti-Müllerian hormone (AMH) levels and body weight as the indicator for initiating dose unlike the current FSH preparations. This reduces the possibility of hyperstimulation in the patients even without using other preventive modalities.

I. Corifollitropin alfa (Elonva®) is the first hybrid FSH molecule which demonstrated sustained follicle-stimulating activity. The beta subunit of this molecule contains the carboxy-terminal peptide of HCG, which alters the pharmacokinetic profile of the molecule. It demonstrates a longer circulation half-life and extended time to peak levels when compared with recombinant FSH (rFSH). Like rFSH, it lacks LH activity and binds specifically to the FSH receptor in vitro. Clinical trials show that corifollitropin alfa is able to sustain multiple follicular growth for a week, with a similar ovarian response and safety profile as rFSH. A single injection of corifollitropin alfa can replace seven daily injections of rFSH during the 1st week of ovarian stimulation in gonadotropin-releasing hormone antagonist protocols.
J. Luveris is the recombinant LH available delivers 75 IU of GT. Addition of LH, in conjunction with FSH, is necessary for follicular development when used in patients suffering from hypogonadotropic hypogonadotropism who have profound LH deficiency. It can be used as add back therapy to improve ovarian response especially in poor responders.
K. Pergoveris has recombinant FSH and LH in 2:1 ratio (150 IU FSH + 75 IU LH).
L. Recombinant HCG is available as 250 µg with the added benefit of consistency and better tolerability. 250 µg is equal in efficacy to 5,000 IU of urinary preparation.

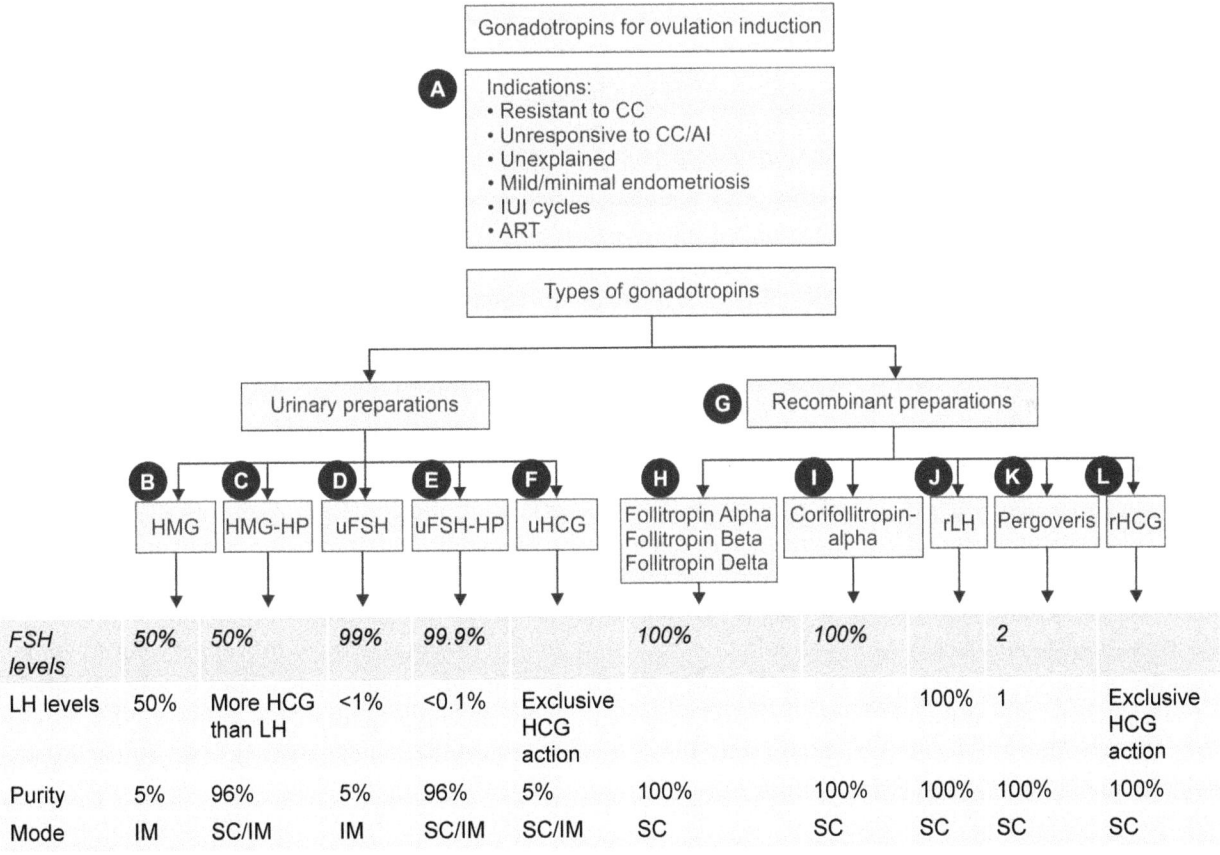

(ART: assisted reproductive technique; CC: clomiphene citrate; HCG: human chorionic gonadotropin; HMG: human menopausal gonadotropin; HMG-HP: highly purified HMG; IM: intramuscular; IUI: intrauterine insemination LH: luteinizing hormone; FSH: follicle-stimulating hormone; rHCG: recombinant HCG; r-LH: recombinant LH; SC: subcutaneous; uFSH: urinary FSH; uHCG: urinary HCG; AI: aromatase inhibitors)

CHAPTER 26
Ovulation Induction: Adjuvants in Polycystic Ovarian Syndrome

Bhavana Mittal, Poonam Goyal

Adjuvants are drugs that enhance the effectiveness of another pharmacological agent. The absence of a perfect ovulation induction agent demands the need of adjuvants in ovulation induction.

POLYCYSTIC OVARIAN SYNDROME

Introduction: Polycystic ovarian syndrome (PCOS) is characterized by insulin resistance at both prereceptor and postreceptor level leading to hyperinsulinemia. Insulin increases the levels of intraovarian androgens effecting the follicular development. Reducing insulin resistance reduces the levels of circulating androgens thus proposed to improve rates of ovulation in both induced and spontaneous cycles. All the adjuvants used in polycystic ovarian syndrome are used to improve hyperinsulinemia or reduce the levels of circulation/intraovarian androgens.

A. Metformin, a biguanide, is not only the most commonly used adjuvant in PCOS worldwide but also probably the only agent that has evidence backing its efficacy. It lowers the levels of both circulating and free androgen levels improving rates of ovulation in women with PCOS who are clomiphene citrate (CC) resistant, with anovulatory infertility and no other infertility factors, to improve ovulation and pregnancy rates. Concurrent use of metformin when using gonadotropin for ovarian stimulation reduces the incidence of ovarian hyperstimulation syndrome (OHSS). It may be noted that testing for insulin resistance is not mandated before stating metformin therapy. Body mass index (BMI) more than or equal to 25 kg/m^2, clomiphene resistance, letrozole resistance, need to start gonadotropins, and metabolic syndrome are considered some indications for starting metformin therapy to improve metabolic outcome. Metformin therapy can be stopped at the time of the pregnancy test or menses unless the metformin therapy is otherwise indicated. Start at lower doses and titrate at 500 mg/day to a maximum of 2,500 mg. Long-term therapy results in Vitamin B12 deficiency and further leading to elevation of homocysteine levels in a dose dependent manner. Hence it is of utmost importance to supplement Vitamin B12 for all women on long term metformin therapy. Levels less than 150 pg/mL require therapy with intramuscular preparation thrice a week for two weeks. Values may be tested every 6 months.

B. Inositol is a nutritional supplement existing in nine different stereoisomers, two of which have been shown to be secondary messengers for insulin action: myo-inositol (MI) and D-chiro-inositol (DCI). As of now MI supplementation is considered experimental for reducing total required dose of gonadotropin, improving rate of ovulation, improve the quality of embryos and clinical pregnancy rate in infertile women undergoing ovulation induction. Women who are nontolerant to metformin may be offered MI preparation as insulin sensitizers.

C. Pharmacological antiobesity agents should be considered an experimental therapy in women with PCOS for the purpose of improving fertility, with risk to benefit ratios currently too uncertain to advocate this as fertility therapy.

D. Dexamethasone affects the pituitary gland and reduces the adrenal source of androgen synthesis, thus improving the follicular growth. Use of dexamethasone may be considered in cases of elevated adrenal androgens like dehydroepiandrosterone sulfate (DHEAS).

E. During treatment with hormonal contraceptives, serum concentrations of follicle-stimulating hormone (FSH), luteinizing hormone (LH), and estradiol decrease. After stopping oral contraceptive pills (OCPs), both pituitary and ovarian activity will recover. The LH levels remain low for a longer time (21–28 days), as compared to FSH, which recovers in 5–7 days after stopping the OCP. There is also a reduction of the endometrial thickness, and the pinopod expression is delayed in women using OCP as compared to normally cycling women or those using CC. When given for a shorter duration, and if controlled ovarian stimulation (COS) is started after a washout period, OCP pretreatment might have a beneficial effect on ovulation rates. A 5-day washout period after OCP is optimal before the initiation of COS. There was no difference in the assisted reproductive technique (ART) outcome noted if the pills were administered only for 12–16 days and there was a washout period of 5 days.

Ovulation Induction: Adjuvants in Polycystic Ovarian Syndrome

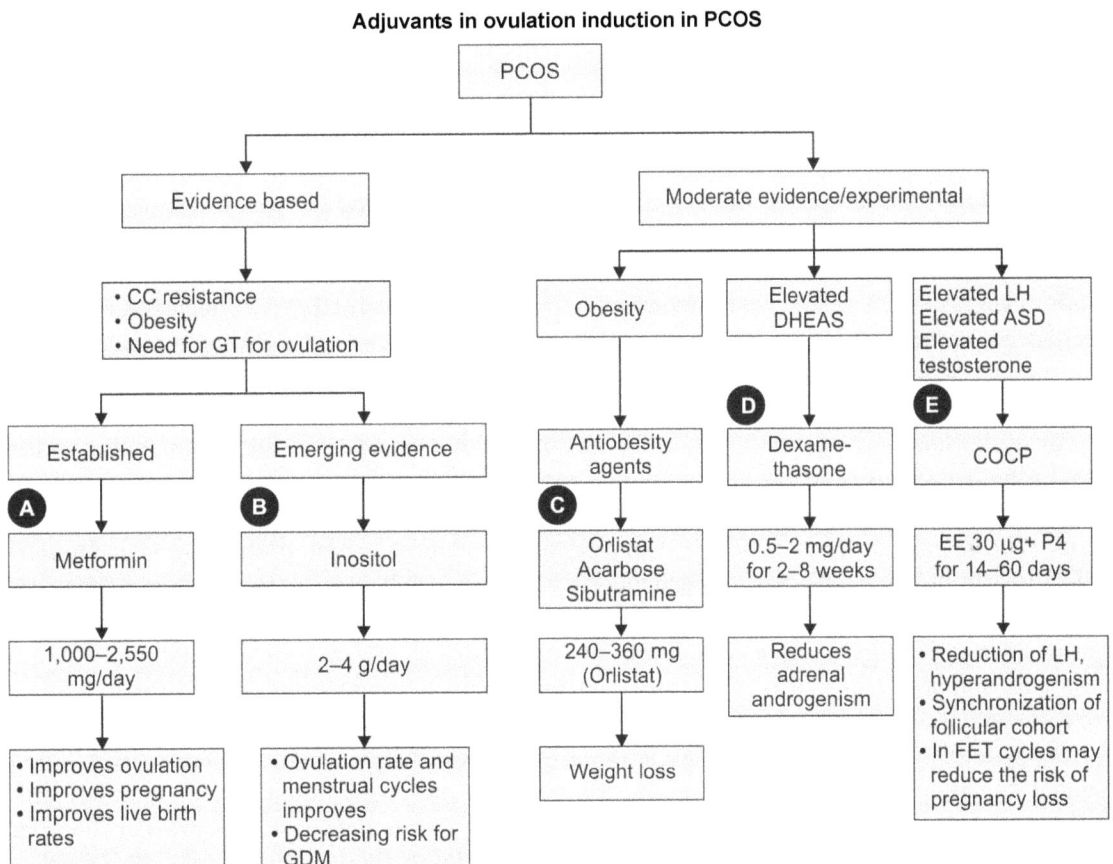

(ASD: androstenedione; CC: clomiphene citrate; COCP: combined oral contraceptive pill; DHEAS: dehydroepiandrosterone sulfate; EE: etinyl estradiol; FET: frozen embryo transfer; GDM: gestational diabetes mellitus; GT: gonadotropins; LH: luteinizing hormone; PCOS: polycystic ovarian syndrome)

CHAPTER 27

Ovulation Induction: Adjuvants in Poor Ovarian Reserve

Rajeev Agarwal, Apoorva Pallam Reddy

ADJUVANTS IN OVULATION INDUCTION

Adjuvants are drugs that enhance the effectiveness of another pharmacological agent. The absence of a perfect ovulation induction agent supports the need of adjuvants in ovulation induction.

POOR OVARIAN RESERVE

Introduction: Women with poor ovarian reserve are predicted to have a poor ovarian response to controlled ovarian stimulation. In this scenario, adjuvants are used to increase the total number of oocytes obtained.

A. The *addition of estradiol in the luteal phase* [E_2 (4 mg/day) from day 20 until next cycle day 2] with or without the simultaneous use of gonadotropin-releasing hormone (GnRH) antagonist is shown to increase the total number of oocytes obtained thus decreasing the risk of cycle cancellation in an in vitro fertilization (IVF) cycle and increasing the chance of clinical pregnancy in poor responder patients. The biological rationale might be that luteal estradiol priming could improve synchronization of the pool of follicles available to controlled ovarian stimulation.

B. Some authors suggested the addition of *recombinant luteinizing hormone* (LH) [75 IU subcutaneously (SC) from day 6 till day of cycle] or *low dose human chorionic gonadotropin (HCG)* (100–200 IU) during gonadotropin stimulation in poor responder patients. However, robust evidence supporting increase in clinical pregnancy rate is lacking.

C. Use of *growth hormone (GH)* 2 IU SC from day 1 stimulation till day of HCG administration, upregulates the local synthesis of insulin-like growth factor-1 (IGF-1). The IGF-1 amplifies the effect of follicle-stimulating hormone (FSH) at the level of both granulosa and theca cells. There is enough evidence from pooled data suggesting that use of GH improves clinical pregnancy rate significantly.

D. *Androgens* [*dehydroepiandrosterone (DHEA)* 75 mg/day orally 1–3 months prior to stimulation *and testosterone gel*], produced primarily by theca cells, play a critical role for an adequate follicular steroidogenesis and for a correct early follicular and granulosa cell development. The androgens produced in the theca cells are converted into estrogen under aromatase action in granulosa cells. Furthermore, androgens increase the expression of FSH receptor on granulosa cells, amplifying the effects of FSH and thus enhancing the responsiveness of ovaries to FSH. Inadequate levels of endogenous androgens are associated with decreased ovarian sensitivity to FSH and low pregnancy rates after IVF. Serum levels of androgen reduces proportional to the age of women. Adequate intraovarian androgen levels are essential for the progression of follicles from preantral to antral stage. Although DHEA is widely used, there is lack of strong evidence supporting its role in either increasing the number of oocytes obtained or clinical pregnancy rate. It may be noted that younger women, with low serum DHEA levels are more suited for management with DHEA supplementation as compared to the older counter parts. On the other hand a meta-analysis of three *randomized controlled trials* (RCTs) has shown that transdermal use of testosterone is associated with increased clinical pregnancy rate and live birth rate although there was no change in the total number of oocytes obtained.

E. Increasing the intraovarian vascularity is associated with improved delivery of gonadotropic hormones or other growth factors required for folliculogenesis. On the other hand, impaired ovarian blood flow could contribute to poor ovarian response. Based on this rationale, enhancing ovarian vascularization with vasoactive substances such as *aspirin* (75–150 mg/day orally from approximately day 15 previous cycle before stimulation till 8–12 weeks of pregnancy) could theoretically improve the ovarian response.

F. Use of varied stimulation protocols like agonist, antagonist, natural cycle, letrozole, etc. is not shown to affect the pregnancy rates.

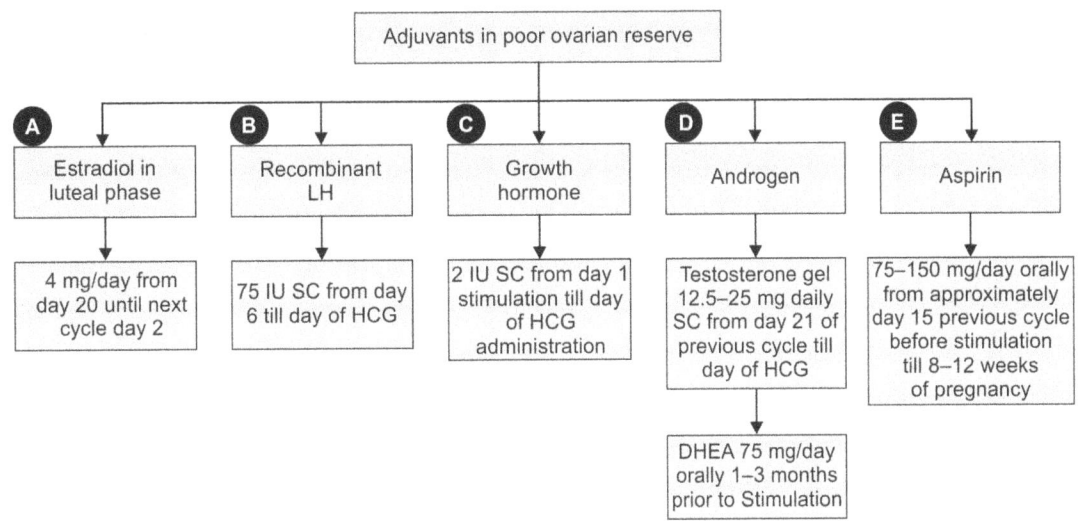

(DHEA: dehydroepiandrosterone; FSH: follicle-stimulating hormone; HCG: human chorionic gonadotropin; LH: luteinizing hormone; SC: subcutaneously)

EXPLANATION

Nutrition affects the biological processes in reproduction. Deficiency of various essential micronutrients can adversely affect the chances of fertility by impacting embryogenesis and placentation. The prophylactic use of micronutrients thus helps in preventing several adverse pregnancy outcomes. Apart from vitamins and minerals, use of antioxidants such as vitamins C and E, *N*-acetylcysteine, insulin sensitization with inositol, and improvement of blood flow in the pelvic organs with the presence of L-arginine help in improving reproductive outcome. Micronutrient supplementation is not only tolerated well but also is cost effective without any serious adverse effects making them a favorable choice for clinician and clients alike. Most women achieve pregnancy with simple measures like awareness of fertile period, lifestyle changes, and a healthy diet accompanied with right micronutrient supplementation. Although larger studies are required to confirm the benefits of universal supplementation, most studies favor the use of micronutrient supplementation.

- Vitamin C, E (400 mg/day)
- Carotene (2,600 IU/day)

- N-acetyl cysteine
- 600 mg thrice/day oral

L-arginine (1,000–3,000 mg/day)

Coenzyme Q 10/ Ubiquinone 50–600/day oral

- Vitamin D3
- 60,000 IU/week × 12 weeks

SECTION 10

Endometriosis and Fibroids

- Endometriosis: Etiology of Infertility in Endometriosis
- Endometriosis: Diagnosis
- Endometriosis: Laparoscopy Staging
- Endometriosis: Fertility Index Staging
- Endometriosis and ART
- Endometriosis: Role of Endoscopy
- Endoscopy for Ovarian Endometrioma
- Fibroids in Infertility
- Adenomyosis and Infertility

CHAPTER 28

Endometriosis: Etiology of Infertility in Endometriosis

Indranil Dutta

INTRODUCTION

The presence of endometrial glands and stroma in an ectopic region outside the uterus is defined as endometriosis. The prevalence can be as high as 50% in infertile women with history of dysmenorrhea (Meuleman et al., 2009). Endometriosis debilitates women of reproductive age at multiple levels, resulting in infertility, pain, and a significant negative impact on psychological and reproductive aspects of a woman's life.

A. Endometriosis may cause both endocrine and ovulatory disorders, resulting in impaired folliculogenesis, luteinized unruptured follicle syndrome, luteal phase defect, and premature LH surge.

B. Women with endometriosis have higher chances of tubal block, hydrosalpinx, impaired fimbrial function, and altered tubal peristalsis that interfere with oocyte transport and sperm capacitation. The peritoneal fluid in endometriosis is said to have ovum capture inhibitor (OCI) which is thought to be responsible for fimbrial failure of ovum capture.

C. By laparoscopy, it is commonly observed that the "pelvic factor" is affected more commonly in patients with severe forms of endometriosis due to pelvic anatomy distortion explaining the infertility. Pelvic and/or peritubal adhesions that disturb the tubo-ovarian liaison and tube patency can interfere with the oocyte release from the ovary, inhibit oocyte pickup by fimbria, or hamper ovum transport. Peritoneal fluid is increased not only in volume but has high levels of activated macrophages, prostaglandins, interleukin-1 (IL-1), tumor necrosis factor (TNF), and proteases.

D. Endometriosis reduces the endometrial receptivity due to the inflammatory behavior of ectopic endometrial implants mediated by a complex system of humoral and cellular immunity factors. Deferred histologic maturation or biochemical disturbances may result in endometrial dysfunction.

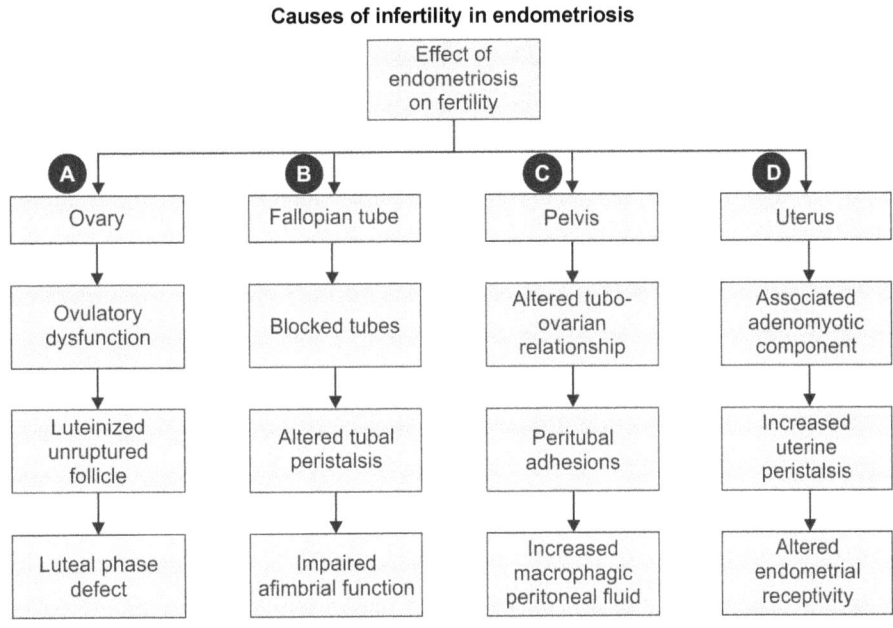

CHAPTER 29

Endometriosis: Diagnosis

Indranil Dutta

A. Diagnosis of endometriosis can be done using multiple modalities. Presence of classic symptoms like chronic pelvic pain, dysmenorrhea, and dyspareunia should raise suspicion of endometriosis. Gynecological symptoms like dysmenorrhea, noncyclical pelvic pain, deep dyspareunia, infertility, and nongynecological cyclical symptoms like painful stools, dysuria, hematuria, rectal bleeding, shoulder pain, intestinal complaints—periodic bloating, diarrhea, or constipation—are also suggestive of endometriosis.

B. Clinical examination should be performed in all women with suspicion of endometriosis. Presence of induration and/or nodules of the rectovaginal wall, or visible vaginal nodules in the posterior vaginal fornix are suggestive of deep endometriosis, whereas painful adnexal mass may be seen in cases of ovarian endometrioma.

C. Serum CA125 is not a useful tool to diagnose endometriosis. If a coincidentally reported serum CA125 level is available, be aware that a raised serum CA125 (i.e. 35 IU/mL or more) may be consistent with having endometriosis. CA125 values may be used to evaluate the severity of active disease or the effect of therapy.

D. Transvaginal ultrasonography (USG) is the most common method to evaluate ovarian endometriosis. Endometrioma are characterized by ground glass echogenicity on USG with or without locules and absence of papillations or vascularity. Occasionally, deep endometriosis involving the bowel, bladder, or ureter can be detected.

E. The use of 3D sonography to detect rectovaginal endometriosis is not well established.

F. Laparoscopy has a higher negative predictive value than positive predictive value for endometriosis. A systematic examination of various pelvic structures including (1) the uterus with bilateral ovaries and tubes, (2) ovarian fossae, vesicouterine fold, pouch of Douglas, and pararectal spaces, (3) the rectum and sigmoid colon, (4) the appendix and cecum, and (5) the diaphragm should be performed to increase the diagnostic value of laparoscopy. Laparoscopy with positive histology is considered the gold standard in diagnosing endometriosis. Histology should be done on the excised tissue including ovarian endometrioma to exclude rare instances of malignancy.

G. Magnetic resonance imaging (MRI) is not yet an established modality for the diagnosis of peritoneal endometriosis. When deep endometriosis is suspected based on history or examination, we should evaluate the involvement of ureter, bladder, and bowel through supplementary imaging, like barium enema, transrectal sonography, and MRI.

H. When diagnosed, it is best to perform operative laparoscopy (excision or ablation of the endometriosis lesions) including adhesiolysis, rather than performing diagnostic laparoscopy alone in women seeking fertility, to increase ongoing pregnancy rates.

I. Before performing laparoscopic surgery for endometriosis, we need to discuss the risks and benefits of surgery. This may include potential benefit future pregnancy prospects, the impact on ovarian reserve, and other alternatives to surgery.

Endometriosis: Diagnosis

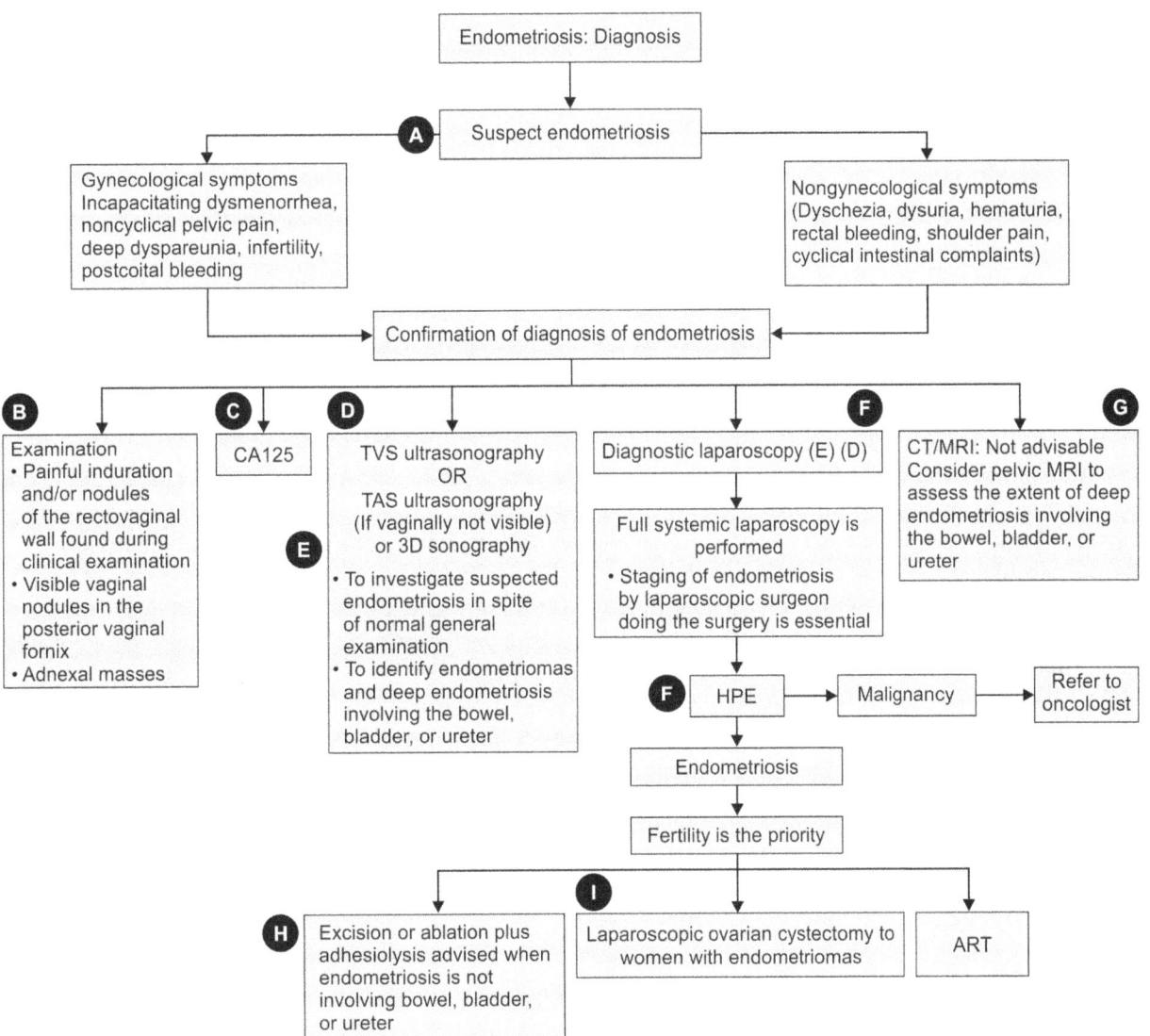

(ART: assisted reproductive technique; CT: computed tomography; HPE: histopathological examination; MRI: magnetic resonance imaging; TAS: transabdominal sonography; TVS: transvaginal sonography)

CHAPTER 30

Endometriosis: Laparoscopy Staging

Priyankur Roy, Shaheen Hokabaj

Laparoscopy with histology is considered the gold standard for diagnosis of endometriosis. A good quality laparoscopy should include systematic checking of—(1) the uterus and adnexa, (2) the peritoneum of ovarian fossae, vesicouterine fold, Douglas and pararectal spaces, (3) the rectum and sigmoid (isolated sigmoid nodules), (4) the appendix and cecum, and (5) the diaphragm. There should also be a speculum examination and palpation of the vagina and cervix under laparoscopic control, to check for "buried" nodules. A good quality laparoscopy can only be performed by using at least one secondary port for a suitable grasper to clear the pelvis of obstruction from bowel loops, or fluid suction to ensure the whole pouch of Douglas is inspected. Staging of endometriosis helps in deciding the further course of management in women seeking fertility.

A. Dysmenorrhea, chronic pelvic pain, deep dyspareunia, cyclical intestinal cramps, fatigue/weariness, and infertility continue to be classical and the leading symptoms of endometriosis.
B. The benefits and risks of laparoscopic surgery for deep endometriosis involving the bowel, bladder or ureter are to be discussed in detail with the patient. Topics to be included in the discussion are—(1) effect on the chance of future pregnancy, (2) possible impact on ovarian reserve, and (3) alternatives to surgery.
C. A scoring system is developed based on the extent of disease spread. This predicts the severity of disease thus predicting future fertility perspectives. Peritoneal lesion: Superficial—(1) <1 cm: 1, (2) 1-3 cm: 2, (3) >3 cm: 4; Deep—(1) <1 cm: 2, (2) 1-3 cm: 4, (3) >3 cm: 6.
D. Ovarian endometriosis: Superficial—(1) <1 cm: 1, (2) 1-3 cm: 2, (3) >3 cm: 4; Deep—(1) <1 cm: 4, (2) 1-3 cm: 16, (3) >3 cm: 20. Score is given for both the ovaries separately. Bilateral involvement will double the score based on superficial or deep involvement. Presence of an ovarian endometrioma is considered deep endometriosis.
E. Cul-de-sac obliteration: Partial—4; Complete—40.
F. Ovarian adhesion: Filmy—(1) <1/3 Enclosure: 1, (2) 1/3-2/3 Enclosure: 2, (3) >2/3 Enclosure: 4; Dense—(1) <1/3 Enclosure: 4, (2) 1/3-2/3 Enclosure: 8, (3) >2/3 Enclosure: 16. Score is given for both the ovaries separately. Bilateral involvement will double the score based on filmy or dense adhesions.
G. Tubal adhesion: Filmy—(1) <1/3 Enclosure: 1, (2) 1/3-2/3 Enclosure: 2, (3) >2/3 Enclosure: 4; Dense—(1) <1/3 Enclosure: 4, (2) 1/3-2/3 Enclosure: 8, (3) >2/3 Enclosure: 16. Score is given for both the tubes separately. Bilateral involvement will double the score based on filmy or dense adhesions.

Addition of all these scores (C + D + E + F + G) clinches the severity of disease. The classification as per ASRM is finally made based on the score:

Stage I	Minimal	1–5
Stage II	Mild	6–15
Stage III	Moderate	16–40
Stage IV	Severe	>40

Endometriosis: Laparoscopy Staging

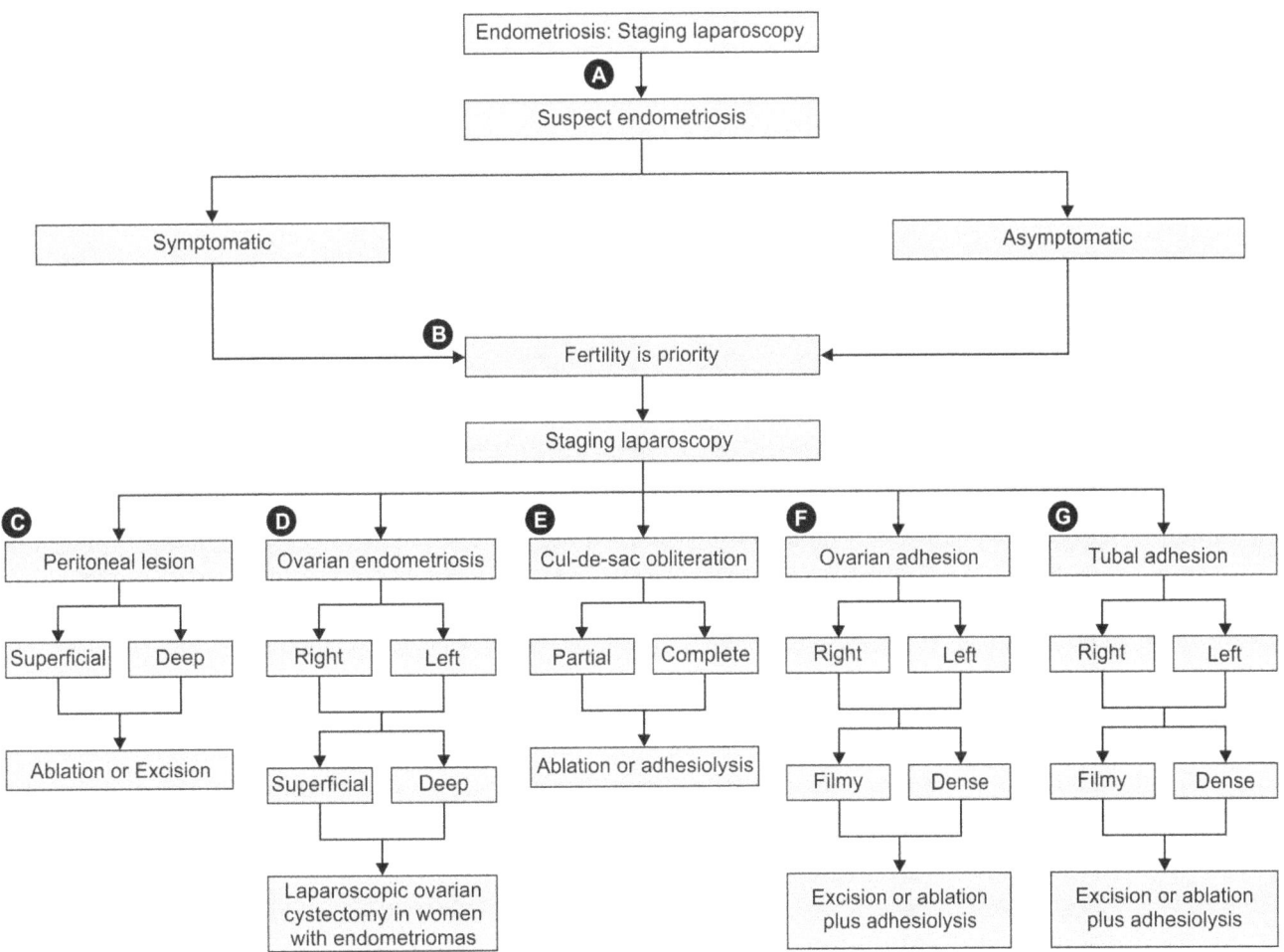

CHAPTER 31
Endometriosis: Fertility Index Staging

Fessy Louise T, Aparna

A. Endometriosis is a debilitating condition ranging from 10% in general reproductive age group women to 25% with chronic pelvic pain to 35% in women suffering from infertility.
B. In 1979, the American Fertility Society (AFS) first proposed a classification system for endometriosis. This was extensively evaluated and modified in 1985 and revised in 1997. Despite these revisions, the currently used revised AFS (r-AFS) system has serious limitations. Chief among them is the relatively poor correlation with pregnancy rate postsurgery.
   For example, According to r-AFS, if pouch of Douglas (POD) is obliterated completely, it directly implies severe (stage IV) endometriosis irrespective of tubes and ovarian status, because in spite of POD obliteration if tubes and ovaries are relatively free pre- or post-adhesiolysis gives better result in pregnancy rate.
C. In 2009, Adamson and Pasta proposed endometriosis fertility index (EFI) score to predict fecundity after endometriosis surgery which combines conception-related factors from history like age, duration of infertility, and prior pregnancy and surgical factors include least function (LF) score, revised AFS endometriosis score, and revised AFS total score.
D. Least function score is the key component of EFI score which provides detailed description of the adnexa—fallopian tubes, fimbria, and ovary on both the sides. The structures are assessed for its dysfunction and graded as normal, mild, moderate, severe, and non-functional with scoring for each grade. *The lowest score among both the sides is summed up and LF score is given.* If an ovary is absent on one side, the LF score is obtained by doubling the lowest score on the side with the ovary.

		Descriptions of least function terms
Structure	Dysfunction	Description
Tube	Mild	Sight injury to serosa of the fallopian tube
	Moderate	Moderate injury to serosa or muscularis of the fallopian tube; moderate limitation in mobility
	Severe	Fallopian tube fibrosis or mild/moderate salpingitis isthmica nodosa; severe limitation in mobility
	Non-functional	Complete tubal obstruction, extensive fibrosis or salpingitis isthmica nodosa
Fimbria	Mild	Slight injury to fimbria with minimal scarring
	Moderate	Moderate injury to fimbria, with moderate scarring, moderate loss of fimbrial architecture and minimal intrafimbrial fibrosis
	Severe	Severe injury to fimbria, with severe scarring, severe loss of fimbrial architecture and moderate intrafimbrial fibrosis
	Non-functional	Severe injury to fimbria, with extensive scarring, complete loss of fimbrial architecture, complete tubal occlusion or hydrosalpinx
Ovary	Mild	Normal or almost normal ovarian size; minimal or mild injury to ovarian serosa
	Moderate	Ovarian size reduced by one-third or more; moderate injury to ovarian surface
	Severe	Ovarian size reduced by two-thirds or more; severe injury to ovarian surface
	Non-functional	Ovary absent or completely encased in adhesions

E. Endometriosis fertility index score ranges from 0–10 (0 = poorest prognosis, 10 = best prognosis). It is a useful tool to tailor patient management after surgical management of endometriosis in infertility cases.
   Those with poorer scores 0–3 should be referred directly to fertility specialist for assisted reproductive technique (ART) treatment, as chances of spontaneous conception are only 5–10%.
   Women with scores 4–6 can wait for non-ART treatment conception for 6 months and women with scores 7–10 for 12 months as conception rate is around 30% and 45–50%, respectively. If not conceived in 6 to 12 months, referred for ART treatment.

Endometriosis: Fertility Index Staging

```
Women with history of infertility with endometriosis
                    ↓
After proper evaluation post for laparoscopic surgery
                    ↓
During laparoscopy for endometriosis it is important to restore the anatomy as much as possible and do satisfactory adhesiolysis
                    ↓
At the conclusion of surgery calculate the least function (LF) score for each side of the fallopian tube, fimbria and ovary. *The Final LF score is calculated by adding the lowest score for each side.* If an ovary is absent on one side, the LF score is obtained by doubling the lowest score on the side with the ovary.
```

Least function (LF) score at conclusion of surgery

Score	Description		Left	Right
4	= Normal	Fallopian tube		
3	= Mild dysfunction	Fimbria		
2	= Moderate dysfunction	Ovary		
1	= Severe dysfunction			
0	= Absent or nonfunctional			

To calculate the LF score, add together the lowest score for the left side and the lowest score for the right side. If an ovary is absent on one side, the LF score is obtained by doubling the lowest score on the side with the ovary.

Lowest score: [Left] + [Right] = [LF score]

Total historical score is calculated by using historical factors like age, duration of infertility, and prior pregnancy details.
Total surgical score is calculated using surgical factors like final LF score, r-AFS endometriosis score and r-AFS total score calculate the *EFI score.*

Endometriosis fertility index (EFI)

Historical factors			Surgical factors		
Factor	Description	Points	Factor	Description	Points
Age	If age is ≤ 35 years	2	LF score		
	If age is 36 to 39 years	1		If LF score = 7 to 8 (high score)	3
	If age is ≥ 40 years	0		If LF score = 4 to 6 (moderate score)	2
Years infertile				If LF score = 1 to 3 (low score)	0
	If years infertile is ≤ 3	2	AFS endometriosis score		
	If years infertile is > 3	0		If AFS endometriosis lesion score is < 16	1
Prior pregnancy				If AFS endometriosis lesion score is ≥ 16	0
	If there is a history of a prior pregnancy	1	AFS total score		
	If there is no history of prior pregnancy	0		If AFS total score is < 71	1
				If AFS total score is ≥ 71	0
Total historical factors			**Total surgical factors**		

EFI = Total historical factors + total surgical factors: [Historical] + [Surgical] = [EFI score]

Final *EFI* score is calculated by adding the total historical score and the total surgical score. Then the patient management is tailored based on the *EFI* score as follows

EFI score 0–3	EFI score 4–6	EFI score 7–10
Directly refer patient to Fertility specialist for ART	Can wait for spontaneous conception or induce superovulation ± IUI for 6 months	Can wait for spontaneous conception or induce superovulation ± IUI for 12 months
	↓	↓
	If not conceived in 6 months	If not conceived in 12 months
	↓	↓
	Refer for ART	Refer for ART

(ART: assisted reproductive technique; IUI: intrauterine insemination; r-AFS: revised American Fertility Society)

CHAPTER 32

Endometriosis and ART

Shaweez Faizi, Pratap Kumar

A. In early endometriosis, there might just be a suspicion of the disease as ultrasonography (USG) would not reveal much. In such cases, more often than not, laparoscopy might be done as a diagnostic procedure or for establishing tubal patency. After laparoscopy the severity of endometriosis can be assessed with higher precision.
B. EFI or endometriosis fertility index was established in 2010 by identifying the most predictive variables for pregnancy postsurgery. It is used as a clinical tool to counsel patients on the approach toward fertility postsurgery. It is a staging system for predicting the possibility of non-ART pregnancy [spontaneous/controlled ovarian stimulation (COS) + timed intercourse (TI)/intrauterine insemination (IUI)] after endometriosis surgery. It considers, age, duration of infertility, prior pregnancy, functional score of ovaries, fimbria, and fallopian tube unlike the older revised American Fertility Society (r-AFS) score. The EFI score is given from 0 to 10 with higher numbers being predictive of higher chances of pregnancy over the next 3 years.
C. Women with advanced stages of endometriosis (Stage III and IV) have extremely low probability of spontaneous conception and benefit from assisted reproductive technique (ART). In some conditions laparoscopy may be considered to improve the conception rate.
D. When considering in vitro fertilization (IVF), the following points need to be considered:
    - Are the ovaries accessible vaginally for oocyte pickup (OPU)? If not, abdominal route for OPU may need to be planned and patient counseled for reduced number of oocytes being obtained than what is being seen on follicular scan.
    - Is there concomitant adenomyosis? If so, then management of the same needs to be planned by way of prolonged gonadotropin-releasing hormone (GnRH) agonist downregulation/cabergoline 0.5 mg twice weekly/or surgery.
    - Would you prefer a long protocol or an antagonist protocol?
    - The ovarian reserve may be compromised in endometriosis thus quantity and quality of oocytes may be poor. Counseling of the couple is important.
    - Would you perform a fresh embryo transfer (ET)? If there are high estradiol (E2) levels and risk of ovarian hyperstimulation syndrome (OHSS) and endometrium–embryo asynchrony or if progesterone levels are more than 1.4 ng/mL, then frozen transfer is better. If there is adenomyosis then again downregulation with GnRH agonists and then frozen transfer is better. If however the E2 values are less than 2,500, progesterone value is less then 1.2 ng/mL and the number of quality of embryos is poor, then one may consider a fresh embryo transfer.
E. The only valid indications for laparoscopy in endometriosis associated infertility are:
    - Excessive pain
    - Endometriotic cyst obstructing access to follicles during OPU
    - Rapid growth of endometriotic cyst
    - Mere presence or size of endometriotic cyst is not by itself a criterion for removal.
F. Gonadotropin-releasing hormone agonists and antagonists are similar in terms of implantation rate and clinical pregnancy rates but GnRH agonists produce more metaphase II (MII) oocytes and embryos. The agonist protocol should be preferred for women with good ovarian reserve. In women with poor ovarian reserve GnRH antagonist (Cetrorelix and Ganirelix) can be used so as to avoid pituitary suppression and thus facilitate follicular recruitment.

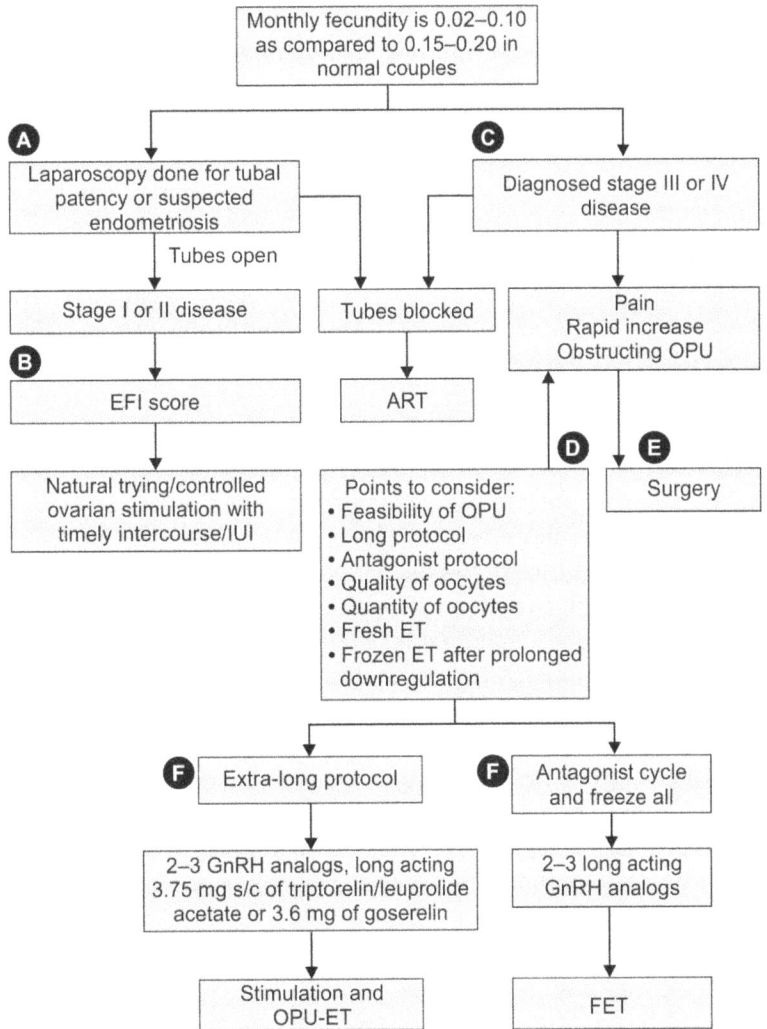

(ART: assisted reproductive technique; EFI: endometriosis fertility index; ET: embryo transfer; FET: frozen-thawed embryo transfer; GnRH: gonadotropin-releasing hormone; IUI: intrauterine insemination; OPU: oocyte pickup; s/c: subcutaneous)

CHAPTER 33

Endometriosis: Role of Endoscopy

Priyanka Pipara, Bhaskar Pal

A. Endometriosis is a progressive disease and has detrimental effects on the reproductive outcome at multiple levels. The prognosis in fertility is directly proportional to the stage of the disease, age of diagnosis, and other associated subfertility factors. The early stages of endometriosis (Stage I-II superficial endometriosis) can be diagnosed only after performing a diagnostic laparoscopy in a suspected case or as a part of routine evaluation. In this subset of women with early stages of endometriosis, performing laparoscopic excision or ablation of endometriotic lesion with adhesiolysis, concurrently at the time of diagnosis, increases the pregnancy rate significantly and is preferred to expectant management. If not for laparoscopy, most cases would go undiagnosed. Hence, laparoscopy may be considered especially in cases of unexplained infertility with or without symptoms of dysmenorrhea/dyspareunia.

B. In order to improve the time to conception, women with stage I/II endometriosis are suggested to undergo intrauterine insemination (IUI) with controlled ovarian stimulation within 6 months after surgical treatment. The results are considered superior to expectant management. The number of cycles of IUI depends on multiple factors like age of female partner, ovarian reserve, married life, tubal functionality, associated male factor, and last but not the least the patient preference. Women who fail to conceive through IUI are advised to proceed for assisted reproductive techniques (ART).

C. Higher stages of endometriosis are associated with poorer prognosis compared to lower stages. In cases of stage III/IV endometriosis, performing operative laparoscopy is considered beneficial compared to expectant management to increase the rate of spontaneous conception. For women seeking fertility, there is no role of using hormonal suppression either in the form of oral contraceptive pill (OCP) or gonadotropin-releasing hormone (GnRH) agonists postsurgery. This is not associated with improved fertility rate.

D. Presence of an ovarian endometrioma categorizes the patient directly into deep endometriosis. There is constant argument regarding the need to perform an endoscopy on an ovarian endometrioma diagnosed on ultrasonography (USG). Presence of endometrioma alone should not be a criterion for performing either endoscopy or ART. Cysts smaller than 3 cm do not benefit from surgery. Women should be advised for controlled ovarian stimulation with IUI or ART based on associated fertility factors. In infertile women with endometrioma larger than 3 cm, cystectomy may be considered only for pain management or improve accessibility to follicles and there is no evidence that cystectomy prior to treatment with assisted reproductive technologies improves pregnancy rates.

E. When the decision to operate is taken on an ovarian endometrioma, excision of the capsule has higher possibility of increasing the rates of spontaneous conception as compared to drainage of endometrioma. Risk factors should be evaluated before surgery and the patient should be counseled regarding possibility of reduced ovarian function after surgery and the possible loss of the ovary.

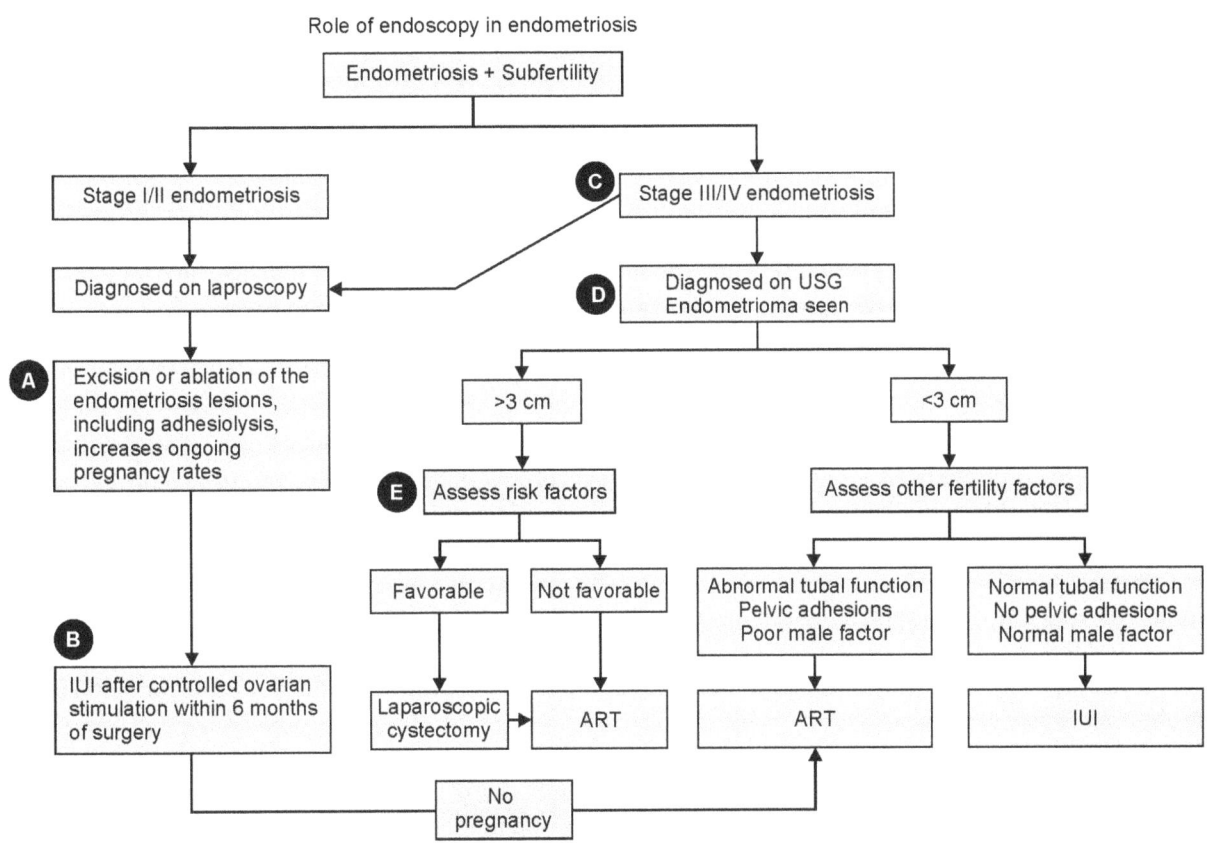

Characteristics	Favors surgery	Favors ART
Previous interventions	None	≥ 1
Ovarian reserve	Good	Poor
Pain	Present	Absent
Growth	Rapid	Stable
Bilaterality	Unilateral	Bilateral
Sonographic features of malignancy	Present	Absent

Expert Advice:
- Use of GnRH analogs before or after surgery is NOT associated with increased pregnancy rate.
- Use of GnRH analogs before ART for 3 months might increase pregnancy rate.

(ART: assisted reproductive technique; GnRH: gonadotropin-releasing hormone; IUI; intrauterine insemination; USG: ultrasonography)

CHAPTER 34

Endoscopy for Ovarian Endometrioma

Apoorva Pallam Reddy, Aruna Siddharth

INTRODUCTION

When a decision to operate an ovarian endometrioma is taken, laparoscopic approach is the best possible method.
A. A three-port laparoscopic technique is preferred when opting for surgical management of ovarian endometrioma. Endometriomas are often stuck compactly to adjacent structures like the fallopian tube, the posterolateral aspect of the uterus, and lateral pelvic wall with or without involving the bowel. When dense adhesions are suspected, it is advised that the surgeon considers the possibility of ureteric stenting to prevent inadvertent damage. Before cystectomy, it is advised to separate the ovary with endometrioma from other pelvic structures by adhesiolysis.
B. If the cyst ruptures during adhesiolysis, extend the opening in the cyst wall adequately to expose the cyst cavity and excision of the cyst wall may be attempted. Turning the cyst inside out may ease the process of cyst wall excision. Multiple incisions and excessive opening should be avoided to reduce the damage to the ovarian cortex, functional ovarian tissue, and the hilum.
C. Suturing to reconstruct the ovary is required only after excision of large endometriomas. Approximation and hemostasis are best achieved with monofilament sutures. Most small endometriomas approximate spontaneously and hence do not require suturing. Reduce the exposure of suture material on the surface of the ovary to reduce the risk of adhesion formation.
D. When the ovary is not adherent, the incision should ideally be over the thinnest part of the ovarian endometriotic surface or, if this is not visible, on the antimesenteric border.
Irrigate and aspirate thoroughly to check for hemostasis and to remove any remaining cyst fluid or blood clots from the abdominal pelvic cavity.
E. Once the cleavage plane is delineated, gentle traction and countertraction are used to dissect the cyst capsule from the ovarian parenchyma during the initial part of the dissection. Use of excessive force to separate a highly adherent cyst from the ovary may cause tearing of ovarian tissue and result in excessive bleeding.
F. When used, laser should be operated in an ablative setting that destroy the endometriotic tissue and at the same time prevent any damage to the underlying healthy tissue. Aim to vaporize the endometriotic cyst lining only until hemosiderin pigment-stained tissue is no longer visible (until the color changes from reddish to yellow-white).
G. For large endometriomas, instead of a single sitting, a two- or three-step procedure can be considered.
  1. The first step encompasses opening and draining the endometrioma as described in the initial stages section. Inspect the cyst cavity and take a biopsy.
  2. Administer 3 months of gonadotropin-releasing hormone agonist (GnRHa) therapy postsurgery, during which time the thickness of the cyst wall significantly decreases, with atrophy and reduction in stromal vascularization of the cyst (Donnez et al., 1996).
  3. Complete the surgery with a second laparoscopy in the form of either cystectomy, CO_2 vaporization, bipolar diathermy, or plasma ablation of the cyst wall lining.

Endoscopy for Ovarian Endometrioma

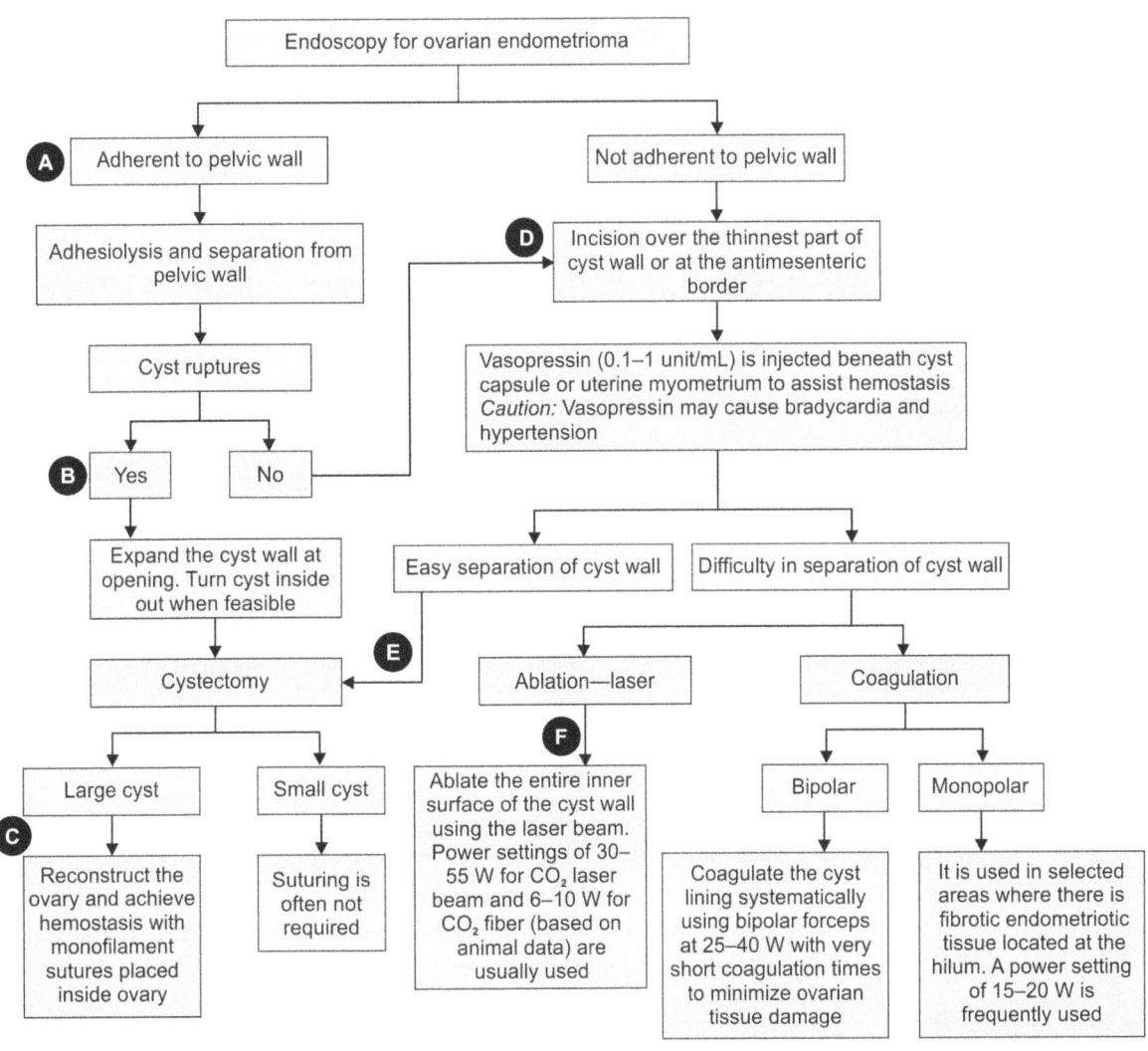

CHAPTER 35

Fibroids in Infertility

Jiteeka Thakkar, Nandita Palshetkar

A. Uterine fibroids are the most common benign tumors in women and may be symptomatic or asymptomatic.
B. Ultrasound is the most important diagnostic tool for accurate fibroid mapping, i.e. description of size, location, and nature of fibroids. Both transabdominal and transvaginal methods are effective in assessing fibroids. Whenever feasible both routes should be used to increase the sensitivity of picking up fibroid.
C. Saline infusion sonography (SIS) can be used to rule out submucosal involvement.
D. Hysteroscopy is extremely useful in the diagnosis of submucous fibroids and their management as well.
E. The routine use of magnetic resonance imaging (MRI) for diagnosis of fibroids is not warranted. It should be reserved for complex cases, to differentiate from adenomyosis or assess junctional zone. Having said that MRI is extremely sensitive in picking up the number, size, and location of the fibroids.
F. Based on the position fibroids are classified into 8 types:

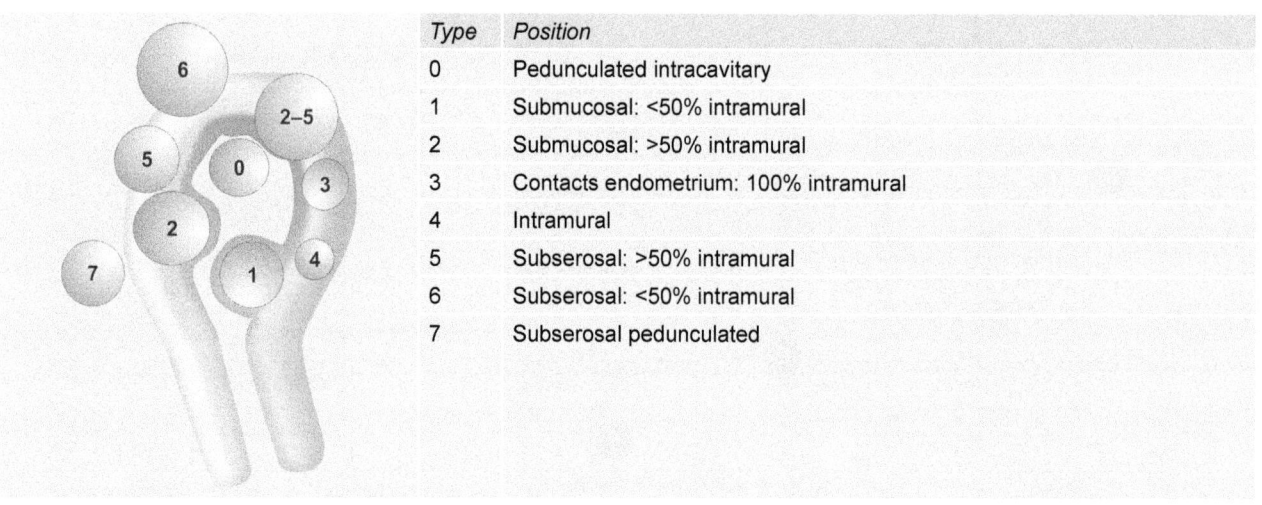

Type	Position
0	Pedunculated intracavitary
1	Submucosal: <50% intramural
2	Submucosal: >50% intramural
3	Contacts endometrium: 100% intramural
4	Intramural
5	Subserosal: >50% intramural
6	Subserosal: <50% intramural
7	Subserosal pedunculated

G. As the subserous fibroids are located far from the endomyometrial junction, they do not seem to affect fertility outcome and hence there is no need of further management.
H. Intramural fibroids are proposed to alter the myometrial contractibility, distort the pelvic cavity or in cases of large fibroids, alter the tubo-ovarian morphology impacting fertility. Fibroids that are touching the endometrium (type 3) may be considered for myomectomy before assisted reproductive technique (ART) after discussing the pros and cons with the patient.
I. In case of recurrent implantation failure or recurrent pregnancy loss, even type 4 fibroids can be considered for myomectomy.
J. The route of myomectomy does not seem to impact the fertility potential. The route of surgery should depend on the location, size of fibroids, and expertise of the operating surgeon.
K. There is reasonable evidence to support the statement that myomectomy does not impair reproductive outcomes (clinical pregnancy rates, live birth rates) following ART (Grade B). Despite lacking robust evidence, there is reasonable consensus that women can get pregnant after 3 months of myomectomy if there was a breach in the endometrial cavity and within 2 months of surgery if there was no breach in endometrial cavity.
L. Medical therapy, uterine artery embolization, MRI-high intensity focused ultrasound (HIFU) are not recommended for routine practice in women seeking fertility. A short course of gonadotropin-releasing hormone (GnRH) analogs may be used to reduce the vascularity and control bleeding prior to procedure.

Fibroids in Infertility

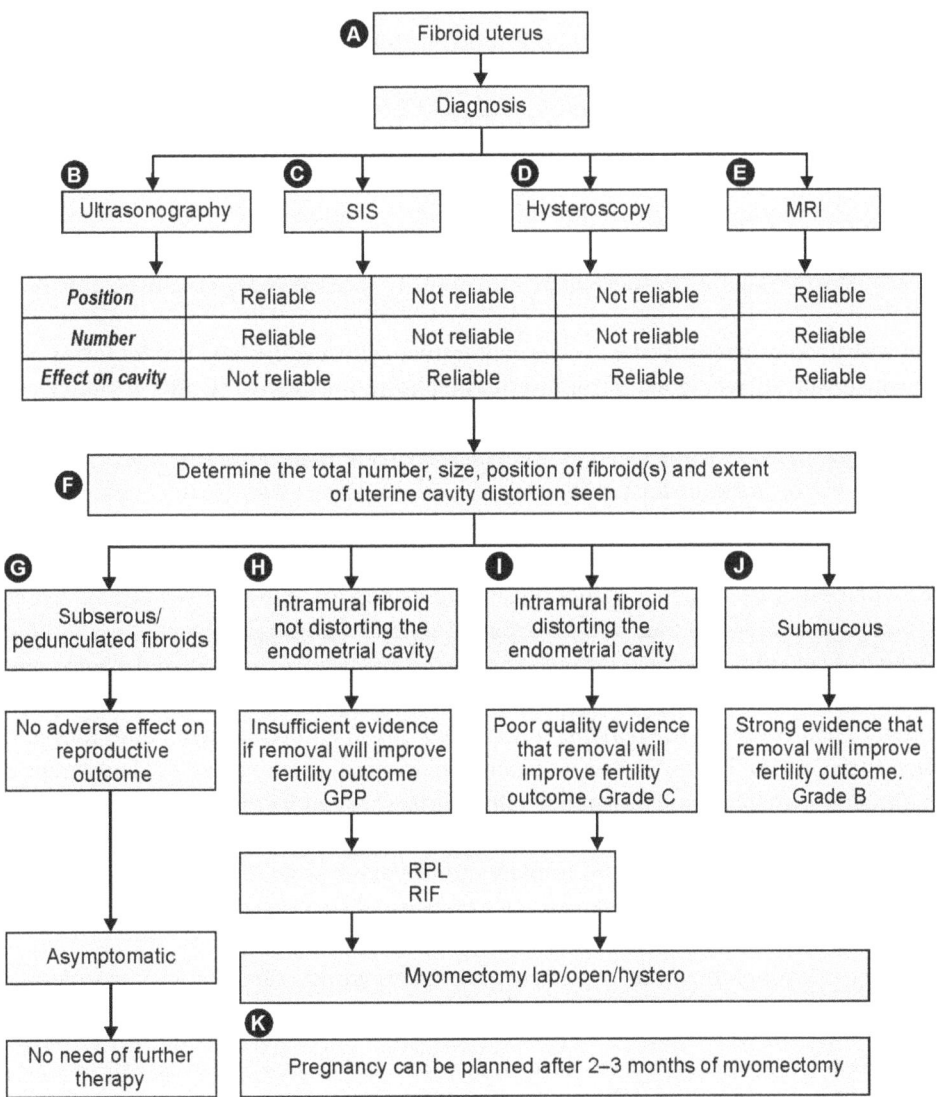

(GPP: Good practice principle; MRI: magnetic resonance imaging; RIF: recurrent implantation failure; RPL: recurrent pregnancy loss; SIS: saline infusion sonography)

CHAPTER 36

Adenomyosis and Infertility

Basab Mukherjee, Anurag Mallick

A. Adenomyosis (AD) is the disease of the endomyometrial junction characterized by the infiltration of heterotopic endometrial glands and stroma into the myometrium. This can be associated with varying degree of muscular hypertrophy resulting in a bulky appearance of the uterus.

B. Although the gold standard for diagnosis of AD is through histopathology, the increased resolution of transvaginal sonography (TVS), three-dimensional transvaginal sonography (3D-TVS), and magnetic resonance imaging (MRI) has made it possible to achieve an image diagnosis of AD as well as clearly display the endomyometrial junction. Most common image features of AD comprise heterotopic endometrial tissue and accompanied with unequal myometrial hypertrophy. TVS, 3D-TVS, and MRI features of AD are listed. AD often coexists with endometriosis in younger women.

C. Adenomyosis effects fertility by not only reducing natural conception rate but also reduces the success rates of assisted reproductive technique (ART) procedures. There is increasing evidence indicating decreased implantation and increased early abortions in the presence of AD. The rate of successful pregnancies is directly proportional to the extent of AD.

D. Younger women with good ovarian reserve, no coexisting subfertility factors, and milder forms of the disease can be managed more conservatively with gonadotropin-releasing hormone agonist (GnRHa) therapy. Once spontaneous ovulation is restored, conception can be planned immediately. GnRHa treatment diminishes the size and demarcation of adenomyotic lesions, and with a positive effect on endometrial implantation marker.

E. Younger women with severe and more focal adenomyosis can be advised for surgical resection after counseling the risk of uterine rupture. Suturing postresection has to be done meticulously in multiple layers by overlapping the residual seromuscular layer (flaps) in two or three layers.

F. Optimal thickness of the uterine wall, for conception and prevention of rupture after cytoreductive surgery, may range from 9 mm to 15 mm. Thickness less than 7 mm increases the risk of uterine rupture.

G. Older women with poor ovarian reserve and coexisting subfertility factors should be advised to opt sooner than later for ART to increases the chances of live birth rates.

H. Niu et al. analyzed the outcomes in AD patients undergoing frozen embryo transfer after long-term suppression of the endometrium with GnRHa therapy before hormone replacement therapy. In GnRHa pretreated women, clinical pregnancy, implantation, and ongoing pregnancy rates (PRs) were significantly higher compared with women not pretreated with GnRHa. The study suggested that long term (3–6 months) suppression of the hypothalamo-pituitary-ovarian axis produces a window of enhanced implantation. Women with AD in their late reproductive years, with reduced ovarian reserve, prolonged time to pregnancy because of GnRHa therapy or surgery should be counseled before initiating therapy.

I. Women experiencing recurrent miscarriage, recurrent pregnancy loss, and significantly bulky uterus may be counseled for surrogacy for better fertility rates.

Trivia: Ulipristal acetate and Dienogest are not yet recommended for reducing adenomyosis-related fertility implications.

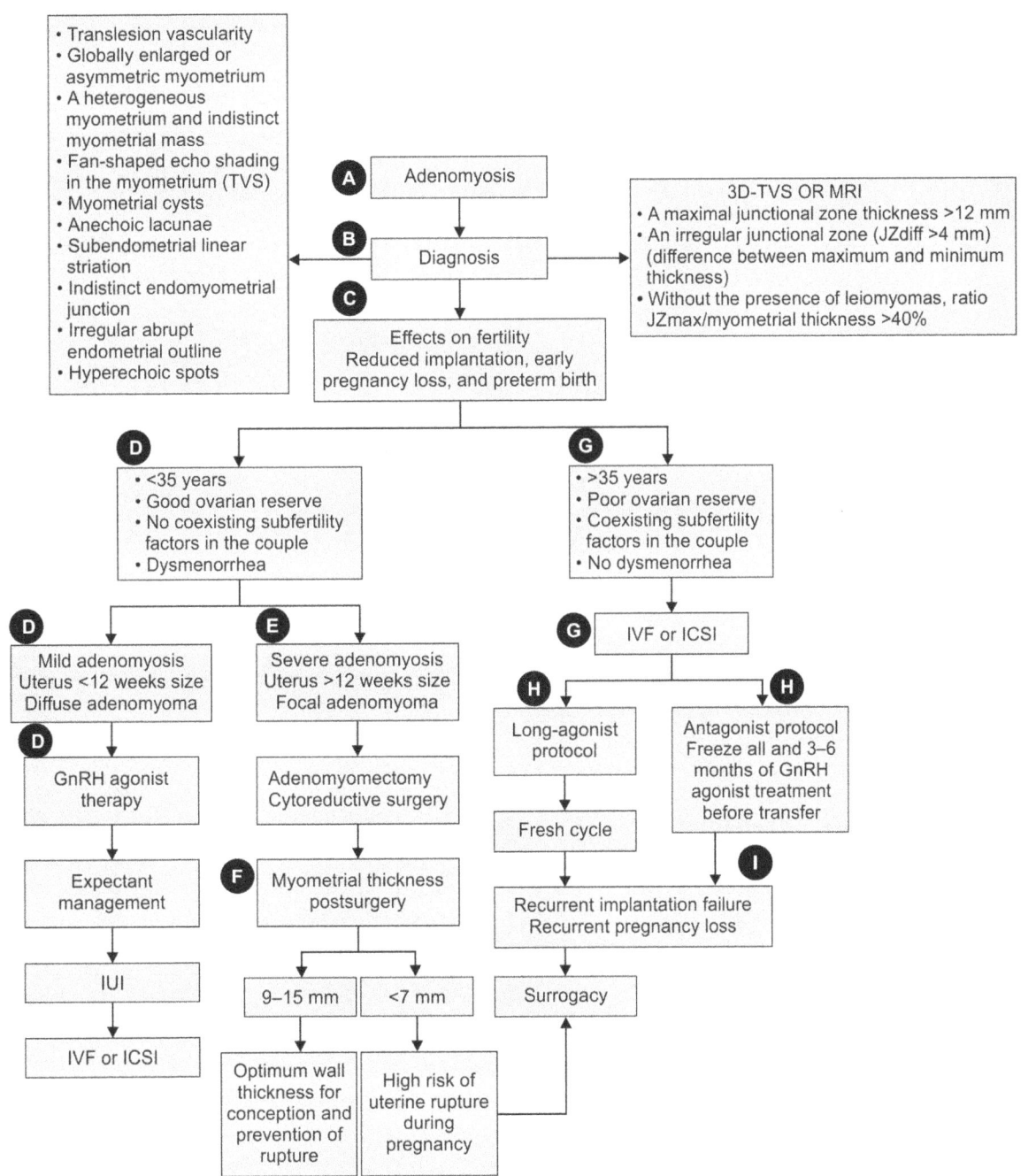

Section 10: Endometriosis and Fibroids

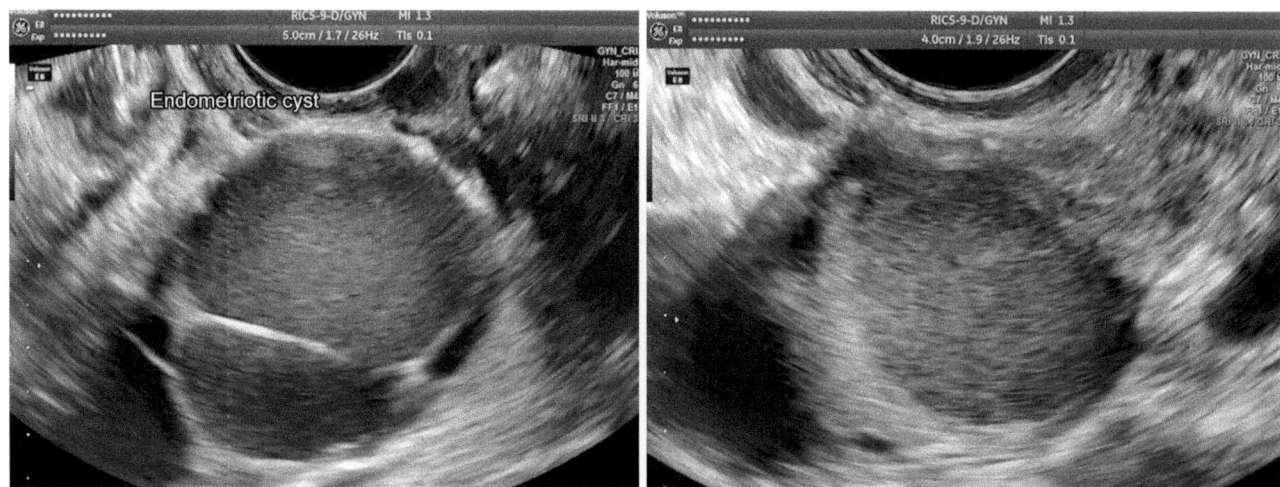

Endometriotic cyst- ground glass appearance on 2D ultrasonography (USG)

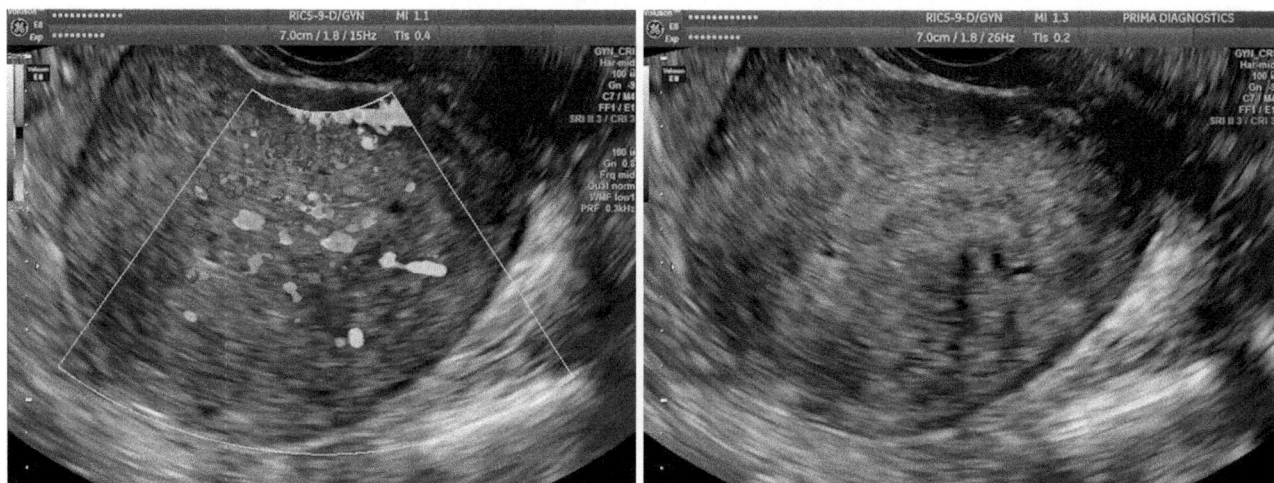

Adenomyosis: increased vascularity of the myometrium. Posterior uterine wall larger than anterior uterine wall

SECTION 11

Infection in Infertility

- Vaginal Infections
- Pelvic Tuberculosis- Diagnosis
- Pelvic Tuberculosis- Management

CHAPTER 37

Vaginal Infections

Shally Gupta

INTRODUCTION

Vaginitis constitutes symptomology like abnormal vaginal discharge, odor, vaginal irritation, and itching with or without burning sensation.

A. In women of reproductive age complaining of vaginal discharge, the most common cause is physiological especially during the periovulatory period. However, presence of itching, odor, or persistent symptoms should prompt elimination of infective or other causes (e.g. foreign body, cervical ectopy). The noninfectious causes accounting for 5–10% of vaginitis cases are due to atrophic, irritant, allergic, and inflammatory vaginitis. Treatment of noninfectious vaginitis should aim at managing the underlying cause. Atrophic vaginitis is usually seen in the perimenopausal to menopausal age group and treated with hormonal and nonhormonal therapies. Inflammatory vaginitis can be treated with topical clindamycin and/or steroid application.

B. The most common causes of infective vaginitis are bacterial vaginosis (BV), vulvovaginal candidiasis, and trichomoniasis. BV accounts for 40–50% of cases, with vulvovaginal candidiasis for 20–25% of cases, and trichomoniasis for 15–20% of infective cases. The diagnosis is made using not just laboratory testing but an amalgamation of symptoms, physical examination findings, and/or office-based testing.

C. Bacterial vaginosis has characteristically thin copious fish smell discharge. There is no complains of itch or inflammation. Gram stain is the diagnostic standard. BV is treated with oral metronidazole, intravaginal metronidazole, or intravaginal clindamycin. It is noteworthy that BV is not sexually transmitted; hence, treatment of partner is not warranted.

D. Candidiasis is second most common infective cause. It has thick curdy white vaginal discharge with itching and erythema, soreness, and inflammation. The diagnosis is made with clinical signs and symptoms of curdy white discharge and visualization of hyphae on microscopy using potassium hydroxide treated vaginal smears. Definitive diagnosis of most organisms causing vaginitis can be done using real-time polymerase chain reaction (PCR) technique of vaginal swabs. Management of vulvovaginal candidiasis comprises of oral fluconazole or topical azoles therapy. However, only topical azoles are recommended during pregnancy.

E. Trichomoniasis is a sexually transmitted infection (STI) and it leads to profuse thin yellowish discharge treated with oral tinidazole or metronidazole. To prevent recurrence, treatment of the active sexual partner is always advised.

F. Cervicitis is usually due to gonococcal and chlamydial infection and is an indication for suspecting upper genital tract infection especially when associated with lower abdominal pain and dyspareunia.

Vaginal discharge is the most common symptom in gynecological outpatient department (OPD) and should not be ignored or taken lightly. It has definite significance in infertile women too. It is suggestive of underlying acute or chronic pelvic pathology. That may be a manifestation of diseases causing infertility, and hence guide in management. It can rarely lead to contamination of cumulus-oocyte complex (COC)/follicular fluid that is aspirated in oocyte pickup (OPU). Vaginal discharge, cervical mucous, and any bleeding due to cervicitis can plug or block the embryo transfer catheter tip and jeopardize the crucial embryo transfer. Cervicitis can lead to difficult embryo transfer that is very critical. Therefore, for women undergoing assisted reproductive technique (ART) procedures, evaluation of vaginal discharge is part of mandatory initial treatment.

Vaginal Infections

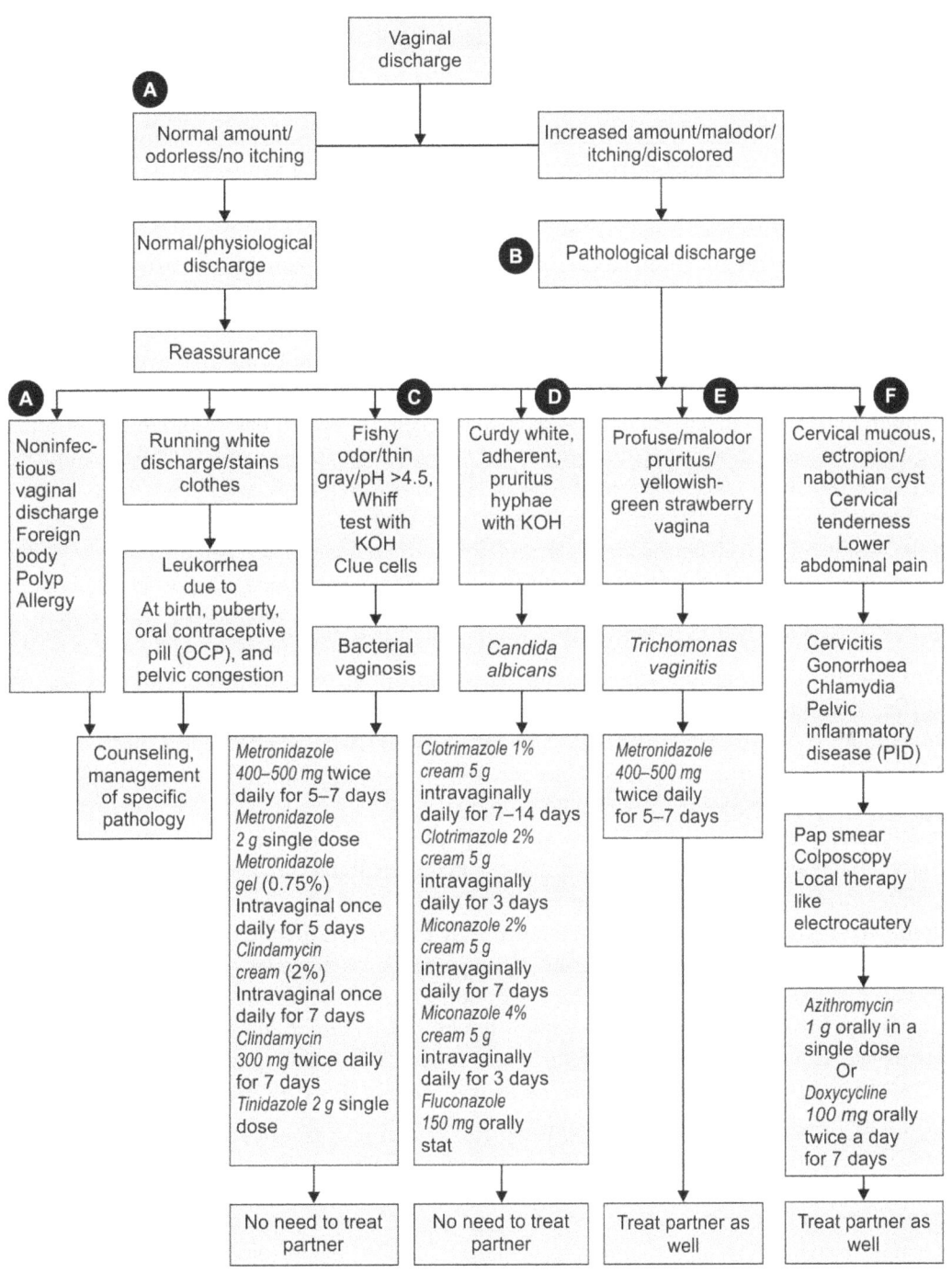

(KOH: potassium hydroxide)

CHAPTER 38

Pelvic Tuberculosis- Diagnosis

Sonia Malik, Vandana Bhatia

A. Tuberculosis (TB) is one of the most common diseases in India and the incidence of genital TB in infertility is as high as 17–20%. The appearance of the disease may vary among different women based on site and stage of the disease.
B. A patient may present with an active form of disease whereby the most common symptoms are menstrual disturbances, chronic pelvic pain, excessive vaginal discharge, mass in abdominal cavity or nonspecific symptoms like general ill-health, anorexia, and low-grade fever.
C. On the contrary, few patients may totally be asymptomatic and may come with complaint of infertility, recurrent pregnancy loss or repeated implantation failures. The possibility of these patients having underlying dormant genital tuberculosis should always be considered, especially in patients who come from an area where TB is endemic, a patient with her own past or family history of exposure to TB, or a patient with some proven extragenital manifestations of the disease. Chronic pelvic inflammatory disease refractory to standard antibiotic therapy should arouse high degree of suspicion of female genital tuberculosis (FGTB).
D. Unlike extrapulmonary tuberculosis, genital tuberculosis is very difficult to diagnose and remains undetected in most cases. Being a paucibacillary disease, demonstration of *Mycobacterium tuberculosis* (MTB) may not be possible in all cases. Though there are batteries of tests available, there is no single diagnostic test available to confirm the diagnosis. The biggest dilemma is whether all infertile women should be subjected to investigations routinely.
E. High degree of suspicion with elaborate history taking, specially taking into account the risk factors like endemicity, past history of tuberculosis or exposure to tuberculosis, low socioeconomic background, patients having human immunodeficiency virus (HIV) or drug abusers should be subjected to battery of tests. This is followed by detailed systemic examination to rule out tubercular focus elsewhere in the body—especially any evidence of lymphadenopathy, abdominal examination, local examination of genitalia, per speculum examination to look for cervical tuberculosis, per vaginal bimanual examination to rule out adnexal masses. All patients should have complete blood count (CBC), erythrocyte sedimentation rate (ESR), Mantoux (Mx) test, and chest X-ray as a baseline. Chest X-ray can be normal in FGTB and Mx test is also nonspecific and is of limited utility in countries like India where Bacillus Calmette-Guérin (BCG) vaccination is done routinely.
F. The two basic imaging techniques—(1) hysterosalpingography (HSG) and (2) ultrasonography (USG) are routinely done for every patient and can prove to be useful in the diagnosis for FGTB. HSG evaluates the internal structures of female genital tract and sometimes even nonspecific changes like tubal dilatation, hydrosalpinx, occluded tubes, irregular uterine contour, synechiae, cavity obliteration may be pointers toward the disease. Similarly USG may vary from normal scan to findings like distorted uterine cavity, presence of endometrial fluid, calcifications and synechiae in uterine cavity, thin endometrium, hydrosalpinx, pyosalpinx and these may suggest the need for further evaluation.
G. Though laparoscopy is an invasive procedure yet it is the most reliable tool for diagnosing FGTB. It helps in visual inspection of pelvic cavity, uterus, ovaries, fallopian tubes, biopsy of the suspected lesions if any and cytology/adenosine deaminase (ADA) of any fluid in the peritoneal cavity. Combining this with hysteroscopy offers added advantage of getting more information about endometrial involvement and sending endometrial tissue for histopathological examination (HPE), polymerase chain reaction (PCR), and acid-fast bacilli (AFB) smear, culture, and GeneXpert. Ideally endometrial sampling should be done in late secretory phase when possibility of finding classic giant cells is maximum.
H. Magnetic resonance imaging (MRI), computed tomography (CT), and positron emission tomography (PET) are advised in the presence of abdominal or adnexal masses on USG.
I. Though HSG, USG, and laparoscopy may strongly suggest the possibility of FGTB, they are not sufficient to diagnose and treat the same and have to be supported by HPE or bacteriological confirmation. Demonstration of caseous epithelioid granuloma on HPE or making mycobacterial smear using Löwenstein-Jensen (LJ) medium or BACTEC 460 or *Mycobacterium* growth inhibitor tube (MGIT) and specific gene probes can help in rapid identification of the

tubercular bacilli and hence diagnosis of the disease. PCR is a sensitive and specific method for detecting mycobacterial DNA and can detect less than 10 bacilli/mL including dead ones within 8–10 hours and therefore more sensitive than HPE and standard culture (which may take 6–8 weeks) but it can be false positive and false negative. Therefore patients should not be started on anti tubercular therapy only on the basis of positive PCR and it should be correlated with clinical evidence or with laparoscopic findings.

J. *GeneXpert*: This is a cartridge-based nucleic acid amplification test (NAAT), a form of PCR, that has been recommended by World Health Organization (WHO) as the test for rapid diagnosis of all forms of tuberculosis—pulmonary or extrapulmonary. However, published data on endometrial samples is scant hence its use is still debatable in FGTB. Advantages are:
   - Rapid test with a turnaround time of 2.5 hours
   - Specific for *Mycobacterium tuberculosis*, no false positives
   - Sensitivity similar to culture
   - Detection of rifampicin (RIF)-resistance via rpoB gene.

K. The patient is subjected to antitubercular therapy only if more than one test is positive or a single gold standard test is positive. Once diagnosed, medical treatment using directly observed treatment, short course (DOTS) strategy for adequate time is the mainstay of treatment.

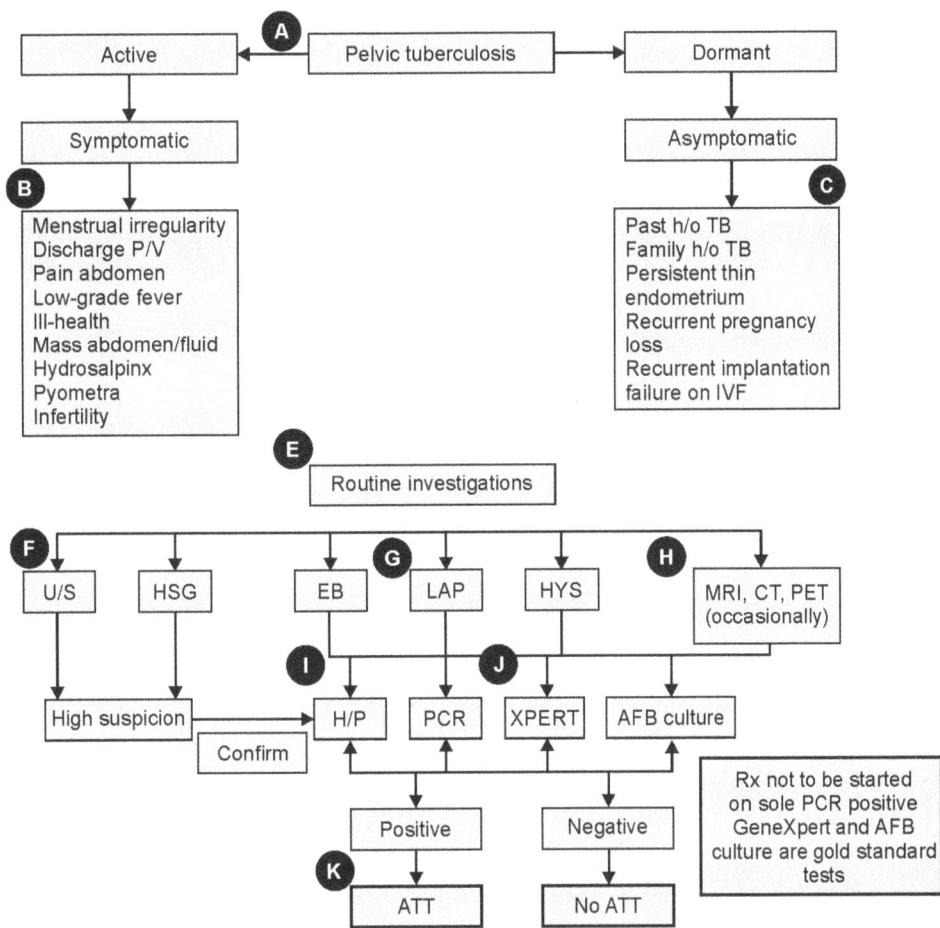

(AFB: acid-fast bacilli; ATT: antitubercular therapy; EB: endometrial biopsy; H/P: histopathological examination; HSG: hysterosalpingography; HYS: hysteroscopy; IVF: in vitro fertilization; LAP: laparoscopy; PCR: polymerase chain reaction; PET: positron emission tomography; TB: tuberculosis; U/S: ultrasound; Rx: treatment; P/V: per vaginally; h/o: history of)

CHAPTER 39

Pelvic Tuberculosis- Management

Sonia Malik, Vandana Bhatia

In the past before the advent of antitubercular drugs, surgical treatment was the mainstay therapy, but now regular intake of multiple drug therapy, to which the organism is susceptible, for adequate period of time, is the mainstay of treatment for female genital tuberculosis (FGTB). According to World Health Organization (WHO):

Standard therapy: A daily therapy of rifampicin (RIF), isoniazid (INH), pyrazinamide (PZA), and ethambutol (EMB) for 2 months followed by INH and RIF daily for 4 months is the recommended treatment.

Alternate therapy: Initial 2 months of four drugs followed by alternate day combination of RIF and INH for 4 months can be given. A course of 6–9 months is effective for treatment of FGTB.

Relapse or failure of treatment: An addition of intramuscular injections of streptomycin thrice weekly together with four drugs (RIF, INH, PZA, EMB) for initial 2 months followed by four drugs thrice a week for next 1 month followed by three drugs (INH, RIF, EMB) thrice a week for another 5 months is recommended.

Multidrug Resistant (MDR): Second-line drugs like kanamycin, ofloxacin, ethionamide, and cycloserine need to be added and 18–24 months of therapy is needed to cure the disease.

Surgery: Rarely recommended nowadays and its use is limited for large tubo-ovarian abscesses or pyosalpinx as it is associated with higher complication rates like injury to bowel and other abdominal organs, adhesion formation, and recurrence of infection. Surgery if needed should be followed by antitubercular therapy (ATT) for better results.

Associated infertility: Assisted reproductive technique (ART) after ATT is a good option though the results have to be taken with a pinch of salt, the conception rate being 17–19% which is still higher than after surgical fertility enhancing surgery (4.3%). ART should be offered to women whose uterine cavity/endometrium is not damaged while adoption/surrogacy is the option for those with damaged cavity/endometrium. Infertility after FGTB may be an irreversible event and these women have a very poor prognosis even after ATT and subjecting these patients to repeated ATT is futile and not recommended.

Safety in pregnancy: It is safe to get pregnant while on the first-line medication. Streptomycin, kanamycin, amikacin, capreomycin, and fluoroquinolones are contraindicated in pregnancy.

Pelvic Tuberculosis- Management

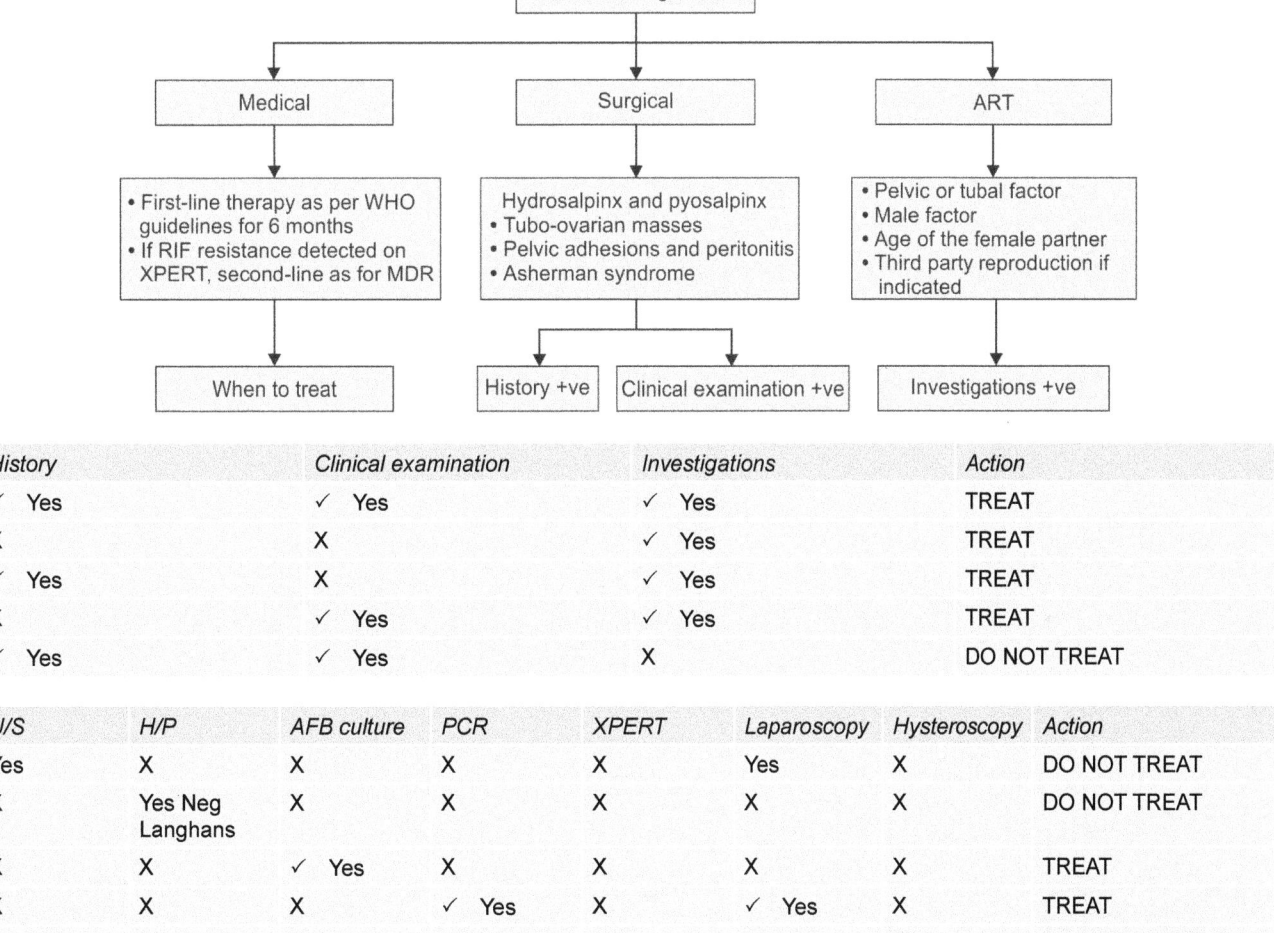

History	Clinical examination	Investigations	Action
✓ Yes	✓ Yes	✓ Yes	TREAT
X	X	✓ Yes	TREAT
✓ Yes	X	✓ Yes	TREAT
X	✓ Yes	✓ Yes	TREAT
✓ Yes	✓ Yes	X	DO NOT TREAT

U/S	H/P	AFB culture	PCR	XPERT	Laparoscopy	Hysteroscopy	Action
Yes	X	X	X	X	Yes	X	DO NOT TREAT
X	Yes Neg Langhans	X	X	X	X	X	DO NOT TREAT
X	X	✓ Yes	X	X	X	X	TREAT
X	X	X	✓ Yes	X	✓ Yes	X	TREAT
X	X	X	✓ Yes	X	X	X	DO NOT TREAT
X	X	X	X	✓ Yes	X	X	TREAT
X	X	X	✓ Yes	✓ Yes	✓ Yes	✓ Yes	TREAT

(AFB: acid-fast bacilli; ART: assisted reproductive technique; FGTB: female genital tuberculosis; H/P: histopathological examination; MDR: multidrug resistance; PCR: polymerase chain reaction; RIF: rifampicin; U/S: ultrasound; WHO: World Health Organization)

SECTION 12

Poor Ovarian Response

- Poor Ovarian Response: Diagnosis
- Poor Ovarian Response: Medical Management
- Newer Modalities to Improve Poor Ovarian Response

CHAPTER 40

Poor Ovarian Response: Diagnosis

Nayana Patel, Molina Patel

A. *Poor ovarian reserve*:
   Definition: As of date, there is no accepted definition of "poor" ovarian reserve (POR) and it may refer to three related but different parameters: (1) the oocyte quality, (2) the oocyte quantity, and (3) the oocyte reproductive potential. All the ovarian reserve tests (ORTs) predict the probable response of the patient for an assisted reproductive technique (ART) cycle and are not prognostic indicators of conception rates.
B. *Diagnosis for POR*: The Bologna's criterion proposed by European Society of Human Reproduction and Embryology (ESHRE) is the most widely used system for identifying a poor ovarian response. Presence of at least two of the following three features is suggestive of a poor response:
   i. Advanced maternal age (≥ 40 years) or any other risk factor for POR
   ii. A previous POR (≤ 3 oocytes with a conventional stimulation protocol)
   iii. An abnormal ovarian reserve tests [i.e. antral follicle count (AFC), 5–7 follicles or anti-Müllerian hormone (AMH), 0.5–1.1 ng/mL]
   Poor response to maximal stimulation on two previous occasions also defines POR.
   Bologna criteria have been criticized mainly because it failed to consider the fact that younger women with poor ORTs have a better prognosis as compared to older women.
C. Recently, the POSEIDON group (**P**atient-**O**riented **S**trategies **E**ncompassing **I**ndividualize **D** **O**ocyte **N**umber) proposed a new stratification of ART in patients with a reduced ovarian reserve or unexpected inappropriate ovarian response to exogenous gonadotropins. Poseidon criterion distinguishes the patients with a low prognosis despite normal ovarian reserve tests (Group 1 and 2) from those with low ovarian reserve tests (Group 3 and 4). In brief, four subgroups have been suggested based on quantitative and qualitative parameters, namely:
   i. Age and the expected aneuploidy rate
   ii. Ovarian biomarkers (i.e. AFC and AMH)
   iii. Ovarian response—provided a previous stimulation cycle was performed.
   The new classification introduces a more nuanced picture of the "low prognosis patient" in ART, using clinically relevant criteria to guide the physician to most optimally manage this group of patients. Fertility peaks before the age of 30 and thereafter, it is believed to decline gradually. In addition to the "natural" age-related decline, factors that may further deplete the ovarian reserve during reproductive years are diverse.
D. Endometrioma, certain pelvic infections, ovarian surgery, all can reduce the ovarian reserve. Endometrioma and its surgical excision is known to cause POR. Genital tuberculosis, even in its latent form, is increasingly being recognized as a cause of POR in Indian women. Chlamydial infection is known to adversely influence the ovarian response in those undergoing ART. Both chemotherapy and radiotherapy are known to affect the ovarian reserve adversely. Obesity and chronic smoking are other factors known to be associated with POR. Altered expression of certain genes in cumulus and granulosa cells have been implicated in the etiology of POR in young women. Follicle-stimulating hormone receptor (FSHR) polymorphism is considered to be an important cause of unexpected poor response in young women undergoing in vitro fertilization (IVF). Certain types of mutations in *FMR1* gene are known to be associated with reduced ovarian functional reserve in young women.
E. FORT (Follicular output rate): FORT, first proposed by Genro, is considered as an effective tool in evaluating ovarian response to controlled ovarian stimulation. It is calculated by using the formula: Pre-ovulatory follicle (16–22 mm in diameter) count (PFC) on human chorionic gonadotropin (hCG) day × 100/small antral follicle (3–8 mm in diameter) count at baseline. Based on the values, patients can be categorized as poor responders (low FORT <42), normal responders (normal FORT 42–58%) and hyper-responders (high FORT >58%). There is emerging evidence that FORT score correlates to clinical pregnancy rate and thus can be invaluable in patient counseling as well change of future therapeutic strategies.

F. Identification of poor responders helps prognostic counseling as well change of therapeutic strategies to improve the fertility outcome. Hence all patients undergoing an ART procedure should be evaluated for ovarian response.

$$\text{FORT} = \frac{\text{No. of mature follicles (16–22 mm) on the day of trigger}}{\text{No. of antral follicles (3–8 mm) on day 2 of MC}} \times 100$$

Poor responders (low FORT <42),
Normal responders (normal FORT 42–58%)
Hyper-responders (high FORT >58%).

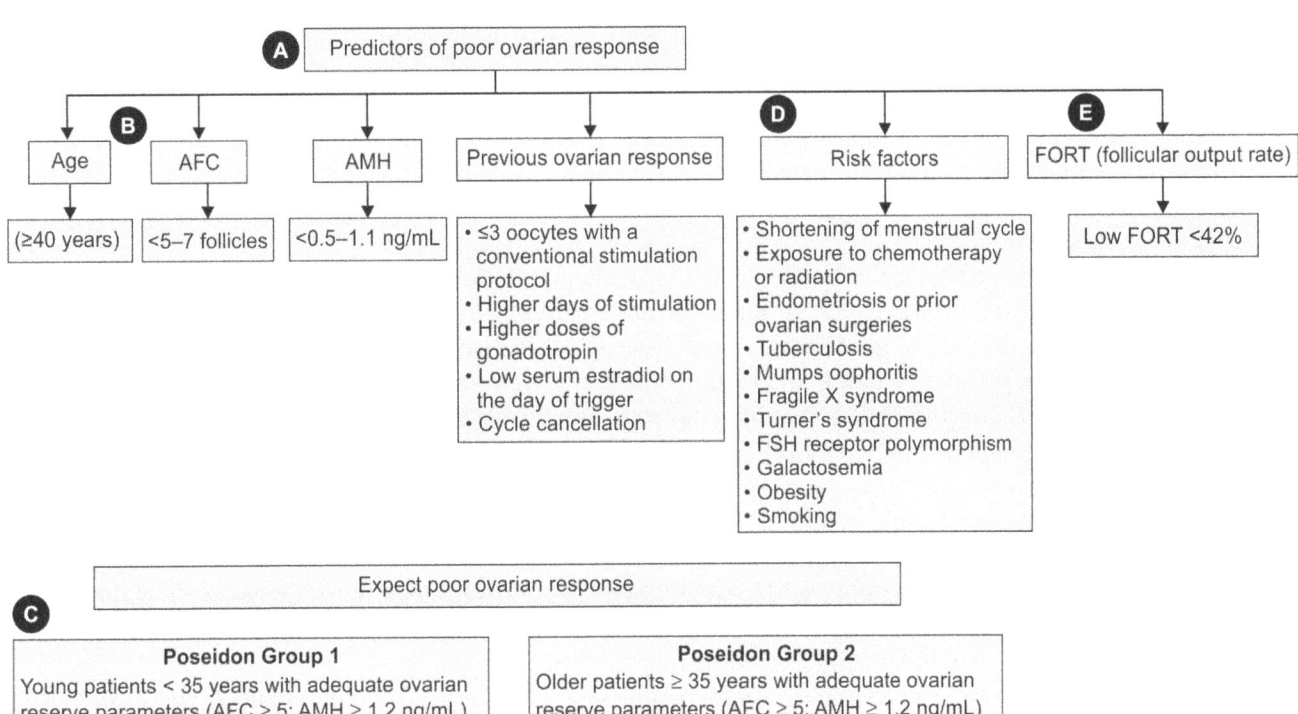

(AFC: antral follicle count; AMH: anti-Müllerian hormone; FSH: follicle-stimulating hormone)

CHAPTER 41

Poor Ovarian Response: Medical Management

Nayana Patel, Molina Patel

Women with poor ovarian reserves, frequently result in a poor response to conventional stimulation protocols. With reduced number of oocytes, the cumulative pregnancy rates take a hit. Multiple strategies have been adopted to improve the quantity and quality of oocytes obtained in women with poor ovarian reserve (POR).

A. *High-dose gonadotropin*: The strategy of using high-dose gonadotropins (GT) in ovarian stimulation in patients with likely poor response is debatable as the response is not dependent on the levels of gonadotropins but on the number of recruitable follicles. Use of higher doses should be judicious to prevent any adverse effect on oocyte quality. Another strategy is to use high-dose gonadotropins in the beginning and then step down in the second part of the cycle without compromising the cycle outcome. Increasing the starting dose to 300 IU may be effective but increase above 450 IU/day may have limited effectiveness. Administration of long-acting gonadotropin, corifollitropin alfa, has also been suggested. Patients with follicle-stimulating hormone (FSH) receptor polymorphism benefit significantly by using higher doses of GT.

B. *Addition of LH stimulations*: Luteinizing hormone (LH) supplementation during the stimulation protocol is known to be useful in poor responders as well as patients of advanced maternal age. It has been seen that sufficient steroidogenesis can occur even if less than 1% of the LH receptors are occupied. Patients with poor response to FSH stimulation especially of advanced age may benefit from LH supplementation from stimulation day 6 to 8 onward when the LH receptors are acquired. This could be because the number of functional LH receptors decreases with age.

C. *Mild ovarian stimulation for in vitro fertilization (IVF)*: Involves using the following agents as monotherapy or in combination: Clomiphene citrate (CC), aromatase inhibitors, low-dose gonadotropins, gonadotropin-releasing hormone (GnRH) antagonists, and late follicular phase human chorionic gonadotropin (hCG)/LH. The recent recommendation states that mild stimulation produces comparative results as that of high-dose or conventional IVF.

D. ACCUVIT (embryo accumulation vitrification) is a protocol of accumulating embryos with serial minimal stimulation cycles, vitrifying the resulting embryos and transferring them in a remote cycle (IVF Lite protocol). Some studies have shown promising results in improving the pregnancy rates.

E. Low-dose aspirin therapy has been demonstrated to enhance blood perfusion to multiple organ systems including the ovary. In patients with poor response, *75–150 mg/day* aspirin is proposed to increase blood flow and responsiveness. In a randomized controlled trial (RCT), specifically done in poor responders, it was concluded that low-dose aspirin failed to improve either blood flow or responsiveness.

F. Dehydroepiandrosterone (DHEA) is supplemented in a dose of around *75 mg/day and started 2 months prior* and continued throughout stimulation. It has been summarized in a review by Gleicher that DHEA supplementation improves ovarian function, increases pregnancy chances, and lowers aneuploidy and miscarriage rates. In a very recent retrospective analysis conducted in Australia of 626 patients, it was observed that the patients with adjuvants of either growth hormone (GH) and DHEA showed better live birth rates which were significant as compared to no adjuvant therapy.

G. AndroGel or testosterone has a role in folliculogenesis in the early phase before the follicle becomes sensitive to gonadotropins. They inhibit the apoptosis and, in gonadotropin sensitive follicles, it enhances the FSH action. With increasing age, the levels of androgens decline. Most commonly used in the transdermal form, testosterone has also shown to have beneficial effects on the poor ovarian reserve patients. It can be administered by gel or spray form. Dose: 25–50 mg of testosterone gel daily from Day 21 of previous cycle or D2 of stimulation cycle is shown to be beneficial.

H. *Growth hormone*: It is proposed that GH improves the outcome in poor responders by increasing the estradiol, insulin growth factor-1 levels which promote better developmental potential, enhanced nucleocytoplasmic maturation and DNA repair mechanisms. The dose varies from *4–8 IU daily or 10–24 IU on alternate days* in patients with diminished ovarian reserve. According to the Cochrane review, the results still need to be interpreted with caution, and the included trials were few in number and small sample size. Therefore, before recommending GH adjuvant in IVF further research is necessary to fully define its role.

I. *Coenzyme Q10/vitamin D3*: Coenzyme Q10, ubiquinol, and vitamin D are seen responsible for maintaining ovarian physiology and its supplementation is seen to improve ovarian reserve.

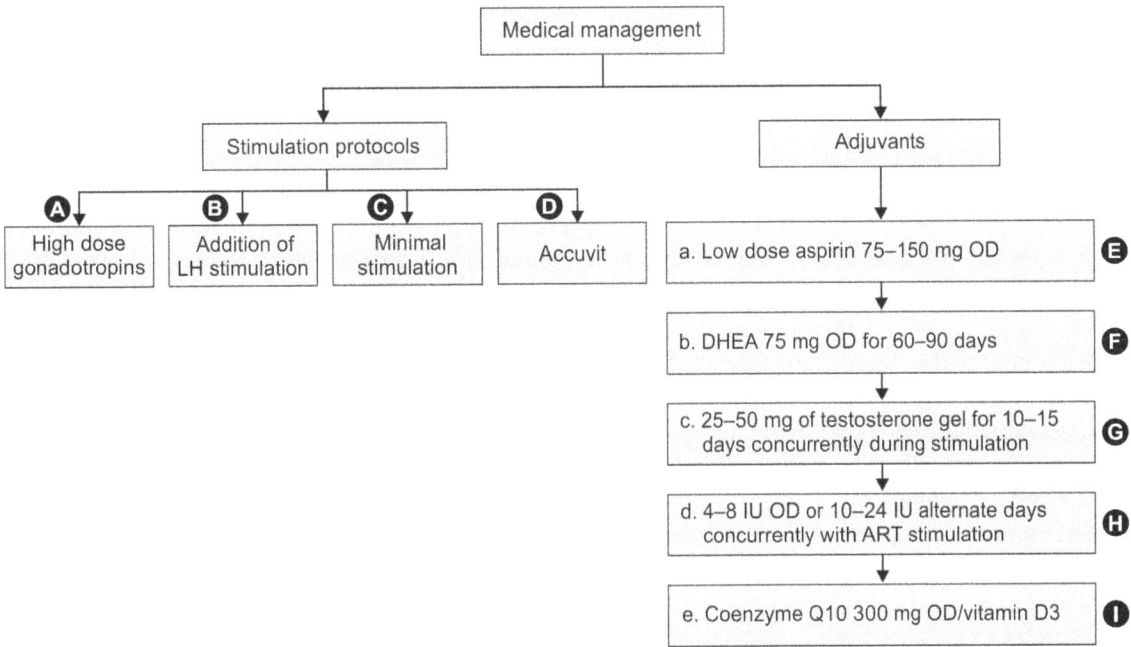

(DHEA: dehydroepiandrosterone; LH: luteinizing hormone; ART: assisted reproductive technique)

CHAPTER 42
Newer Modalities to Improve Poor Ovarian Response

Nayana Patel, Molina Patel

Poor response to gonadotropin stimulation is due to limited number of gonadotropin sensitive antral follicles. However, they might still have a reserve of secondary follicles non-responsive to gonadotropins (GT) stimulation awaiting transition. Most of the newer modalities aim at transformation of secondary follicles into preantral and antral follicles, leading to the increase in the number of retrieved oocytes after ovarian stimulation.

A. *Bone marrow-derived stem cells*: Two live birth have been reported after stem cell ovarian autologous transplantation of mobilized bone marrow-derived stem cells in poor responder women in trial (registration number: NCT02240342) done by Herraiz et al. (2016) and presented at European Society of Human Reproduction and Embryology (ESHRE), 2016.

B. *Platelet-rich plasma:* Sfakianoudis's team has found that platelet-rich plasma (PRP) seems to rejuvenate older ovaries. The team was able to collect oocytes and fertilize them from a woman whose menopause had established 5 years ago, at age of 40. For the treatment, they injected PRP into ovaries of the patient and 6 months after, she experienced her first period since menopause. Thus, PRP is found to be effective in reversal of menopause and initiation of folliculogenesis. Results of the study suggest that autologous stem cell ovarian transplant (ASCOT) optimized the mobilization and growth of existing follicles, possibly related to fibroblast growth factor-2 and thrombospondin-1 within apheresis. The ASCOT improved follicle and oocyte quantity enabling pregnancy in women who are poor responders previously limited to oocyte donation.

C. *Autologous mitochondrion activation:* It is technique of injection of autologous mitochondrial suspension, obtained from ovarian tissue biopsy, along with the sperm into mature oocytes aiming at improving the reproductive outcome.

D. *In vitro activation*: It is hypothesized that inhibition of Hippo signaling in the ovary induces secondary follicular growth. In order to achieve this, ovarian tissue is excised partial from one side of ovary under laparoscopic surgery. Postseparation of the medulla tissues, the ovarian cortex is dissected into 1–2 mm square of ovarian cubes and cultured overnight to suppress Hippo signaling. After culture, these cubes were autotransplanted beneath the serosa of both fallopian tubes. Linear cuttings in the ovarian cortex is also considered to induce physical stimulation in the ovary and activation of secondary follicles.

E. *Triple parenting*: Different investigated methods are apparently helpful to increase the activity of mitochondria in the oocyte cell. The important methods are ooplasmic transfer, mitochondrial injection, nuclear transfer, and mitochondrial deoxyribonucleic acid (mtDNA) injection; however the clinical use of these methods requires further studies. These four methods are known as three-parent in vitro fertilization (IVF) methods because in these, in addition to sperm 2 oocytes cooperate in fertilization; a donor oocyte which has active mitochondria and a recipient in which mitochondria are inactive due to aging or mitochondrial disease.

F. Most of these methods are deemed experimental with varied results and should be offered to patients only after detailed explanation of the possible success rates. If not judiciously used the use of these technologies may result in wastage of resources, time, and emotions.

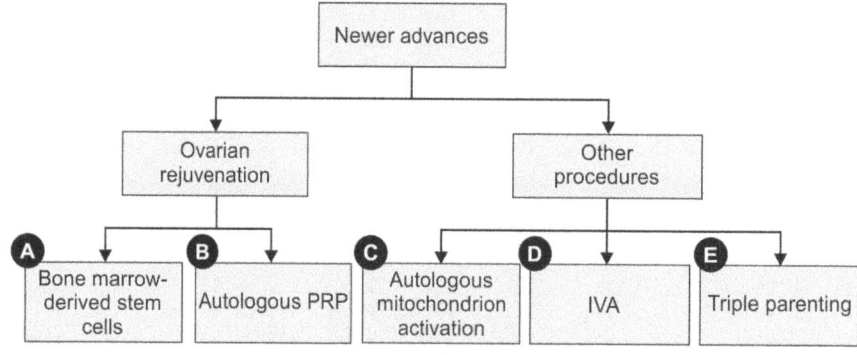

(IVA: in vitro activation; PRP: platelet-rich plasma)

SECTION 13

Andrology: A Gynecologist's View

- Evaluation of the Male Infertility Factors
- Interpretation of Semen Analysis- Macroscopic Parameters
- Interpretation of Semen Analysis- Microscopic Parameters
- Male Hypogonadism
- Azoospermia: Evaluation
- Anejaculation
- Genetic Evaluation of the Infertile Male
- Sperm Deoxyribonucleic Acid Fragmentation
- Varicocele and Male Infertility

Evaluation of the Male Infertility Factors

Sunil Jindal, Anshu Jindal

A. Evaluation of the male partner should be done concurrently along with the female partner if they fail to achieve pregnancy within 1 year of unprotected intercourse. In the presence of a pre-existing risk factor or known sexual dysfunction, an earlier evaluation may be warranted. The initial evaluation constitutes general history along with the reproductive history and two properly performed semen analyses. A detailed evaluation by an andrologist or an urologist should be done if the initial screening brings forward an abnormal semen analysis. Advanced evaluation of the male partner should also be considered in couples with poor reproductive history like unexplained infertility or recurrent pregnancy loss.

B. *Medical history*:
   - A detailed medical and surgical history
   - List of medications used (prescription and nonprescription) and allergies
   - Lifestyle evaluation and exposures and a review of systems
   - Reproductive history of the family, and
   - History of past infections such as sexually transmitted diseases and respiratory infection.

C. *Physical examination*:
   Both the American Urological Association (AUA) and the American Society for Reproductive Medicine (ASRM) recommend the evaluation of following factors in physical examination.
   Apart from the general physical examination, all initial evaluations should ideally include detailed genitalia evaluation:
   - Examine the penis, especially for the opening of the urethral meatus
   - Palpate the testes and measure their size (normal 12–20 cc. Smaller testes indicate hypogonadism)
   - Existence and consistency of both the vasa and epididymides (absence indicates congenital bilateral absence of vas deferens, causes obstructive azoospermia)
   - Presence of a varicocele
   - Secondary sex characteristics including hair distribution body habitus and breast development, and
   - Rectal examination for seminal vesicles, prostatic adenoma, and neoplasia.

D. *Semen analysis*: Semen analysis is the mainstay for the laboratory assessment of the male partner and gives an overview of the fertility potential of male. A systematic assessment with standard instructions for semen collection is the crux for a proper interpretation. The sample is collected by masturbation or by intercourse using special semen collection condoms that do not contain substances detrimental to sperm after a defined period of abstinence of 2–3 days. Although it is ideal to collect the sample at the laboratory, a home collected sample may be accepted after mentioning the same in the report. When collected outside the laboratory, the specimen should be kept at room or body temperature during transport and examined within 1 hour of collection.

   The semen analysis provides assessment of macroparameters like semen volume as well as microparameters like sperm concentration, motility, and morphology. Levels that fall beyond the reference ranges [World Health Organization (WHO)] direct towards a male infertility factor and indicate the need for additional clinical and/or laboratory evaluation. It must be stressed that the reference values for semen variables are not the equivalent to the minimum values needed for conception, and that men with semen parameters outside the reference arrays may still be fertile. On the contrary, patients with levels within the reference range may still be infertile.

E. *Endocrine evaluation*:
   An initial endocrine evaluation should include at least a serum testosterone and follicle-stimulating hormone (FSH). It should be performed if there is:
   - An abnormally low sperm concentration, especially if less than 10 millions/mL
   - Impaired sexual function, or
   - Other clinical findings suggestive of a specific endocrinopathy.

F. *Ultrasound evaluation*: Ultrasound is not done as part of routine investigation of male partner, but is performed only to confirm or rule out a suspected abnormality either on examination or semen analysis. Scrotal ultrasonography (USG) is done to evaluate the scrotal and testicular pathologies like testicular masses, atrophic testis, varicocele, hydrocele, epididymal cysts, etc. Prostate is evaluated using a transrectal ultrasonography (TRUS).

DNA fragmentation index (DFI) and genetic assessment are elaborated in subsequent topics.

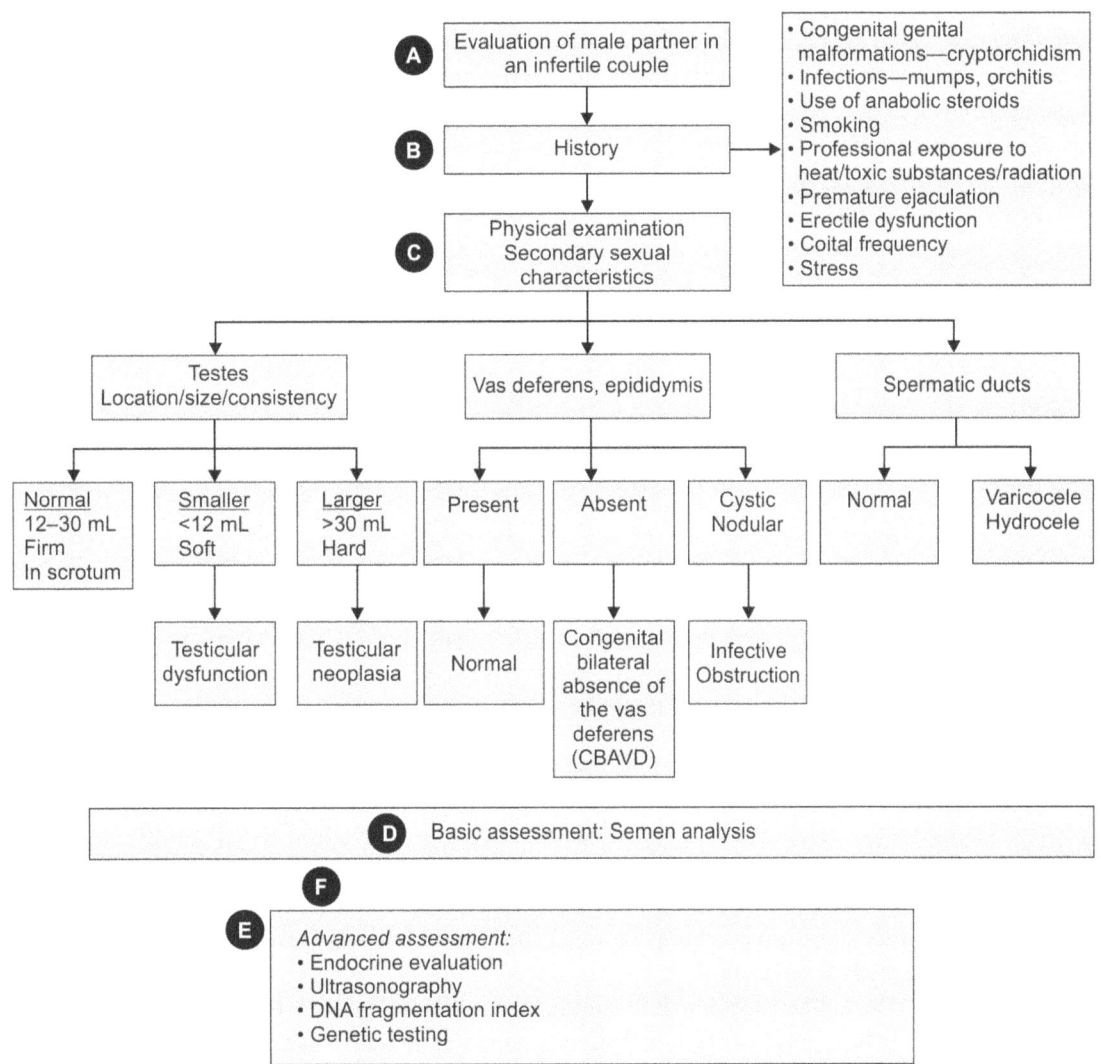

CHAPTER 44

Interpretation of Semen Analysis- Macroscopic Parameters

Aditi Kanungo, Rajeev Agarwal, Apoorva Pallam Reddy

A. Semen analysis is the first step towards evaluation of the fertility potential of the male. It measures the quantity and quality of a man's semen and sperm parameters. The 2010 criterion by World Health Organization (WHO) is the 5th edition of reference values and is the most commonly used reference for evaluating the semen parameters. About 4,500 fertile men (who were able to achieve pregnancy with a normal female partner within 1 year of unprotected intercourse) were evaluated for their sperm parameters. 5th centile of the average semen parameters were taken as the reference point predicting the fertility potential of the male. Values above the reference range are considered to have higher probability of pregnancy and values below this range are considered to have lower probability of pregnancy. It has to be noted that over the years, there has been a progressive reduction even in the references given by the WHO suggesting that these reference values are not sufficient to label a male- fertile or infertile.

Reference values given are 5th centile and are used as lower cutoff limits of normality:

	WHO reference values changed				
	1980	1987	1992	1999	2010
Volume (mL)	ND	≥2	≥2	≥2	≥1.5
Count (10^6/mL)	20–200	≥20	≥20	≥20	≥15
Total count (10^6)	ND	≥40	≥40	≥40	≥39
Motility (%)	≥60	≥50	≥50	≥50	≥40
Progressive (%)	≥2	≥25%	≥25% (a)	≥25% (a)	≥32%
Vitality (%)	ND	≥50	≥75	≥75	≥58
Morphology (%)	80.5	≥50	≥30	(14)*	≥4*
Leukocytes (10^6/mL)	<4.7	<1.0	<1.0	<1.0	1.0

*Strict criteria (Tygerberg); Esteves et al. *Urology* 2012

Analysis can be done in two broad categories—(1) Macroscopic and (2) Microscopic.

B. *Macroscopic analysis*: Macroscopic results sometimes are more relevant for clinical interpretation.
C. *Volume*: Normal volume of semen sample is 1.5–4 mL. Pipetting is a better method of measuring volume. The variation in the volume help us to categorize various disorders, i.e. low volume is associated with improper collection, partial retrograde ejaculation, and congenital absence of vas deferens, obstruction of lower urinary tract whereas hyperspermia is associated with accessory gland infection or prolonged abstinence. In case of suspicion of infection, semen culture followed by antibiotic therapy is warranted.
D. *pH (potential hydrogen)*: Coagulated alkaline fluid coming from seminal vesicle is the main component of semen and the prostatic acidic fluid is the second largest component. Seminal fluid traverses through ejaculatory duct but not the prostatic fluid. Normal semen pH is 7.2–8.2. The alkaline pH of the semen also gives protection to the sperms from the spermiolytic acidic conditions of the vagina. Acidic semen with low volume indicates obstructive azoospermia.
E. *Appearance*: A normal semen sample appears to pearly white and is opaque. Any variation in the physiochemical character, points toward some clinical entity. Most common cause of reddish semen is genital tract trauma or tumor and needs to be evaluated by an andrologist. Yellow color semen either denotes infection or severe jaundice in which case a culture and antibiotic therapy is mandated failing which there is high chance of endometritis during intrauterine insemination (IUI) or infection of culture media during in vitro fertilization (IVF). Thus, the physical variation helps us in the diagnosis of pathology.
F. *Liquefaction time*: The semen is ejaculated in a coagulated state due to the presence of coagulation proteins secreted by the seminal vesicles. This helps in proper deposition of the sperms inside the vaginal cavity. The thinning out of the semen is due to lytic enzymes secreted by the prostate. This thinning (Liquefaction) eases the sperm mobility

into the cervical canal. Normal time is 30–60 minutes. Exact liquefaction time is of no importance until more than 2 hours elapse without change. Failure of liquefaction is a sign of inadequate secretion of the proteolytic enzymes of prostate whereas absence of coagulation points toward ejaculatory duct obstruction or congenital absence of seminal vesicle. In cases of high liquefaction, the sperms are exposed longer to the harsher vaginal environment reducing the possibility of natural conception.

G. *Viscosity*: Viscosity is defined as the resistance of seminal fluid to flow. Normal semen coagulates upon ejaculation and liquefy within 15–20 minutes. Nonliquefaction should be differentiated from hyperviscosity. Viscosity is noted after liquefaction. Highly viscous samples reduce the ease of sperm motility through the seminal fluid.

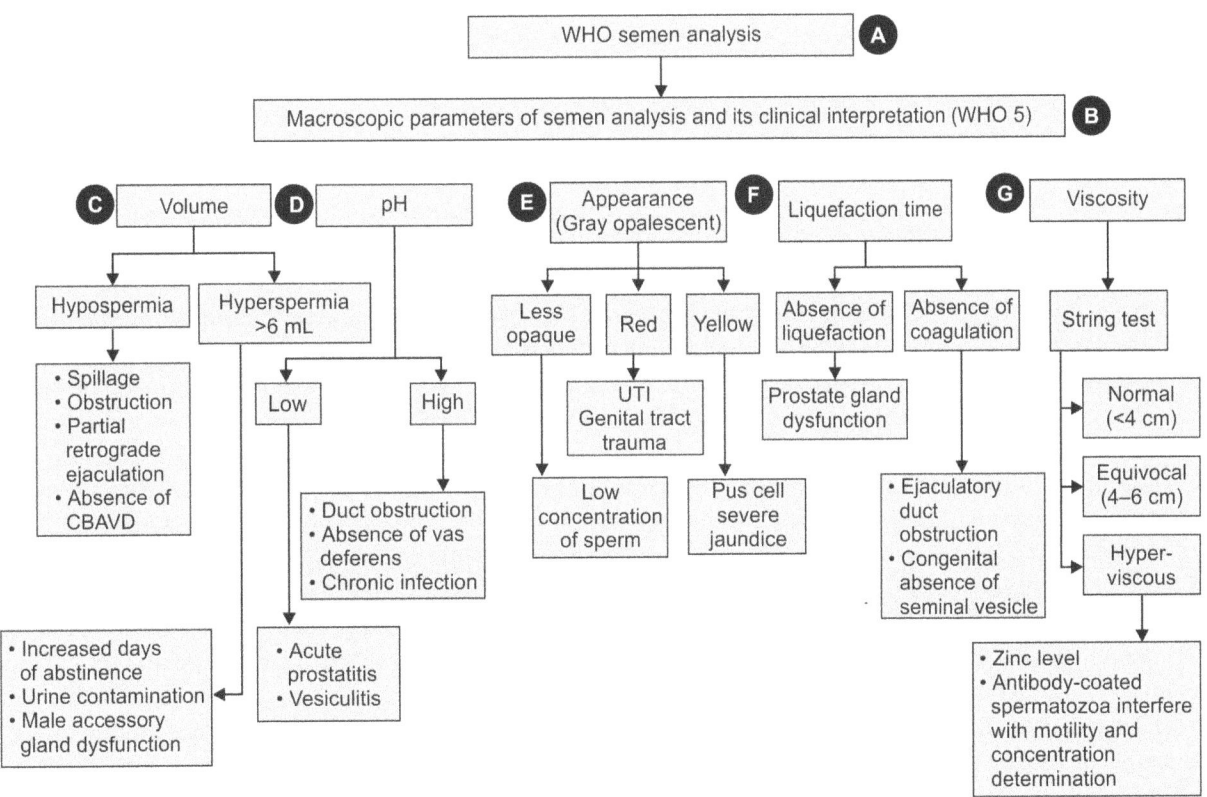

(UTI: urinary tract infection; pH: potential hydrogen; CBAVD: congenital bilateral absence of the vas deferens)

CHAPTER 45

Interpretation of Semen Analysis- Microscopic Parameters

Aditi Kanungo, Rajeev Agarwal, Siddharth

INTRODUCTION

The microscopic examination of semen is carried out after complete liquefaction of the sample using a small drop of it placed over a Mackler's chamber and seen under a phase contrast microscope (40 × magnification).

A. *Concentration and number*: It is a very important prognostic factor for deciding time to pregnancy and conception. Concentration is number of sperm per mL of semen whereas total number is sperm concentration multiplied by total volume. The lower reference number of sperm concentration is 15×10^6/mL and total sperm count is 39×10^6/ejaculate. There are different terminology, i.e. polyzoospermia (>350 million/mL), normozoospermia (>40 million/mL), oligospermia (<20 million/mL), and azoospermia (no sperm in ejaculate). If there is azoospermia, centrifuge the sample at 3,000 rpm for 15 minutes and the pallet should be checked by two observers. In case no sperms are observed even in a centrifuged sample, a tentative azoospermia reporting is given. A confirmation of azoospermia is given only after repeating the assessment a second time a minimum of 2 weeks apart. In case of abnormal result always repeat the test after 2 weeks.

If the count is low than 10 million/mL then follicle-stimulating hormone (FSH) and total testosterone to be measured. Low testosterone may be due to Leydig cell dysfunction or hypothalamic-pituitary-testicular (HPT) axis dysfunction. If total testosterone is also low (<300 ng/dL) then luteinizing hormone (LH), prolactin, and free testosterone measured. With the help of hormonal evaluation we get a vivid idea about the clinical entity responsible for the abnormal result which also helps us to take treatment choices of different assisted reproductive technique (ART) techniques. High FSH is found in testicular failure, Sertoli cell-only syndrome or testicular atrophy. Normal FSH with normal testicular volume needs testicular sampling further to see for spermatogenesis. When spermatogenesis is normal it is mostly due to obstruction to ejaculatory duct where vasovasostomy or vasoepididymostomy can be done or sperm retrieval by testicular sperm extraction/percutaneous epididymal sperm aspiration (TESE/PESA) followed by intracytoplasmic sperm injection (ICSI) to be done and if spermatogenesis is absent it denotes destruction of tubular epithelium. Low FSH or undetectable FSH is indicative of Kallmann syndrome. In case of azoospermia always check for fructose which decides whether it is of obstructive pathology. In severe oligospermia and azoospermia always do genetic evaluation to see karyotyping error or Y chromosome microdeletion. It should be noted that all testicular samplings should be done only in a set up that is capable of freezing any sperms that are identified.

B. *Agglutination*: Agglutination of the sperms is seen for in an unstained sample, it may be sperm versus sperm which can be scored in Grade I (<10 spermatozoa per agglutinate), Grade II (10–50 spermatozoa per agglutinate, some free spermatozoa), Grade III (>50 spermatozoa per agglutinate, some still free), Grade IV (all agglutinate and agglutinates inter connected). This agglutination may be between head to head, tail tip to tail tip, mixed, and tangle. We plan the treatment accordingly; in case of Grade I and Grade II, two to three cycle of intrauterine insemination (IUI) can be done whereas in Grade III and IV better results are obtained by ICSI.

Agglutination may also be between sperm cell with other nonsperm cell (can be quantified by peroxidise activity or CD45). If it is with leukocytes and the leukocyte count is high then it denotes infection, culture the semen sample and treat with antibiotics. If the agglutination is more with immature germ cell then it points toward defective spermatogenesis.

C. *Motility*: The lower reference value for total motility is 40% and progressive motility is 32%. It can be broadly divided in three categories, i.e. rapidly progressive (moving actively in linear or large circle regardless of speed), nonprogressive (all pattern of motility without progression), and immotile. Persistent poor motility is a good prognostic factor for failure of fertilization. When more than 50% are immotile then check for vitality.

D. *Vitality*: It differentiates dead sperm from the live one. It can be done by Eosin-Nigrosin (sperm with intact membrane are alive), hypo-osmotic swelling (HOS) test swollen membrane when placed in a hypo-osmolar medium—HOS tests for the integrity of the sperm membrane. 1 mcl of sperms are added to 250 mcl of hypo-osmolar media available in the market and incubated for 60 minutes at room temperature and a minimum of 100 sperms per slide are observed for swollen tails demonstrating vitality. A vitality >58% is considered normal. The immotile and nonviable sperms denote epididymal pathology whereas immotile and viable sperm shows structural defect in tail of sperm or Kartagener syndrome.

E. *Morphology*: Morphology is scored by World Health Organization (WHO) classification by Kruger's strict criteria classification. The staining differentiates the quantitative normal and abnormal sperm morphological form in an ejaculate. It classifies abnormally shaped spermatozoa in different category on the basis of head, tail, midpiece abnormality from the sperms recovered from postcoital cervical mucus or from surface of zona pellucida. If the sperms fail to meet the strictly defined parameter of normal shape, they fall into the abnormal category. The lower reference value is 4%. It can be head defect (double head, pyriform, absence of acrosome, etc.), midpiece defect (bent neck and asymmetrical insertion into head), tail defect (short tail, hairpin, etc.). Morphology always to be interpreted combining with other criteria and clinical implication is controversial. Teratozoospermic index defined as number of abnormalities present per abnormal spermatozoa. If the value is more than 1.8 the prognosis is poor and need ICSI or intracytoplasmic morphologically selected sperm injection (IMSI).

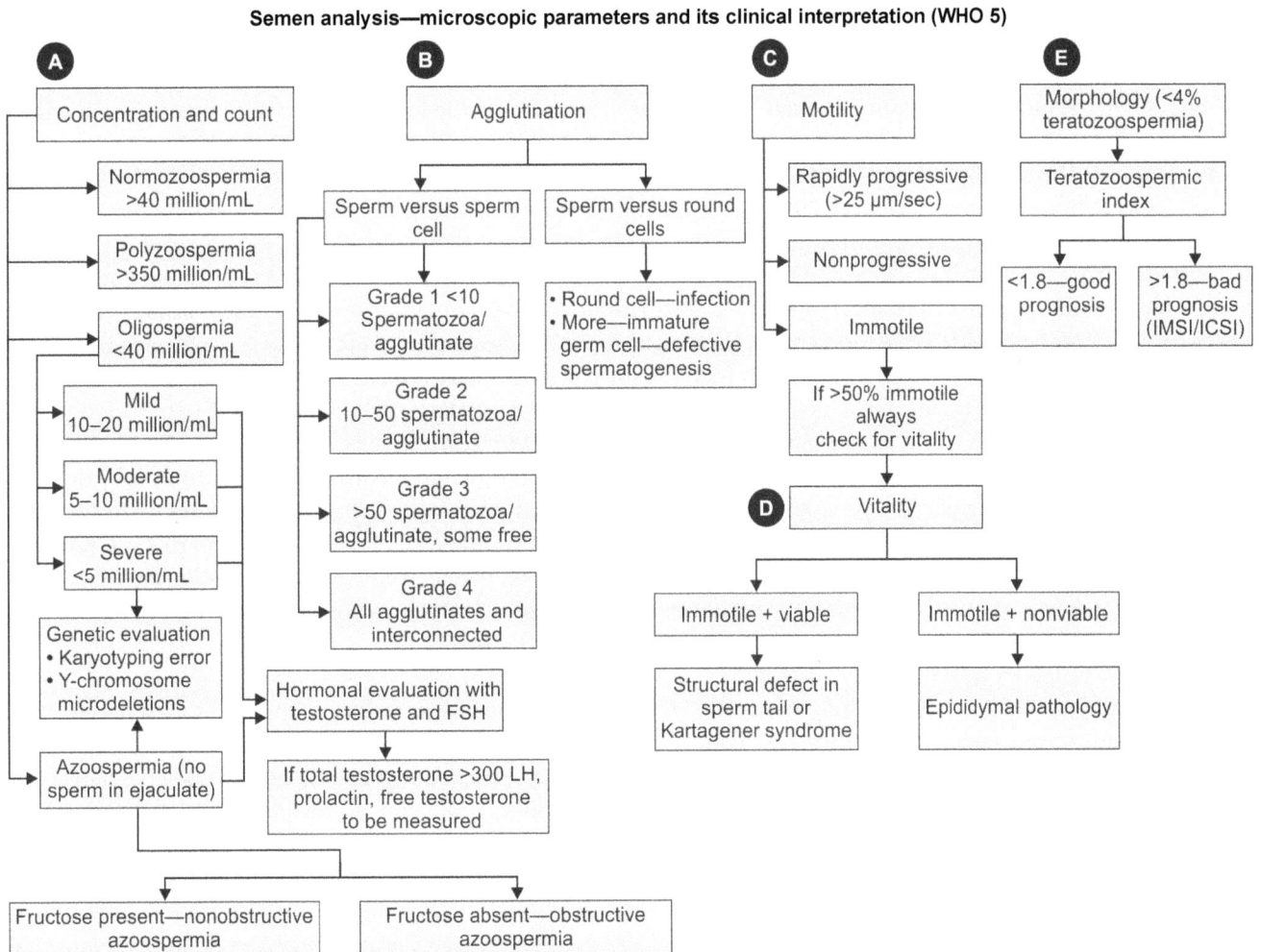

Semen analysis—microscopic parameters and its clinical interpretation (WHO 5)

(FSH: follicle-stimulating hormone; ICSI: intracytoplasmic sperm injection; IMSI: intracytoplasmic morphologically selected sperm injection; LH: luteinizing hormone; WHO: World Health Organization)

CHAPTER 46

Male Hypogonadism

Sunil Jindal, Anshu Jindal

A. The presence of symptoms or signs of testosterone deficiency with or without deficiency of spermatozoa production is defined as as hypogonadism. Normal level of testosterone in a male is required not only for maintaining sperm production, but also is required for routine sexual, cognitive, and body function and development. In men with oligospermia hypogonadism should be suspected. Hypogonadism may be due to primary disorder of the testes (primary hypogonadism) or be secondary to a defect in the hypothalamic-pituitary axis (secondary hypogonadism). The diagnosis and cause of condition is made after assessing serum follicle-stimulating hormone (FSH), and serum luteinizing hormone (LH) along with total (and, when possible, free) serum testosterone levels measured concurrently. To evaluate serum testosterone, blood should be ideally drawn in the morning (before 10:00 am). The total testosterone normally ranges between 300 ng/dL and 1,000 ng/dL (10.5–35 nmol/L).

B. In primary hypogonadism, the testes fail to respond to FSH and LH secreted by the pituitary. This results in reduced production of testosterone and failure of the negative feedback to pituitary inhibiting the production of FSH and LH, leading to elevated FSH and LH levels. Klinefelter syndrome is the most common genetic cause of primary hypogonadism.

C. In secondary hypogonadism either the hypothalamus fails to produce gonadotropin-releasing hormone (GnRH), or the pituitary gland fails to produce enough FSH and LH in response to the hypothalamic stimulation. In secondary hypogonadism, low testosterone levels are seen with either low or borderline levels of FSH and LH.

D. In certain systemic disorders and conditions like cryptorchidism, hypogonadism can affect sperm production more adversely than testosterone levels resulting in normal hormonal profile with abnormal semen parameters.

E. If hypogonadism-associated testosterone deficiency manifests for the first time in adulthood, the manifestations can be varied depending on the degree and duration of the deficiency. Diminished libido, erectile dysfunction; waning in cognitive skills, sleep disturbances; and mood fluctuations are common. Features like gynecomastia, osteopenia, sparse body hair, decreased lean body mass, increased visceral fat, testicular atrophy, etc. typically take months to years to develop. Testosterone deficiency may increase the risk of coronary artery disease and prostate cancer.

F. Childhood-onset testosterone deficiency has few consequences and usually is unrecognized until puberty is delayed. Untreated hypogonadism impairs development of secondary sexual characteristics.

G. To diagnose the origin of secondary hypogonadism, testing should include assessment of serum prolactin level (to screen for presence of pituitary adenoma) and transferrin saturation (to screen for hemochromatosis). Sella imaging with magnetic resonance imaging (MRI) or computed tomography (CT) can be done to rule out pituitary macroadenoma or other mass in men with any of the following: (1) Age less than 60 years with no other identified cause for hypogonadism; (2) Very low total testosterone levels (< 200 ng/dL); (3) Elevated prolactin levels; (4) Symptoms consistent with a pituitary tumor (e.g. headache, visual symptoms).

H. *Treatment:* Testosterone replacement therapy
In primary hypogonadism with complete testicular failure, testosterone replacement therapy (TRT) is mainly given for symptomatic improvement in cognitive, sexual and physical symptoms. However, TRT should be avoided, especially when fertility is a concern, in secondary hypogonadism as exogenous testosterone supplementation impairs endogenous spermatogenesis (unless there is irreversible primary testicular failure). TRT can be considered for men who: (1) Do not show any signs of puberty; (2) Are near age 15; (3) After exclusion of secondary hypogonadism.
They may be given long-acting testosterone enanthate 50 mg intramuscular (IM) once/month for 4–8 months. Testosterone cypionate is given at a dose that is increased gradually over 18–24 months from 50 mg to 100 mg to 200 mg IM every 1–2 week. Older adolescents on high doses of IM testosterone (100–200 mg every 2 week) are best transited to testosterone gel preparations at adult dosages.

I. *Treatment of secondary gonadism:* Therapy begins with replacement of LH and FSH. LH replacement is initiated using human chorionic gonadotropin (hCG) at doses of 1,500 IU subcutaneous (sc) 3 times/for a minimum of 12 weeks. FSH replacement, can be done using human menotropic gonadotropin or human recombinant FSH, at doses of

150 IU 3 times/week. Doses may be adjusted based on the results of periodic testing with semen analysis and levels of serum FSH, LH, and testosterone. Therapy can be continued for a minimum of 6 months to 12 months till sperm production is noticed. Most men who have secondary hypogonadism due to a hypothalamic defect (e.g. idiopathic hypogonadotropic hypogonadism, Kallmann syndrome) become fertile with treatment despite sperm counts that are low (e.g. < 5 million/mL).

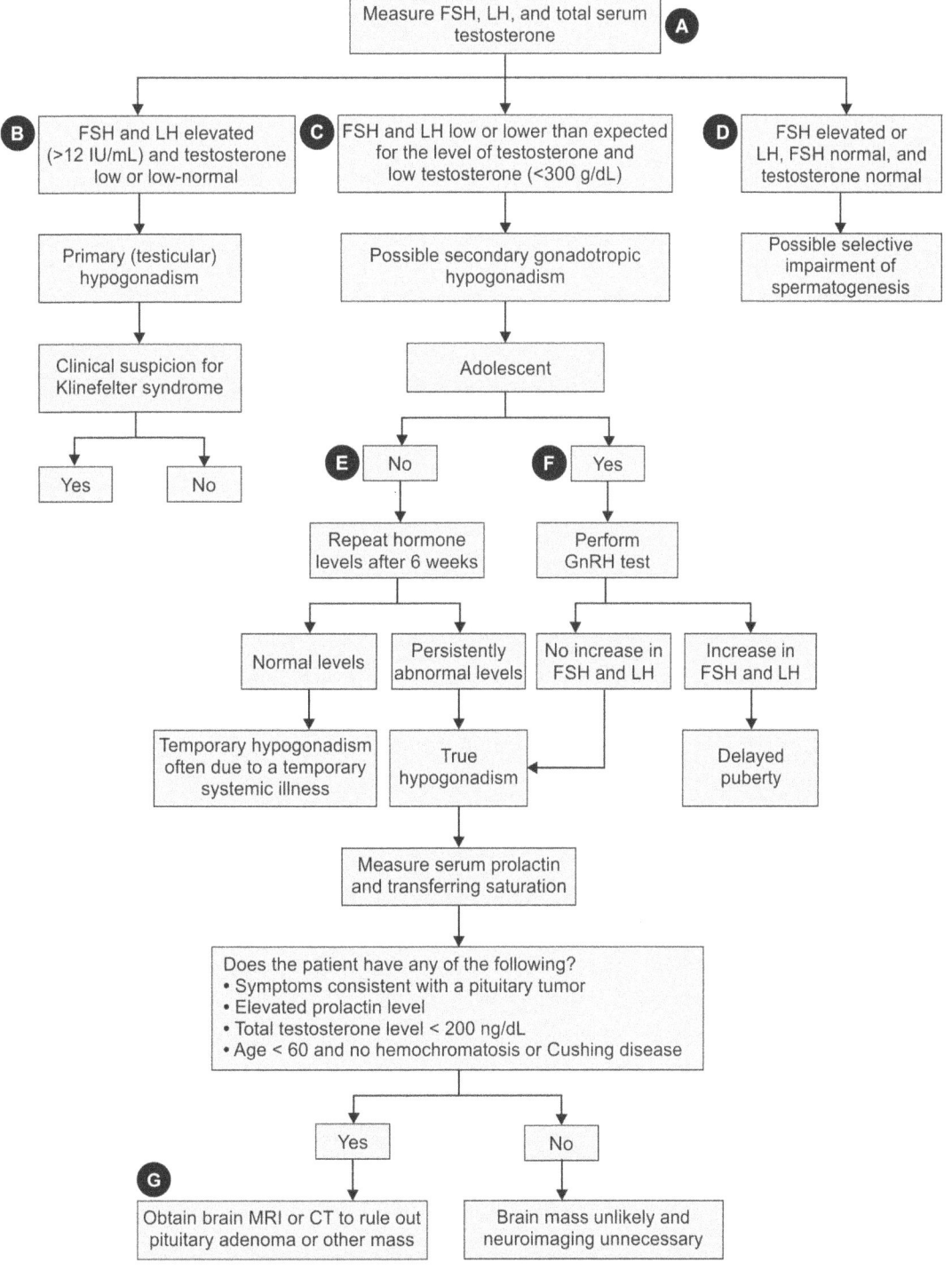

(FSH: follicle-stimulating hormone; LH: luteinizing hormone; GnRH: gonadotropin-releasing hormone)

CHAPTER 47

Azoospermia: Evaluation

KK Gopinathan, Parasuram Gopinath

A. Azoospermia is defined as complete absence of sperms in two semen samples even after centrifugation of semen samples. If sperms are seen after centrifugation, it is called cryptozoospermia and is different from azoospermia. Certain semen samples showing occasional sperms can also be considered azoospermic. Incidence of azoospermia in normal population is around 1 in 100. In infertile population, incidence is as high as 1 in 10.

B. Before making a diagnosis of azoospermia it is essential to exclude any ejaculatory dysfunction. Meticulous and accurate history taking is the best tool to diagnose ejaculatory dysfunctions like anejaculaton and retrograde ejaculation, the former characterized by anorgasmia.

C. Physical examination can give an insight into the cause of azoospermia.
Testes: Look for size and consistency. A soft and small testis point toward testicular failure.
In epididymis and vas deferens look for scarring or dilatation which suggest partial obstruction due to fibrosis and inflammation suggestive of post-testicular obstruction. Secondary sexual characters including body habitus, hair distribution, and gynecomastia.

D. ***Clinical varieties of azoospermia***:
   1. ***Hypogonadotropic hypogonadism (pretesticular)***: It mainly includes endocrinological abnormalities involving the hypothalamus and pituitary or it can be receptor mutations.
   2. ***Hypergonadotropic hypogonadism (testicular)***: It includes the defects that cause testicular failure leading to azoospermia.
   3. ***Normogonadotropic normogonadism (post-testicular or obstructive)***: 40% azoospermic men are normogonadotropic and obstruction of sperm delivery is the main cause.

E. Endocrine tests are the major tools for establishing the cause of azoospermia. Serum follicle-stimulating hormone (FSH) is perhaps the most important investigation to differentiate between various types of azoospermia. Elevated FSH more than 10 IU/L suggests testicular failure. It also has prognostic significance on sperm retrieval for assisted reproductive technique (ART) higher the FSH less chance of sperm retrieval. FSH is markedly low in pretesticular causes like Hypogonadal-Hypogonadism (secondary hypogonadism). FSH are conspicuously unaffected in post-testicular causes—Obstructive azoospermia.

F. Ultrasound, mostly transrectal ultrasound (TRUS) has a role to play when an obstructive pathology is suspected. TRUS should look for presence or absence of vas deferens and seminal vesicle or ejaculatory duct distension.

G. Genetic testing plays a role, especially in nonobstructive cases. Karyotyping to detect chromosomal abnormalities resulting in impaired testicular function (e.g. Klinefelter syndrome), Y chromosomal microdeletions leading to spermatogenic impairment. It helps as a tool to predict sperm retrieval in nonobstructive azoospermia patients. Cystic fibrosis transmembrane conductance regulator (CFTR) mutation testing in congenital bilateral absence of vas deferens, but incidence is low in Asian population.

H. Hypogonadotropic hypogonadism is probably the only group of azoospermic patients that responds well to medical management. The condition can be treated medically by gonadotropins [either human menopausal gonadotropin (hMG), FSH or human chorionic gonadotropin (hCG)] for prolonged duration (1.5-2 years). Prognosis is very good especially in acquired variety, where almost 100% response is achieved. But in congenital variety, response is usually variable. Approximately 30% may respond well and have high chances of natural conception, and around 30% respond with minimal spermatogenesis and may need ART. Another 30-40% may not respond to treatment at all.

I. The obstruction can be proximal to seminal vesicle (rete testis, epididymis, vas) or distal to seminal vesicle (vasal aplasia or ejaculatory duct obstruction). Both distal varieties present with azoospermia, acidic pH of semen, decreased semen volume (< 1 mL). Clinical examination usually differentiates between vasal aplasia (vas absent) and ejaculatory duct obstruction (vas present). Vasography usually has no place in obstructive azoospermia except in case of vasectomy reversal with epididymo vasal anastomosis. Treatment usually involves surgical sperm retrieval. Vasal recanalization

is done in case of postvasectomy. Ejaculatory duct obstruction may be treated with transurethral resection of prostate (TURP).
J. Most acceptable treatment of obstructive azoospermia is percutaneous epididymal sperm aspiration/testicular sperm aspiration (PESA/TESA) with intracytoplasmic sperm injection (ICSI), where there is an almost 100% sperm retrieval rate. The prognosis is usually good owing to retrieval of genetically normal sperms and also because usually the couple with obstructive pathology presents earlier to infertility clinics.
K. Usually no medical or surgical treatment is available or advisable for patients with testicular failure. Only chance to father the child is by attempting to retrieve sperms with the help of TESA/micro testicular sperm extraction (TESE). Despite the possibility of retrieving sperms is low. Micro-TESE has largely improved the sperm retrieval rate in this group of patients, wherein certain studies quote sperm retrieval rates up to 60%. Unfortunately we do not have any test to prognosticate the chance of sperm retrieval. The treatment option, where we do not retrieve sperms on any of these procedures or in couples who cannot afford to do an in vitro fertilization (IVF) treatment, is to go for the use of donor sperms.

Testes	Epididymis	Vas deferens	FSH	Testosterone	Diagnosis	Treatment
Very small to normal size	Normal	Normal	low (<2 mIU/mL)	Less than 4 mg/mL	Hypogonadotropic hypogonadism	Gonadotropin therapy
Normal	Normal or distended	Absent/thickened/beaded/discontinuous	FSH usually low normal around 5 mIU/mL	> 4 mg/mL	Obstructive	PESA TESA Epididymo vasal anastomosis
Soft atrophied to almost normal	Not delineated	Not delineated	high (> 7 mIU/mL)	Testosterone is usually low or normal	Nonobstructive	Micro-TESA

(FSH: follicle-stimulating hormone; PESA: percutaneous epididymal sperm aspiration; TESA: testicular sperm aspiration)

HISTOPATHOLOGICAL TYPES OF AZOOSPERMIA

It is seen in a testicular biopsy specimen.

Normal spermatogenesis
Hypospermatogenesis
Maturation arrest
Sertoli only cell syndrome
Testicular atrophy

However, testicular biopsy from particular site may not represent the total testicular function and is unreliable in predicting the prognosis.

CAUSES OF HYPOGONADOTROPIC HYPOGONADISM (PRETESTICULAR)

Congenital	Acquired
Kallmann syndrome	Trauma
Idiopathic isolated GnRH deficiency	Tumors
	Critical illnesses
Single gene mutations involving GnRH receptor, FSH/LH receptor	Infections, e.g. meningitis
	Infiltrative disorders like sarcoidosis

(GnRH: gonadotropin-releasing hormone)

CAUSES OF NONOBSTRUCTIVE AZOOSPERMIA (TESTICULAR)

- Klinefelter syndrome
- Y chromosome deletions
- Cryptorchidism
- Infections (viral orchitis, tuberculosis)
- Drugs (alkylating agents, antiandrogens)
- Radiation
- Gonadotoxins

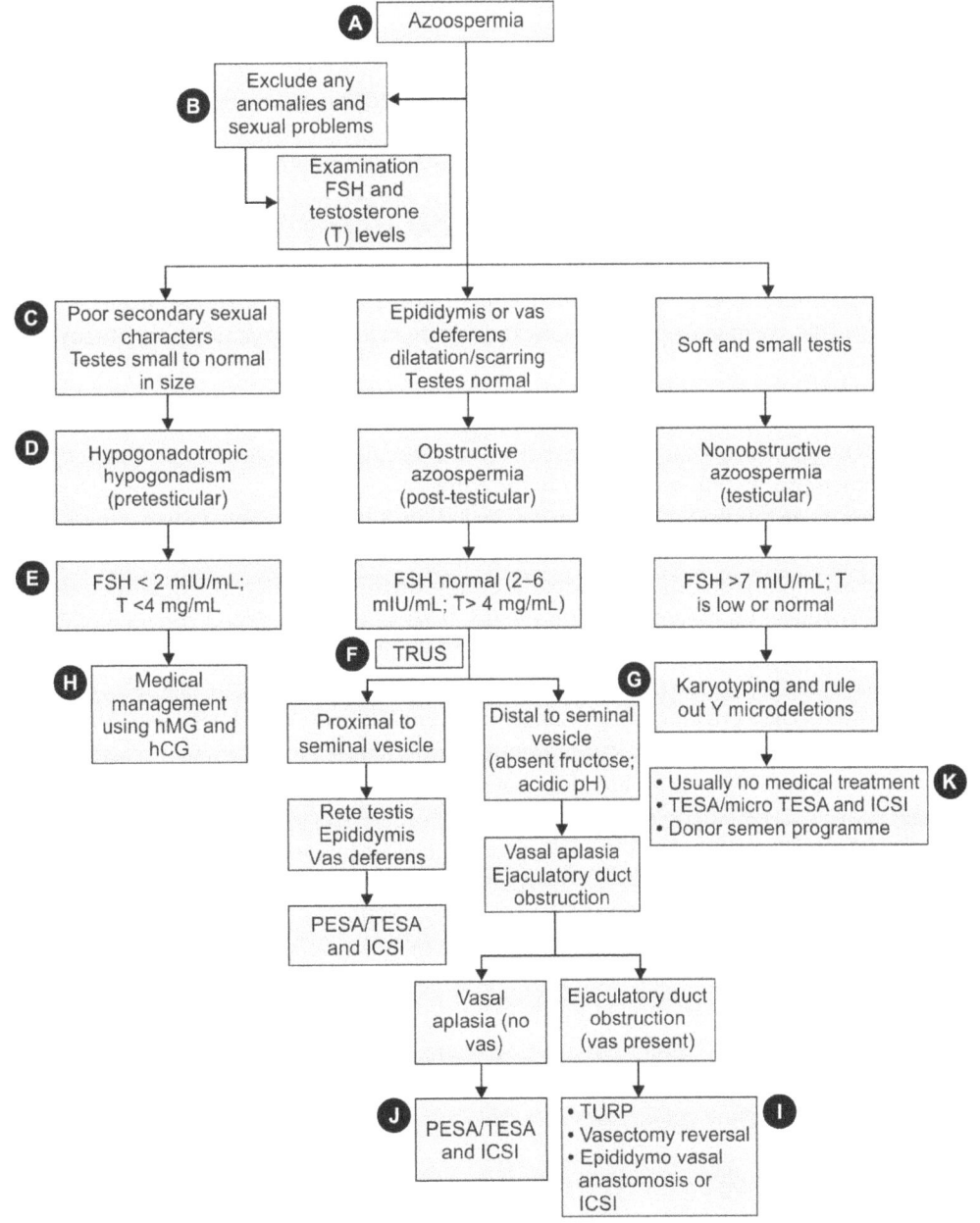

(FSH: follicle-stimulating hormone; ICSI: intracytoplasmic sperm injection; PESA: percutaneous epididymal sperm aspiration; TESA: testicular sperm aspiration; TRUS: transrectal ultrasound; TURP: transurethral resection of the prostate)

CHAPTER 48

Anejaculation

Neharika Malhotra Bora, Chand Mohammad

A. Anejaculation is a clinical entity which may result from both organic and psychological causes. Anejaculation is defined as complete absence of ejaculation during sexual activity, despite normal erections or nocturnal emissions.
B. Anejaculation should be differentiated from retrograde ejaculation by analyzing the post ejaculation urine. Anejaculation can be classified as:
   - Orgasmic (organic) anejaculation
   - Anorgasmic (psychogenic/idiopathic) anejaculation
   - Situational anejaculation.
C. We can encounter different types of situational anejaculation:
   - Clinic anejaculation (can collect semen at home, but has anejaculation in clinic)
   - Periovulatory anejaculation (unable to ejaculate at ovulation, but can ejaculate on other days)
   - Unexpected anejaculation (first time failure of ejaculation on day of ovulation)
   - Masturbatory anejaculation (ejaculates during intercourse, but not by masturbation)
   - Intercourse anejaculation (ejaculates by masturbation, but not during intercourse).
D. Situational anejaculation mostly means existence of ejaculation by masturbation, but not during sexual intercourse and it can be because of performance anxiety or hostility toward the partner or psychosexual development, and unconscious desire to avoid pregnancy but as of now there is no evidence to support these theories.

MANAGEMENT OF ANEJACULATION ON THE DAY OF OPU

Anxiety most likely plays a major role in these reported cases. Acute ejaculation failure can occur in patients who previously had no problems with semen production on demand in the clinic.

E. Sildenafil citrate (Viagra) has been recommended after failed trials of more than 1 hour to produce semen.
F. A prior proper history and counseling is important to diagnose such problems. Each clinic should discuss the possible difficulties associated with sperm procurement with the couple on initial medical consultations and also during the in vitro fertilization (IVF) counseling session with andrologist. If a problem is detected, the possibility of cryopreserving sperm for backup use should always be offered.
G. Anejaculation, or lack of ejaculation, can occur in men with pelvic nerve damage from diabetes mellitus, retroperitoneal surgery, multiple sclerosis, spinal cord injury, or psychosocial causes. The use of penile vibratory stimulation (PVS) or rectal probe electroejaculation (EEJ) can help to procure a semen sample containing sperm for use with assisted reproductive technique (ART). In particular, PVS, which often does not require general anesthesia, works best in men with complete spinal cord injuries above T10, with up to 86% of patients able to achieve ejaculation with PVS. On the other hand, only 0–15% of men with spinal cord injuries below T10 were able to achieve ejaculation with PVS. In men with anejaculation from other etiologies or after failure with PVS, EEJ is preferred and can produce ejaculation in 92% of men with anejaculation from spinal cord injury. Of note, since both PVS and EEJ can cause autonomic dysreflexia in men with spinal cord injuries at or above T6, blood pressure monitoring and premedication with nifedipine should be considered.
H. If noninvasive methods to obtain a sperm sample fail, invasive techniques should be used with caution and cryopreservation of oocytes can be also offered as last resort. If invasive method is required for sperm collection, testicular sperm aspiration should be preferred means of extraction. Performing a percutaneous epidymal sperm aspiration from a normal epididymis might not only be difficult but also has lower probability of obtaining sperms and higher chances of damaging the epididymes.

Trivia:
The first case report of rectal probe EEJ was in 1931 by Learmonth.
Conservative community males have higher risk of anejaculation.
In the flowchart we are discussing only anejaculation on the day of oocyte pickup (OPU).

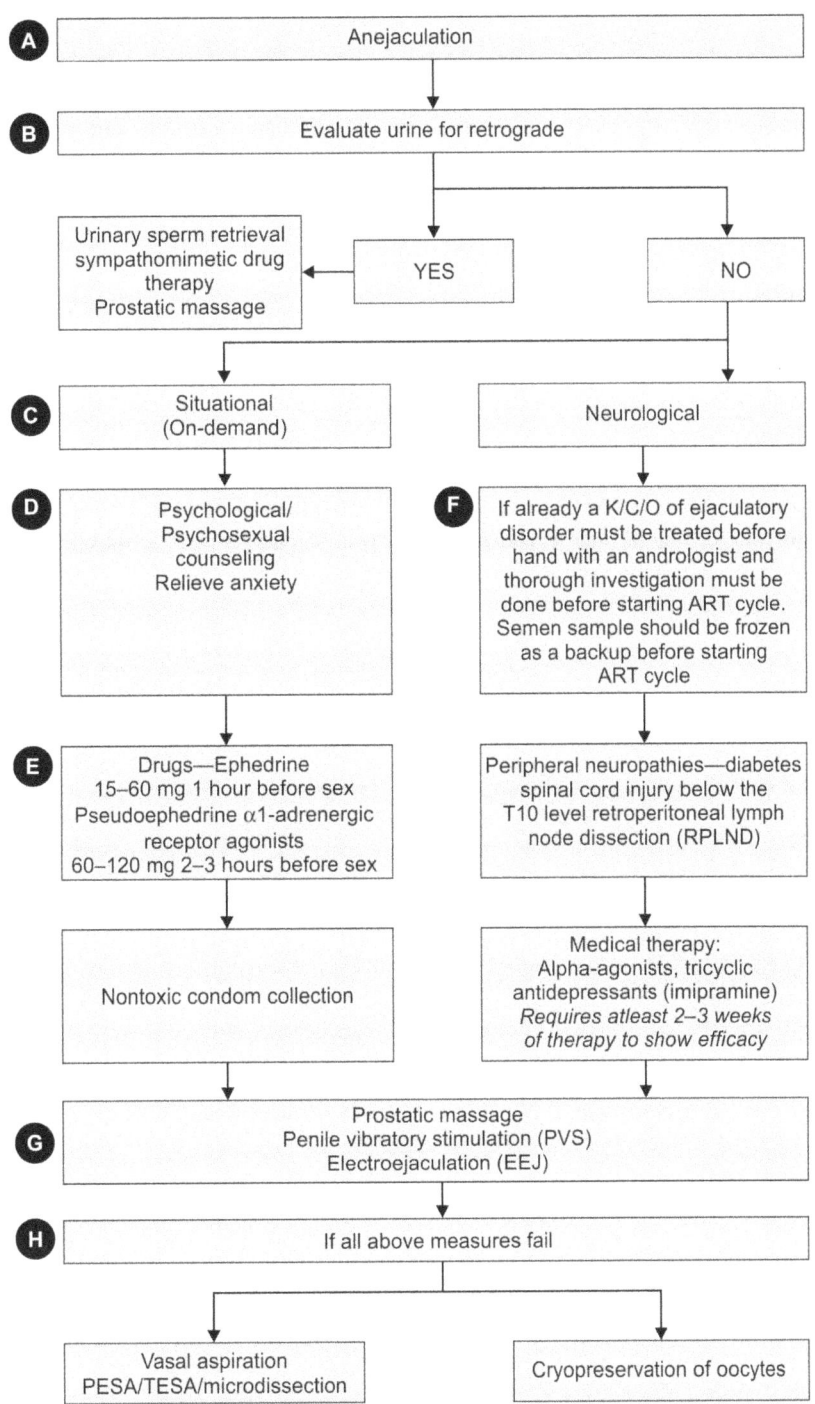

CHAPTER 49

Genetic Evaluation of the Infertile Male

Kamini Patel, Vani Patel

1. The male partner is evaluated for fertility potential using a physical examination combined with a meticulous semen analysis. Genetics plays a very important role in male fertility. Paternal genetics are responsible not only for good sperm production, but the vertically transmitted genes in the fetus are important for a successful and healthy growth of the fetus. Severe abnormality in the sperm parameters or poor reproductive history are triggers for evaluating the genetic profile of the male partner.
2. Multiple pregnancy loss after having normal semen analysis is the trigger for abnormal genetic conditions like Robertsonian translocation.
3. Karyotyping of the patients is important for the couple suffering from multiple pregnancy loss, low semen count, low semen volume, and low motility.
4. Medications like Co-Q helps in improving the quality of the semen or sperm, if the condition is triggered by environmental condition.
5. If the problem still persists after the medication, genetic analysis is important.
6. If any of the genetic analysis turns out to be positive, patient must be assisted for genetic counseling of the possibility of vertical transmission of a similar genetic variation to the off spring and/or the probability of successful reproductive outcome.

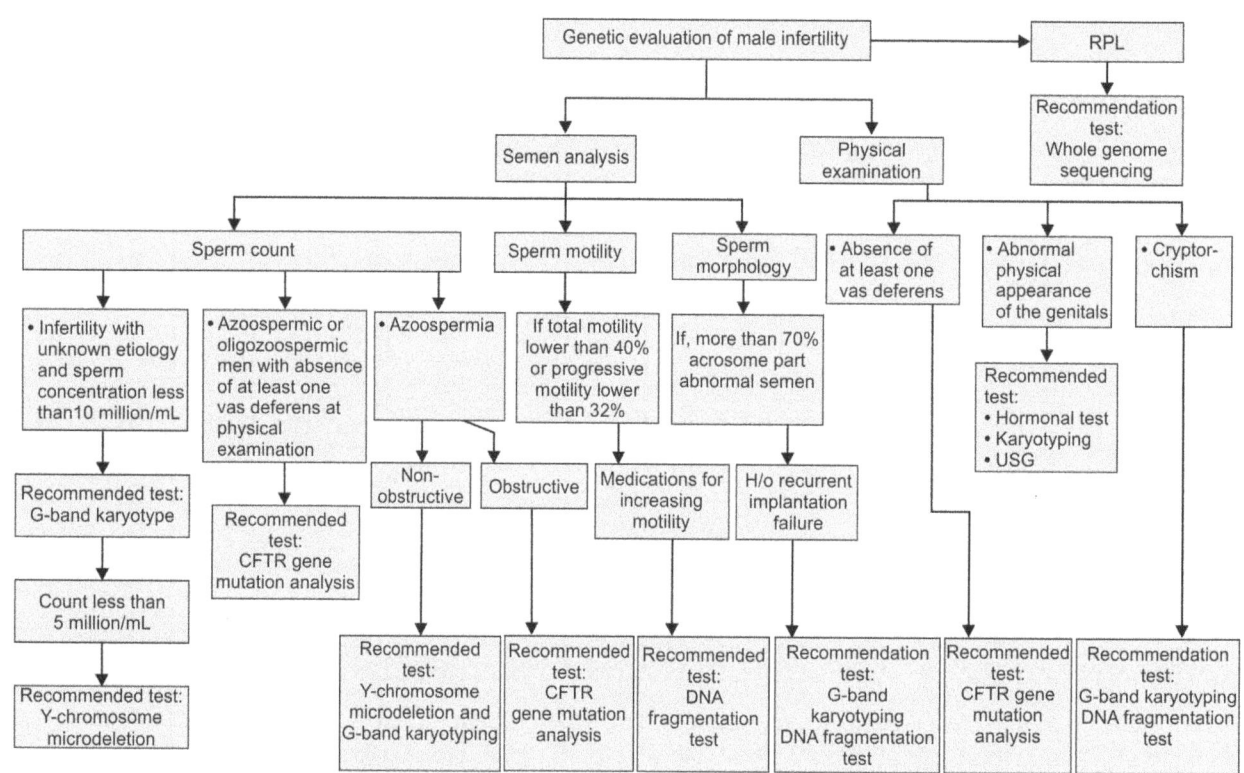

(USG: ultrasonography; H/o: history of; CFTR: cystic fibrosis transmembrane conductive regulator; RPL: recurrent pregnancy loss

CHAPTER 50

Sperm Deoxyribonucleic Acid Fragmentation

Saroj Agarwal, Rajeev Agarwal

The sperm is essential a carrier for the genetic inheritance of the male partner constituting for 50% of the genetic makeup of the embryo. The genetic integrity of the spermatozoon is crucial for the healthy development of the embryo. The deoxyribonucleic acid (DNA) constitutes a double-helical structure and any breakage in this continuity results in elevated levels of sperm DNA fragmentation (SDF). Above the critical threshold, a high SDF, will significantly compromise the possibility of a successful pregnancy.

A. High SDF does not appear to affect possibility of fertilization or even the first or second embryo cleavage stages.
High SDF can affect embryo cleavage once the paternal genome is switched on, and subsequent blastocyst development. Studies have shown that SDF levels during assisted reproductive technique (ART) procedures [intrauterine insemination (IUI), in vitro fertilization (IVF), and intracytoplasmic sperm injection (ICSI)] are directly proportional to the miscarriage and pregnancy rates. Although a normal semen analysis does not ensure a normal SDF level, men with poor semen parameters have higher probability of high DNA fragmentation. Significantly, higher rate of multinucleation is seen among the embryo cohorts of high SDF groups. SDF seems to affect embryo postimplantation development in ICSI procedures: high SDF can compromise "embryo viability", resulting in pregnancy loss postimplantation.

B. *Etiology of sperm DNA damage*: There are many different degrees of sperm's defective genomic material like protein defects in DNA compaction, DNA integrity defects, DNA breaks (both single- and/or double-stranded) or sperm chromosomal aneuploidies (Perreault et al. 2003). Human oocyte has the ability to repair the DNA damage of the sperm to an extent that depends on the quality of sperm and oocyte which is inversely proportional to the paternal and maternal age (Wells et al. 2005).
The etiology of sperm DNA damage is multifactorial.
- Abnormal chromatin packaging, abortive apoptosis
- Varicocele, genital tract infections (leukocytes), and immature sperms (cytoplasmic droplet)
- Laboratory factors, radio- and/or chemotherapy
- Lifestyle factors (obesity, age, cell phones, and nicotine), environmental toxicants
- *Majority of DNA damage is associated with reactive oxygen species (ROS)*: Small levels of ROS are essential for normal sperm functions (capacitation, acrosome reaction, and sperm-oocyte fusion). Balance between ROS production and scavenging system is important. In 25% of infertile men, high ROS levels have been detected in their semen.

C. *DNA fragmentation tests*:
- *Sperm chromatin structure assay (SCSA)*: It measures the intensity of acridine orange (AO) fluorescence using flow cytometry.
- *Terminal deoxynucleotidyl transferase-mediated deoxyuridine triphosphate nick end labeling (TUNEL) assay*: It detects both single- and double-stranded DNA breaks microscopically or using flow cytometry.
- *Single cell gel electrophoresis (COMET) assay*: It involves embedding spermatozoa in agarose on a glass slide, applying electrophoresis, and evaluating DNA migration in comet tails.
- *Sperm chromatin dispersion (SCD) test*: Sperm with fragmented DNA fail to produce a characteristic halo of dispersed DNA loops that is observed in sperm with nonfragmented DNA following acid denaturation and removal of nuclear proteins. Halo sperm kit.

D. The Georgetown Male Factor Infertility Study established the statistical ranges of excellent [≤15% DNA fragmentation index (DFI)], good (>15 to <30% DFI), and fair to poor (≥30% DFI) sperm DNA integrity. In 2000, they found that in vivo patients (n = 215) (with no previous knowledge of their fertility status) showed a declining pregnancy outcome when their DFI was more than 20% and negligible pregnancies when the DFI approached 40%.

NORMAL SPERM DEOXYRIBONUCLEIC ACID FRAGMENTATION VALUES

DNA fragmentation index less than 30%, treatment by IUI or IVF. IUI infertility patients with 30% DFI have as good a statistical probability of obtaining a pregnancy/delivery as in vivo presumably fertile couples with the same DFI.

ABNORMAL SPERM DEOXYRIBONUCLEIC ACID FRAGMENTATION VALUES

DNA fragmentation index more than 30%, patient is advised to go for an ICSI procedure. Reducing the oxidative stress by changing the lifestyle (stop smoking, reduce obesity, and exercise) and improved diet may help reduce the levels of SDF in some cases. Supplementing antioxidants for a duration of 2–3 months can help in improving the DFI only in case of single-strand breakage in the DNA. If breakage is at the level of both the strands in the double-helical structure, therapy with antioxidants is not beneficial. Management of the cause of high SDF like treatment of infections, varicocele repair, etc. has been shown to reduce DNA fragmentation. Most reports suggest that DNA damage occurs at the posttesticular level, so that testicular sperm is hypothesized to have a healthier DNA integrity than ejaculated sperm. Sperms with high SDF should be processed using magnetic-activated cell sorting (MACS) procedure or microfluidics.

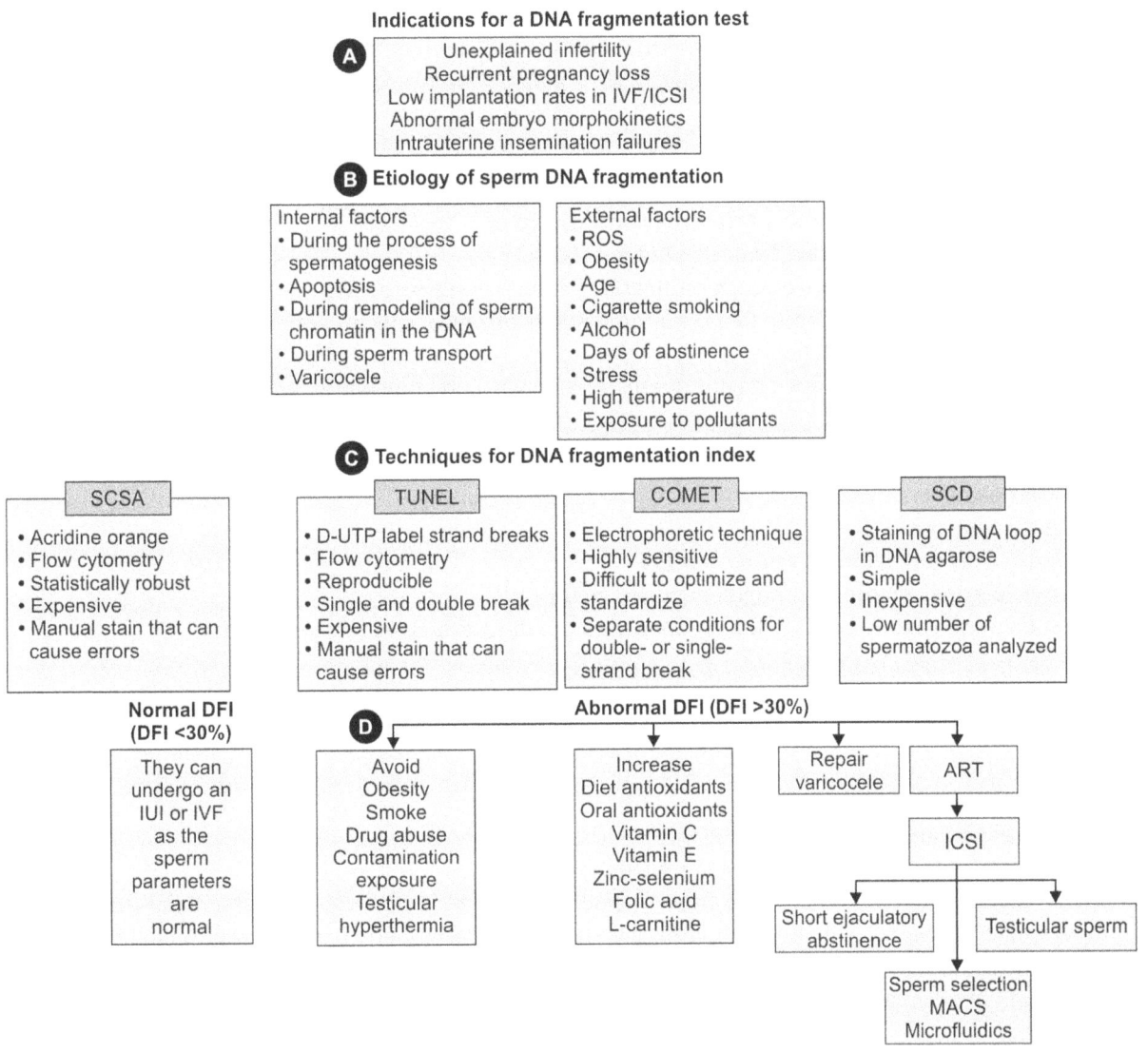

(ART: assisted reproductive technique; DFI: DNA fragmentation index; DNA: deoxyribonucleic acid; ICSI: intracytoplasmic sperm injection; IUI: intrauterine insemination; IVF: in vitro fertilization; MACS: magnetic-activated cell sorting; ROS: reactive oxygen species; SCD: sperm chromatin dispersion; SCSA: sperm chromatin structure assay; TUNEL: terminal deoxynucleotidyl transferase-mediated deoxyuridine triphosphate nick end labeling; D-UTP: deoxyuridine triphosphate)

CHAPTER 51

Varicocele and Male Infertility

Suchetna Sengupta, Rajeev Agarwal

Varicocele: Varicocele is a vascular abnormality of the testicular venous drainage system. It is an abnormal dilation of internal spermatic veins and pampiniform plexus that drain blood from testis.

Incidence: 15% of adolescent boys and adult men; 90% on left side; 50% bilaterally and 2–5% on right side alone; 40% of men evaluated in a male fertility clinic will have a varicocele.

Risk factors: Taller men with lower body mass index (BMI) with history of affected first-degree relatives (especially brothers).

Diagnosis: The diagnosis of fertility impacting Varicocele is almost always made on physical examination. It should be noted that scrotal ultrasonography (USG) is not an alternative for physical examination. Incidental finding of varicose veins on USG has no impact on fertility.

Investigations: (1) Physical examination—(bag of worms), use Valsalva maneuver to elicit; (2) Semen analysis—two or three samples—reduced total count, impaired sperm motility (> 50% motility); (3) Scrotal USG with color flow Doppler imaging; (4) Serum follicle-stimulating hormone (FSH) (+/- gonadotropin-releasing hormone (GnRH) stimulation); (5) Serum testosterone.

Clinical grades of varicocele:
Subclinical—clinical examination—no varicocele, but present on USG Doppler
Grade 1—Not visible or palpable at rest. Elicited only on Valsalva
Grade 2—palpable intrascrotal venous distension but not visible
Grade 3—bulging venous plexus seen through scrotal skin which is easily palpable.
G. *Pathogenesis:* Presence of varicocele increases the reactive oxidative species and oxidative stress thus impairing testicular and spermatozoal function.
H. *Management:* Surgery includes open repair, laparoscopic repair, percutaneous embolization.

Indications for treatment of a varicocele: Treatment to be offered to male partner of subfertile couple when all these factors are present:
1. Varicocele is palpable
2. Couple has documented infertility
3. Female partner has correctable or normal fertility
4. Male partner has one or more abnormal semen parameters
5. Treating subclinical varicocele based merely on ultrasound diagnosis is NOT recommended.

Preoperative predictors of seminal improvement after varicocelectomy:
1. High grade varicocele (grade 3)
2. Lack of testicular atrophy
3. Normal FSH
4. Total motility more than 60%
5. Total motile sperm count more than 5×10^6
6. Positive gonadotropin-releasing hormone-stimulation test.

Varicocele repair may be considered as the primary option in a man with varicocele and suboptimal semen parameters and a normal female partner in a subfertile couple because improvement in sperm parameters occur following treatment, fertility increases, and also because risks of varicocele treatment are small.

After treatment of a varicocele, semen analysis should be done at approximately 3-month interval for a year or until pregnancy occurs.

Surgical varicocelectomy improves sperm parameters as well as pregnancy rates in patients with palpable varicocele and abnormal semen parameters. Sperm can return to ejaculate in 39% of azoospermic men with a varicocele after surgical repair.

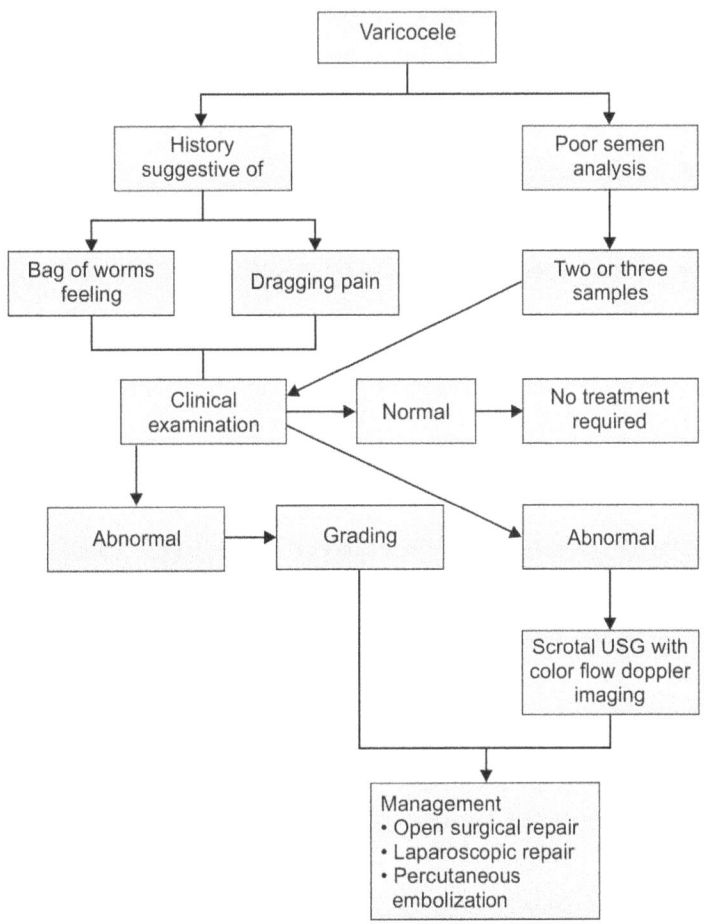

(USG: ultrasonography)

SECTION 14

Intrauterine Insemination

- Ovulation Induction in IUI—Oral Ovulogens
- Ovulation Induction in IUI—Gonadotropins
- Follicular Monitoring in IUI
- Doppler in Follicular Monitoring
- Doppler in Endometrium Evaluation
- Ovulation Trigger in IUI
- 10 Steps to Successful IUI
- Artificial Insemination: Donor
- Luteal Phase Support in IUI

CHAPTER 52

Ovulation Induction in IUI—Oral Ovulogens

Bebu Seema Pandey, Apoorva Pallam Reddy

Optimal ovarian stimulation protocol in intrauterine insemination (IUI) should maximize the probability of conception (ideally expressed as singleton live birth at term) and in the meantime minimize the risk of multiple pregnancies and the occurrence of ovarian hyperstimulation syndrome (OHSS).

A. The most commonly used oral ovulogens include clomiphene citrate (CC) and letrozole.
B. The choice of oral ovulogens used for ovarian stimulation depends on the condition of the female partner. In women with polycystic ovary syndrome (PCOS) and endometriosis letrozole is considered as the drug of choice. Letrozole reduces the local estrogen effect and improves the symptoms in endometriosis and adenomyosis.
C. In women undergoing IUI because of male subfertility or unexplained infertility, either clomiphene citrate or letrozole can be used as the first line of drugs for ovulation induction.
D. Oral ovulogens (OO) should always be the first line of drugs for ovulation induction in IUI. For women not responding to oral ovulogens or women who have failed more than one cycle of IUI stimulated with oral ovulogens or when multi folliculogenesis is desired gonadotropins (GT) can be supplemented with OO or used exclusively for ovulation induction. IUI cycles stimulated with Gonadotropins have higher probability of pregnancy as compared with OO alone. However, all cycles stimulated with GT require more frequent monitoring, are expensive and carry risks of hyperstimulation and multiple pregnancy. Hence, the decision to stimulate with GT should be taken with caution.
E. The starting dose of the drug should be decided based on the age, body mass index (BMI) and more importantly keeping in mind the previous response of the patient. Older and obese women require a higher dose of the drug compared to younger and leaner women. The previous response of a women to medication is extremely important in determining the future therapy. If a patient fails to respond to a particular dose and drug in the previous cycle, then the dose of the drug is increased to the maximum threshold or the drug should be changed in the subsequent cycle unless there has been significant reduction in the BMI. This change of dose/drug reduces the number of anovulatory cycles associated disappointment.
F. All IUI cycles should be followed-up for follicular monitoring. If ovulation is achieved, ovulation trigger is given and IUI is performed as per schedule. If ovulation is not achieved then the dose of the drug is increased in the subsequent cycle. The main advantage of a GT stimulated cycle is that the dose can be increased till ovulation is achieved thus ensuring 100% ovulation. There have been reports of achieving successful pregnancies after a slow GT stimulation even up to 20 days.
G. Although increasing dose of CC can achieve ovulation, this is not favored because of the low pregnancy rates with high doses of CC. Higher doses of CC have higher negative impact on the endometrium, cervical mucous, hypersecretion of luteinizing hormone (LH) and effect on granulosa cells. In view of the same use of CC shouldn't be prolonged beyond 5 days as it can affect the implantation.
H. On the contrary, letrozole can be used for up to 10 days as it does not have any negative effect on the endometrium.
I. Stimulated IUI cycles have a higher probability of pregnancy than natural IUI cycles. Hence a judicious ovarian stimulation is the first step towards achieving an optimum pregnancy in IUI.

Ovulation Induction in IUI—Oral Ovulogens

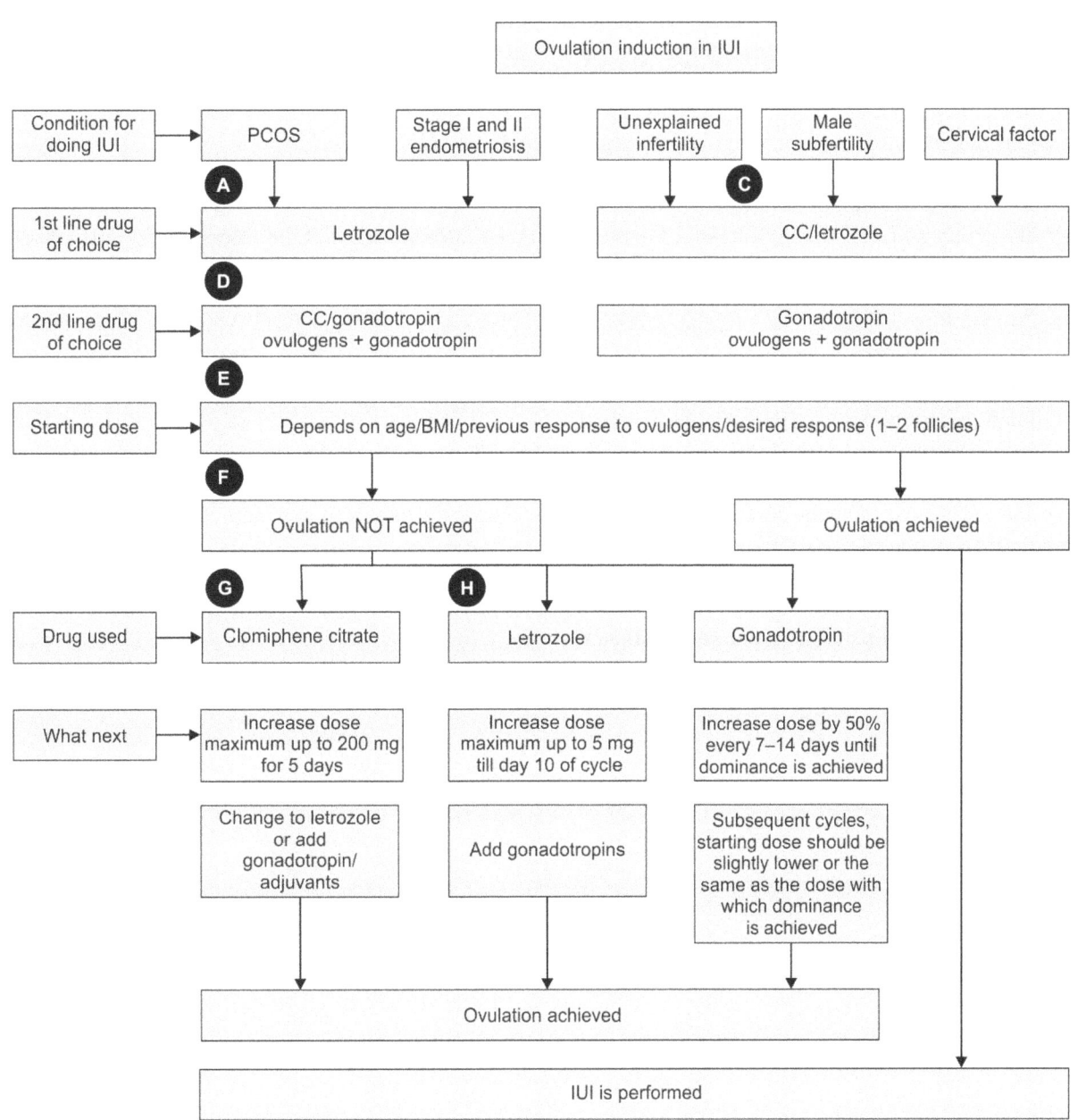

CHAPTER 53

Ovulation Induction in IUI—Gonadotropins

Sheetal Sawankar, Pinky R Shah

A. Ovulation induction with gonadotropins (GT) and subsequent intrauterine insemination (IUI) has higher chances of pregnancy as compared to ovulation induction with oral ovulogens. However, it also carries the risks of multiple pregnancy, increased risk of ovarian hyperstimulation syndrome (OHSS), increased number of visits to the clinic for a stricter follicular monitoring and higher cost. If more than four follicles start to achieve dominance then it is advised either to convert it to an assisted reproductive technique (ART) cycle or cancel the cycle.

B. The patient is called for a baseline scan on day of a spontaneous or induced menstrual cycle. Downregulation is confirmed by the absence of any ovarian simple cysts or unresolved corpus luteal cysts and a thin endometrium. In case of doubt, a serum estradiol level may be suggested to confirm the same. If the values are less than 50 pg/mL, stimulation can be started even in the presence of a simple cyst.

C. The various protocols used are:
   I. *Step-up protocol*: Conventional/low dose/chronic low dose. Started with low doses of GT and increased based on the growth of the follicle.
   II. *Step-down protocol*: Exclusive GT stimulation. Started with higher doses of GT and reduced once the follicle-stimulating hormone (FSH) threshold is reached.
   III. *Sequential regimen*: 5 days of oral ovulogens followed by GT.

D. On the follow-up scan, if there are one or more follicles showing trends of dominance (≥ 14 mm), continue the same dose and call for scan after one day (D9). A healthy follicle grows at the rate of 2 mm per day. Continue GT till complete dominance is achieved (> 18 mm).

E. If there is no follicle showing trends of dominance (≥ 14 mm), dose of GT is increased by 37.5–75 IU every 7–14 days with continued follicular monitoring every 2–3 days. Increase in dose is stopped either if dominance is reached or if there are more than four growing dominant follicles.

F. Ovulation trigger is given as soon as dominance is confirmed in one or more follicles. IUI is scheduled 36 hours from the ovulation trigger.

Ovulation Induction in IUI—Gonadotropins

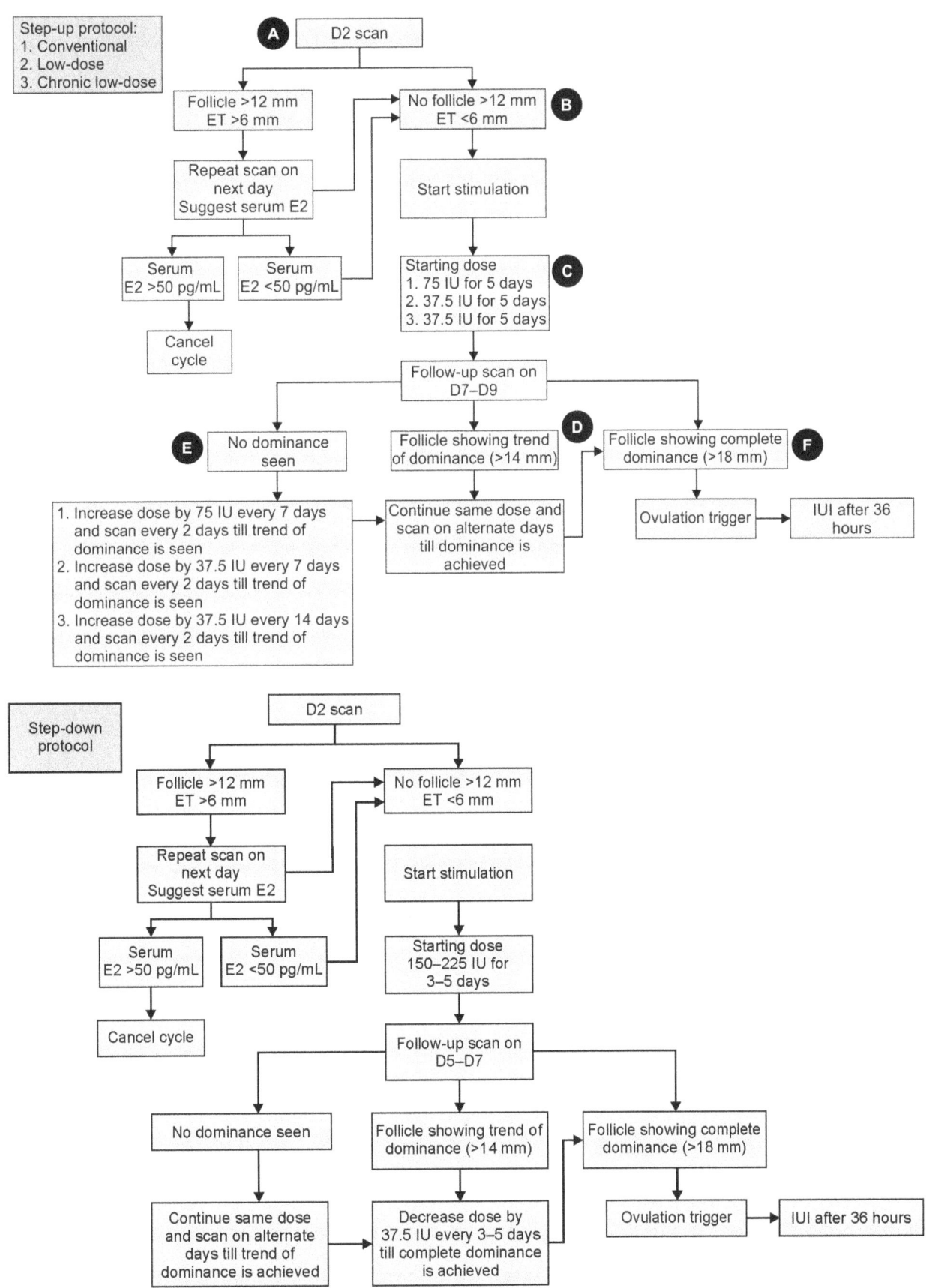

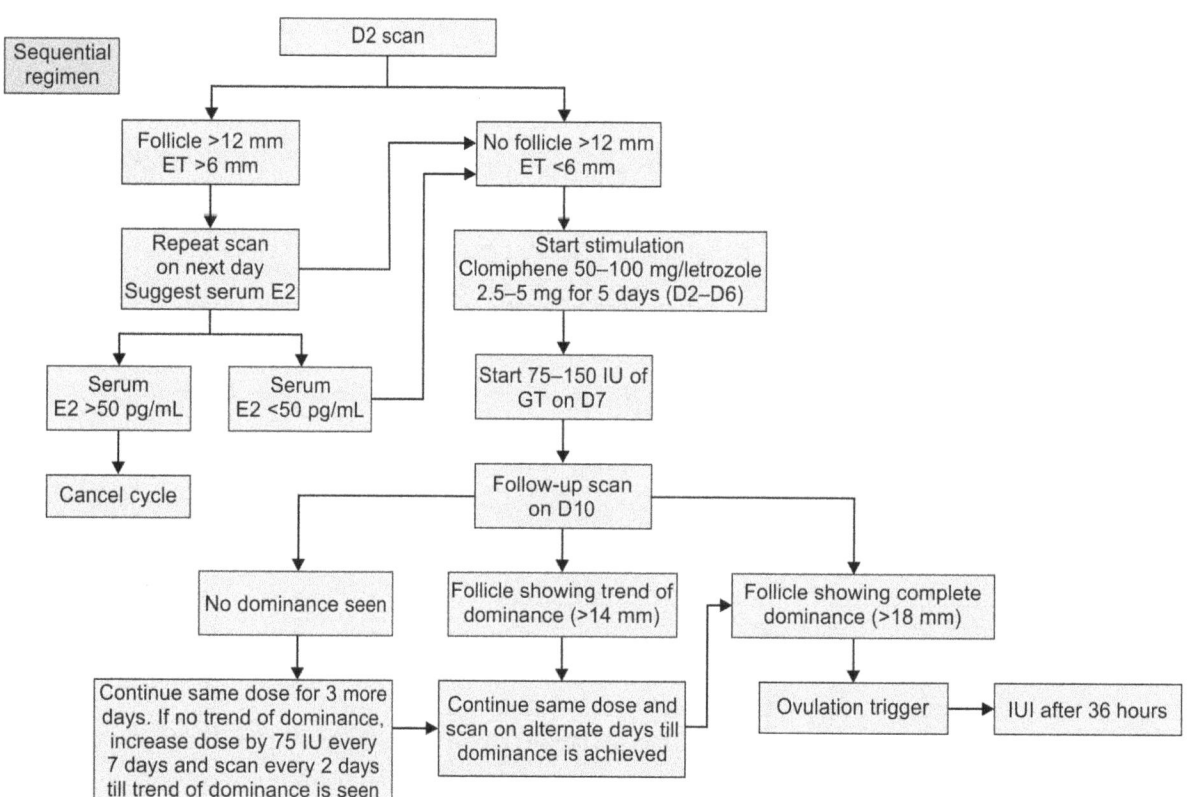

(E2: estradiol; ET: endometrial thickness; IUI: intrauterine insemination; GT: gonadotropins)

CHAPTER 54
Follicular Monitoring in IUI

Shilpa A Reddy

A. Follicular monitoring basically employs a simple technique for assessing ovarian follicles and uterine endometrium at regular intervals and documenting the pathway to ovulation. Follicular study is a vital component of fertility treatments. Route of scan is mainly transvaginal. Adding color or power Doppler and three-dimensional (3D) to follicular assessment improves the result.

B. **Baseline scan of uterus and uterine artery Doppler:** Endometrium should be thin, normal in shape with intact endomyometrial junction. Assess uterocervical length. Subendometrial flow if present on baseline scan indicates either high basal estrogen or inflammation of the endometrium leading to increased vascularity.

C. *Ovarian baseline scan (Day 2-5):* Check for antral follicle count and ovarian volume and ovarian stromal vasculariy. Antral follicles are small follicles measuring 2-10 mm in diameter. Antral follicles help in quantitative assessment of ovarian response. Functional and persistent cysts should not be present at baseline scan.

D. Once the baseline scan is normal, ovulation induction can be started using the various options available.

E. The day of call back for subsequent scan depends on the type of ovulogen used. Gonadotropin stimulation require a closer and more frequent monitoring as compared to oral ovulogens. A follicle which is more than 12-14 mm is called dominant follicle. It grows at a rate of 2 mm/day. Increase in granulosa cell thickness is directly related to the health and growth of the follicle. Endometrium increases in thickness by 1-2 mm daily in proliferative phase. It is noteworthy that the endometrium starts demonstrating triple line pattern 6 days prior to ovulation.

F. **Features of a mature follicle in pre-human chorionic gonadotropin (pre-hCG) scan:** Diameter of atleast least 18-22 mm, volume 3-7 cc (measured by 3D), sonolucent halo, seen 24 hours prior to ovulation, cumulus like shadow is seen 36 hours prior to ovulation, presence of cumulus increases the surety of presence of mature ovum in the follicle. Separation and folding of follicle lining 6-10 hours prior to ovulation, perifollicular color or power Doppler—vascularity surrounding at least 3/4th of the follicle more than 10 cm/s, and resistivity index (RI) 0.4-0.48. Perifollicular peak systolic velocity (PSV) and RI are more important in decision making than the size of follicle alone. Follicular PSV goes as high as 45 cm/s an hour prior to ovulation.

G. **Features of mature endometrium in pre-hCG scan:** Endometrial thickness of 7-12 mm is ideal for implantation. Endometrium decreases by 0.5 mm on the day of luteinizing hormone (LH) surge. Endometrial peristalsis can be detected in cervicofundal direction in preovulatory period. Endometrial grading can be done based on morphology and vascularity; Grade A—multilayered with low level echogenicities in intervening area; Grade B—multilayered with hypoechoic intervening area; Grade C—isoechoic and homogeneous. Applebaum classification according to zones of vascularity; Zone 1—vascularity seen only at endomyometrial junction; Zone 2—vessels penetrate through the hyperechogenic endometrial edge; Zone 3—vessels reach intervening hypoechogenic zone; Zone 4—when they reach the endometrial cavity. Endometrial volume (measured by 3D)—4.28 +/- 1.9 mL is most favorable for implantation. Subendometrial flow more than 5 cm/s at the time of hCG is favorable for implantation.

H. **Pre-hCG uterine artery Doppler and spiral artery power Doppler:** As hCG leads to increased resistance uterine artery Doppler should be evaluated prior to administering hCG. Normal uterine artery—pulsatility index (PI): 2.22-3.16, RI: 0.6-0.8. Spiral artery RI: 0.49-0.59, PI: 1.1-2.3.

I. Once functional maturity of the follicle is established through Doppler and 2D findings, ovulation trigger is given.

J. **Secretory phase:** Check for presence of corpus luteum and hyperechogenic secretory pattern of endometrium. There is further increase by 2 mm in endometrial thickness during luteal phase. Uterine and ovarian artery perfusion demonstrate a significant correlation with histological and hormonal markers of uterine receptivity and may aid in assessment of luteal phase. Corpus luteum is characterized by typical Fire of Ring appearance and low velocity flows. Corpus luteal—PSV: 10-15 cm/s, RI: 0.35-0.50, PI: 0.7-0.8. Uterine artery—PI: 2-2.5, PSV: 15-20 cm/s. Spiral artery PI is much lower than uterine artery PI (0.8-1 vs 2.4-3.4, spiral artery RI: 0.48-0.52).

Follicular Monitoring in IUI

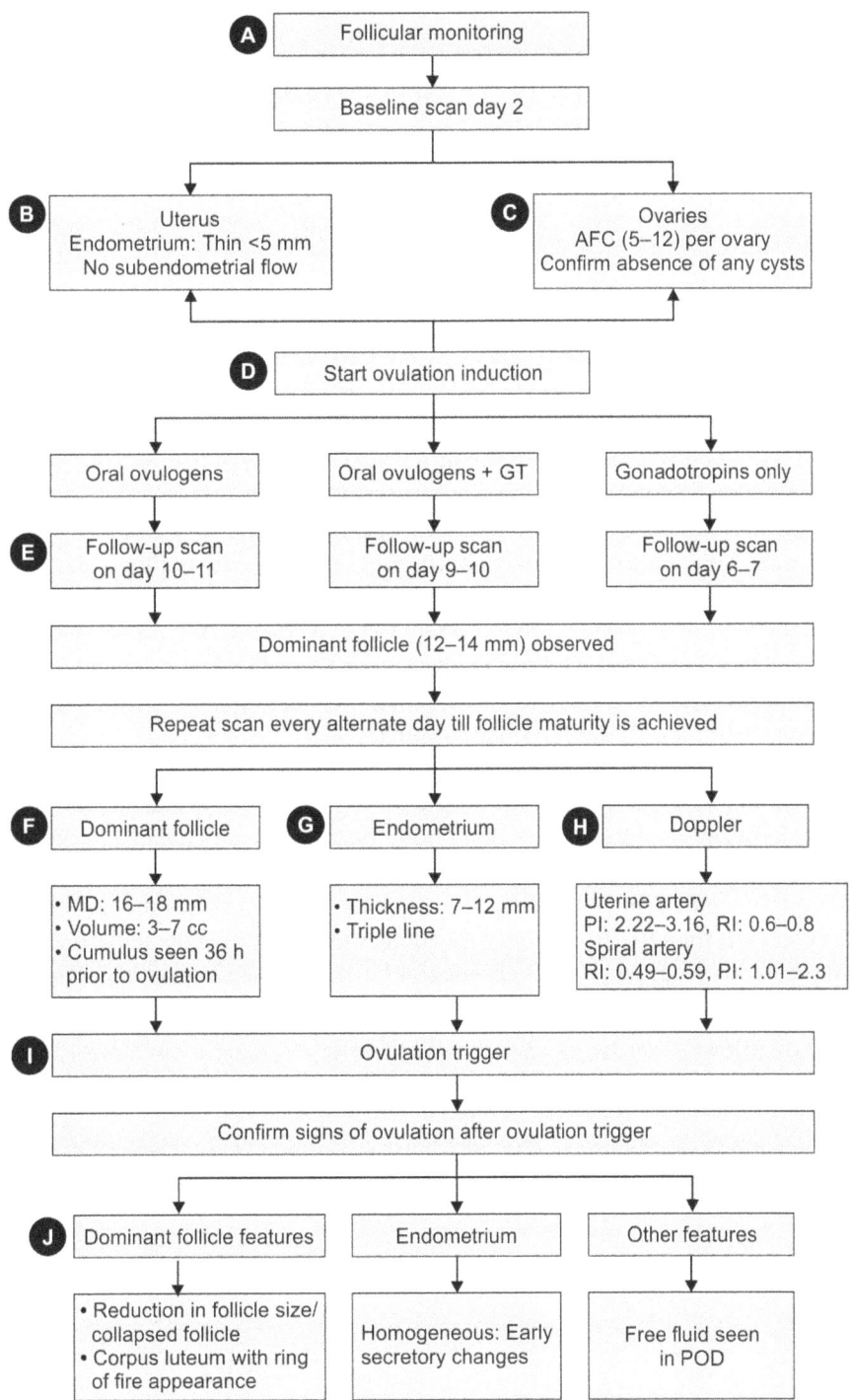

(AFC: antral follicle count; GT: gonadotropins; PI: pulsatility index; POD: pouch of Douglas; RI: resistive index; MD: mean diameter)

CHAPTER 55
Doppler in Follicular Monitoring

Rishab Bora, Jaideep Malhotra

ROLE OF COLOR DOPPLER IN FOLLICULAR MONITORING

The advent of transvaginal color Doppler sonology has added a new dimension to the diagnosis and treatment of infertile female. Color Doppler innovation is a unique noninvasive technology to investigate the circulation to organs like uterus and ovaries. Dynamic vascular changes occurring through the menstrual cycle in a reproductively active female can be picked up very well by transvaginal color Doppler and definite conclusions can be drawn regarding the diagnosis, prognosis, and treatment of infertile patients.

A. Although the structural maturity of the follicle is determined by the size of the dominant follicle (18-22 mm), the functional maturity of the oocyte is proposed to be assessed better using Doppler.
   Resistance index (RI) and *peak systolic velocity (PSV) of the perifollicular vascularity* give a measurement of the functional maturity of the oocyte in the follicle.
   PI (pulsatility index) is not shown to represent the functional capacity of the oocyte.

B. *Baseline Doppler:* Ovarian stromal PSV—5–10 cm/sec, stromal RI—0.6–0.7. Elevated RI or lower PSV indicates that high doses of gonadotropins will be required for achieving optimal ovarian response.

C. *Preovulatory follicle:* At the beginning of luteinizing hormone (LH) surge, the perifollicular PSV is ideally more than 10 cm/sec. The follicular PSV goes as high as 45 cm/sec 1 hour before ovulation under the effect of rising LH. Follicle is said to be functionally mature only when the PSV more than 10 cm/sec. The pulse repetition frequency settings for color Doppler are set at 0.3 and wall filter at the lowest. The perifollicular vessels are only those that obliterate the follicular wall with color. A rising PSV and low RI are suggestive of impending ovulation. This is the best time for administration of surrogate human chorionic gonadotropin (HCG).

D. *Ovulatory follicle:* Fall in perifollicular RI starts 2 days before ovulation, reaches nadir at ovulation, remains low for 4 days, and then with gradual rise reaches 0.5 in midluteal phase. It has been quoted in a study by Nargund et al. that embryos produced by fertilization of the ova obtained from the follicles, which had a perifollicular PSV of less than 10 cm/sec, are less likely to be grade 1 embryos and also have higher chance of chromosomal malformations. In the same study, it has been shown that the probability of developing a grade 1 or 2 embryo is 75%, if PSV was more than 10 cm/sec, 40% if PSV was less than 10 cm/sec, and 24% if there was no perifollicular flow. It is suggested that ovulation trigger may be differed till the Doppler parameters suggest functional maturity of the follicle as well to improve the reproductive outcomes.

E. *Luteal phase changes in ovarian vascularity:* The functional capacity of the corpus luteum is assessed by the low impedance flow and the abundance of vessels around it, mature corpus luteum is a highly vascularized structure with a low RI of 0.44 +/− 0.04. In patients with corpus luteum deficiency, the vascularity is not optimal and the RI is raised to around 0.59, with decreased diastolic flow. If pregnancy occurs then low RI of 0.50 continues.

Doppler in Follicular Monitoring

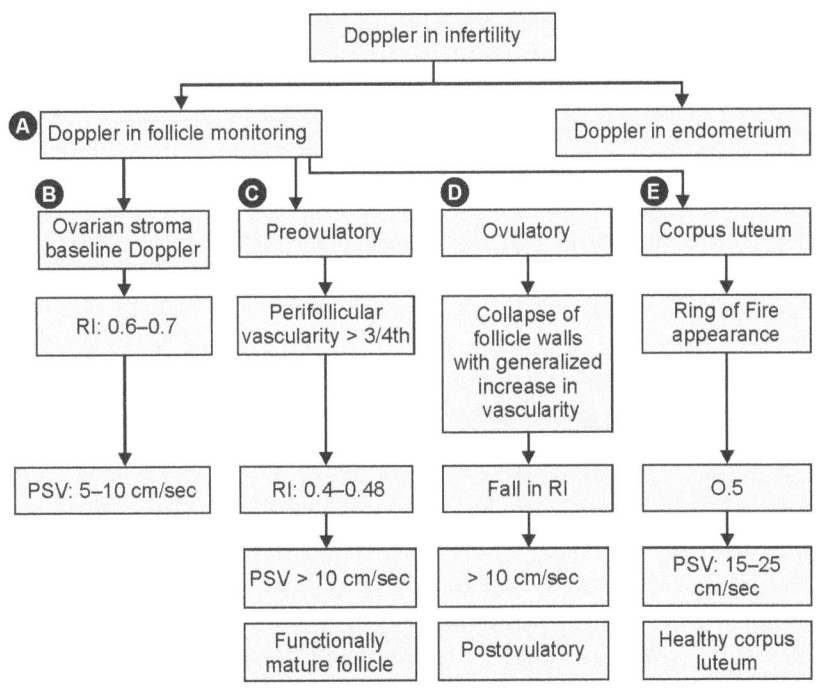

(PSV: peak systolic velocity; RI: resistance index)

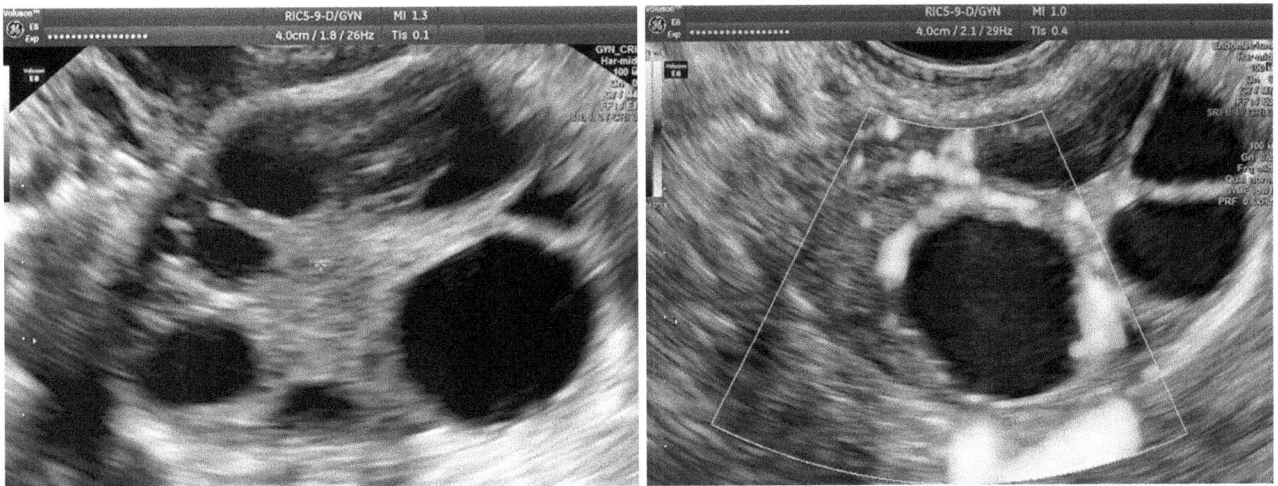

Follicular Doppler

# CHAPTER 56

Doppler in Endometrium Evaluation

Rishab Bora, Jaideep Malhotra

A. Implantation is a crucial step in the process of reproduction. Receptive endometrium increases the probability of pregnancy. Performing an assisted reproductive technique (ART) only when the endometrium is deemed receptive on Doppler increases the possibility of pregnancy and reduces the cycle costs with slightly higher incidence of cycle cancellation.

The Uterine Biophysical Profile—Modified Version of Applebaum Uterine Scoring System

The uterine biophysical profile are a group of sonographic features of the endometrium that have functional predictability. Thus this score can be used as a surrogate to decide for an embryo transfer in ART cycles as well as evaluate the functionality of endometrium.

These include:
1. Endometrial thickness in greatest anteroposterior (AP) dimension of 7 mm or greater (full-thickness measurement)
2. A layered ("5 line") appearance to the endometrium
3. Myometrial contractions causing a wave-like motion of the endometrium
4. Homogeneous myometrial echogenicity
5. Uterine artery blood flow, as measured by pulsatility index (PI), less than 3.0
6. End-diastolic uterine artery flow
7. Blood flow within zone 3 using color Doppler technique
8. Myometrial blood flow seen on gray-scale examination (internal to the arcuate vessels).

All the parameters are given a score based on the value observed. The meta score of all these parameters is used to predict the probability of implantation of the embryo.

Score	Probability of pregnancy
20	100%
17–19	80%
14–16	60%
13 or less	No pregancy

B. Average PI of the uterine artery is higher in nonconception than in conception cycles; most studies reported no conception when PI was more than 2.8–3.
C. Diastolic blood flow may be categorized as full or continuous and discontinuous, i.e. reduced or absent flow velocity. Good uterine perfusion, as shown by full diastolic blood flow with low resistance during the early and midsecretory phases, correlates with conception following assisted reproduction treatment.
D. It has been postulated that a better endometrial and subendometrial vascularity can lead to a better placental development during pregnancy which is associated with a lower risk of miscarriage and a higher chance of live birth.
E. Absent endometrial flow, despite highest values for the other parameters, has always been associated with no conception.

Blood Supply

Zone 1: 2 mm thick area surrounding the hyperechoic outer layer of the endometrium

Zone 2: The hyperechoic outer layer of the endometrium

Zone 3: The hypoechoic inner layer of the endometrium

Zone 4: The endometrial cavity.

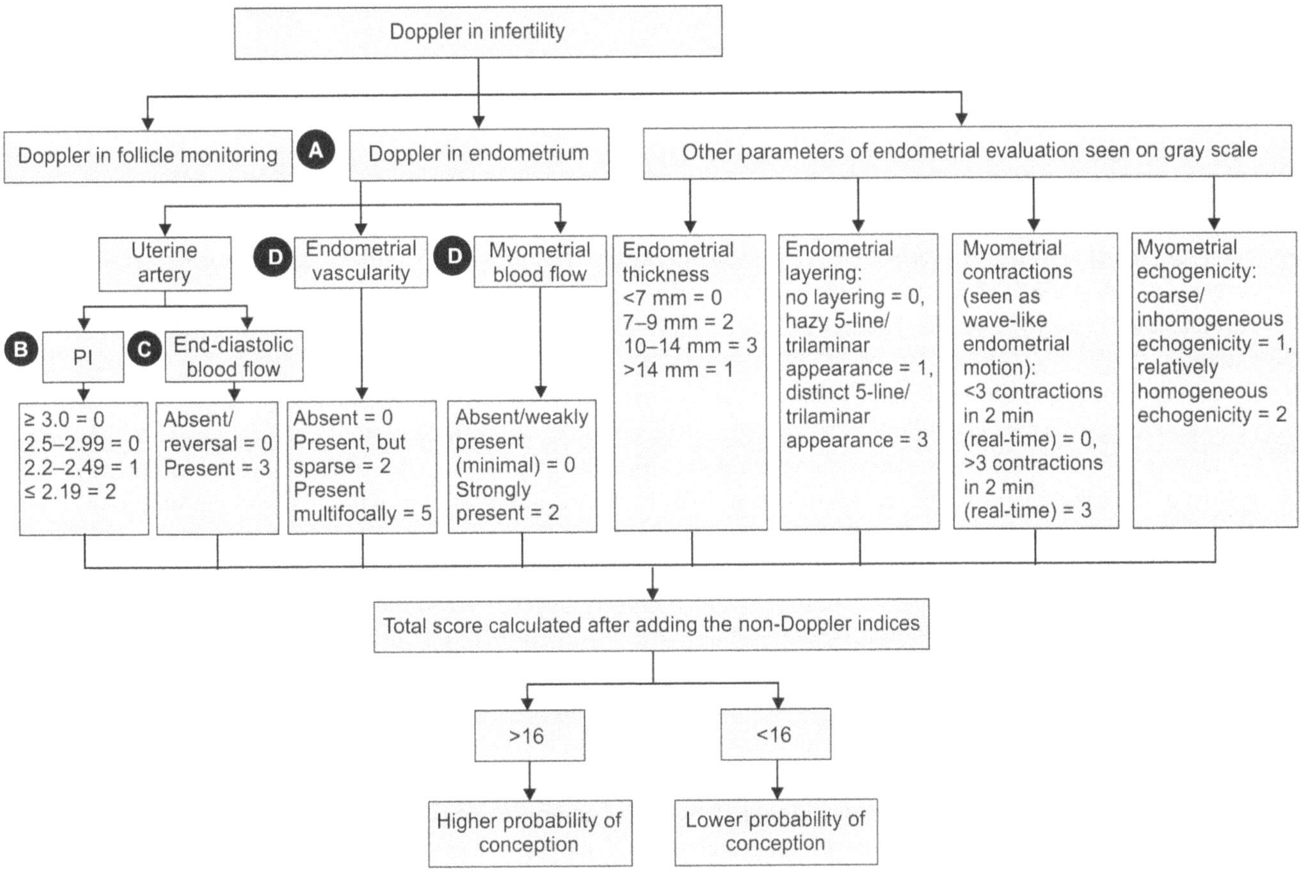

Doppler in Endometrium Evaluation

```
                    Doppler in infertility
                           |
        ┌──────────────────┼──────────────────────────┐
Doppler in follicle    Doppler in endometrium   Other parameters of endometrial
   monitoring  (A)                              evaluation seen on gray scale
```

- **Uterine artery**
  - (B) **PI**
    - ≥ 3.0 = 0
    - 2.5–2.99 = 0
    - 2.2–2.49 = 1
    - ≤ 2.19 = 2
  - (C) **End-diastolic blood flow**
    - Absent/reversal = 0
    - Present = 3
- (D) **Endometrial vascularity**
  - Absent = 0
  - Present, but sparse = 2
  - Present multifocally = 5
- (D) **Myometrial blood flow**
  - Absent/weakly present (minimal) = 0
  - Strongly present = 2
- **Endometrial thickness**
  - <7 mm = 0
  - 7–9 mm = 2
  - 10–14 mm = 3
  - >14 mm = 1
- **Endometrial layering:**
  - no layering = 0,
  - hazy 5-line/trilaminar appearance = 1,
  - distinct 5-line/trilaminar appearance = 3
- **Myometrial contractions** (seen as wave-like endometrial motion):
  - <3 contractions in 2 min (real-time) = 0,
  - >3 contractions in 2 min (real-time) = 3
- **Myometrial echogenicity:**
  - coarse/inhomogeneous echogenicity = 1,
  - relatively homogeneous echogenicity = 2

Total score calculated after adding the non-Doppler indices

- >16 → Higher probability of conception
- <16 → Lower probability of conception

(PI: pulsatility index)

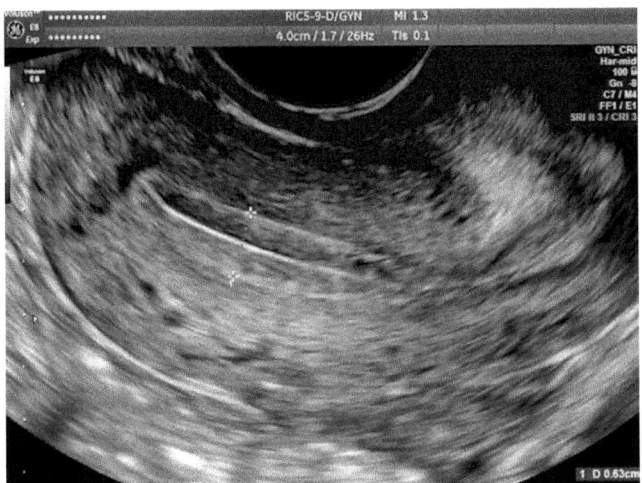

Trilaminar endometrium

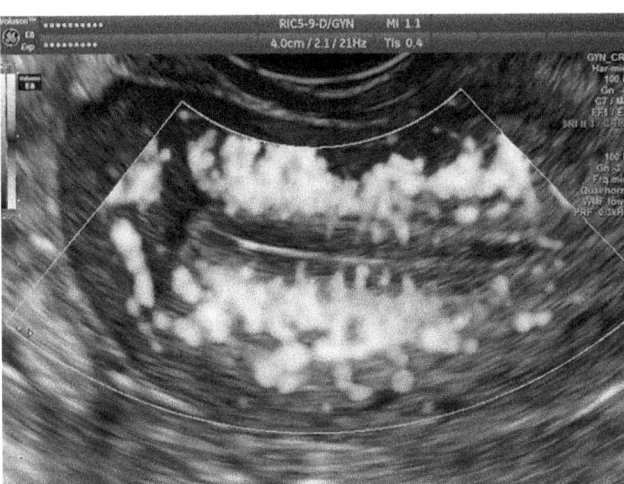

Doppler of endometrium

CHAPTER 57

Ovulation Trigger in IUI

Meenu Handa

Ovulation trigger in controlled ovarian stimulation is a very important aspect in ensuring the final oocyte maturation. It is also imperative to choose the optimum time and type of the trigger to minimize complications of ovarian hyperstimulation and also maximize the yield of mature oocyte. Preovulatory luteinizing hormone (LH) surge plays a very important role in the resumption of meiotic arrest and leading to final maturity of meiosis II oocyte now ready for fertilization.

A. It is imperative to classify the patient based on their age, antral follicular count, anti-Müllerian hormone (AMH), and body mass index (BMI) as normoresponder, expected poor responder or hyper-responder. An optimal stimulation protocol and trigger type can be decided and individualized controlled ovarian stimulation can be provided to every patient.

B. Human chorionic gonadotropin (hCG) shares a striking resemblance to the structural as well as biological molecule of LH and hence is used as standard LH surrogate for triggering. An important difference is prolonged half-life of hCG (>24 hours, LH—60 min) due to delayed degradation caused by the presence of distinct C-terminal sequence.

C. Timing of the trigger in intrauterine insemination (IUI) cycles also depends upon the ovulation induction protocol. With clomiphene cycles, optimum time for trigger is at dominant follicular size of 22–24 mm.

D. In superovulation IUI cycles with gonadotropins, the optimal timing is at dominant follicular size more than 18 mm. IUI procedure can be planned at 36–40 hours of trigger. Adding Doppler to routine follicular evaluation increases the probability of predicting oocyte maturity as compared to just evaluation based on the size of the follicle. Once follicle maturity is confirmed both by size and vascularity, a decision for trigger is taken.

E. Urinary hCG dose should be 5,000–10,000 IU intramuscular. Studies have shown that in comparison to 10,000 IU, lower dose of urinary hCG of 5,000 IU yields the same number of metaphase II (MII) and similar ongoing pregnancy rates and minimizes risk of ovarian hyperstimulation syndrome (OHSS) significantly.

F. Recombinant hCG dose of 250 μg is equivalent to 6,500 IU of urinary hCG. Similar ovulation rates (92% vs 86%) and clinical pregnancy rates are observed with recombinant hCG 250 μg and urinary hCG 5,000 IU administration. Also less local reactions are observed with recombinant hCG. Most natural compound for trigger was recombinant LH. Extremely high doses of recombinant LH 30,000 IU achieved similar clinical pregnancy rates. Not favored for routine clinical use due to significant high cost and low implantation rate.

G. The risk of OHSS and multiple pregnancy increases significantly when the number of dominant follicles (18–22 mm) is more than 3 or when the total number of intermediate follicles (14–16 mm) is more than 5. In such scenarios, the couple is counseled regarding the risk–benefit ratio and given options for either canceling the cycle, performing IUI without trigger after spontaneous ovulation, convert to an in vitro fertilization (IVF) cycle or trigger with gonadotropin-releasing hormone (GnRH) agonist.

H. Gonadotropin-releasing hormone agonist can also be used as a trigger in IVF cycles when using GnRH antagonist protocol. It induces the natural endogenous LH and follicle-stimulating hormone (FSH) surge found to be beneficial on oocyte maturity. It also takes the advantage of shorter half-life of natural LH and completely eliminates the risk of OHSS. Doses used can be 0.2 mg triptorelin, buserelin 0.5 mg or leuprolide 1 mg. It should be emphasized that luteal phase is defective with GnRH agonist trigger, and should be rescued with aggressive luteal support. In addition the pregnancy rates are severely compromised in a GnRH agonist trigger. Hence, it is not used routinely for ovulation trigger in an IUI cycle.

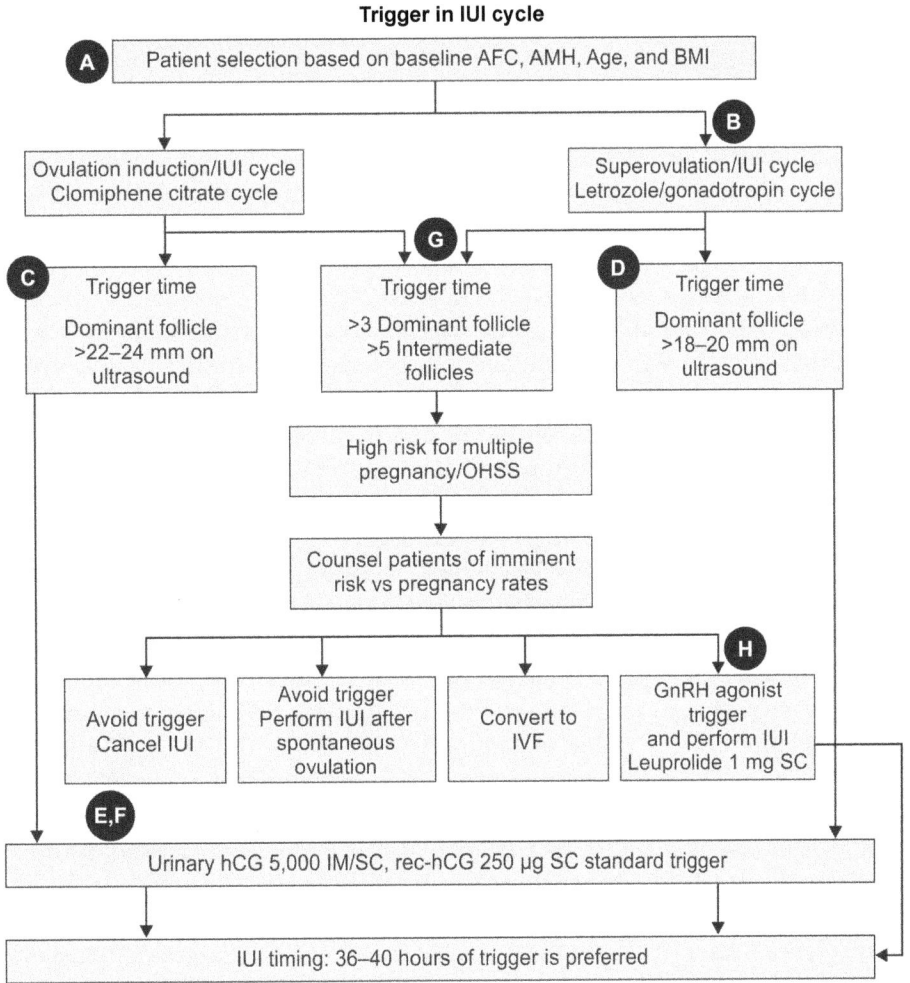

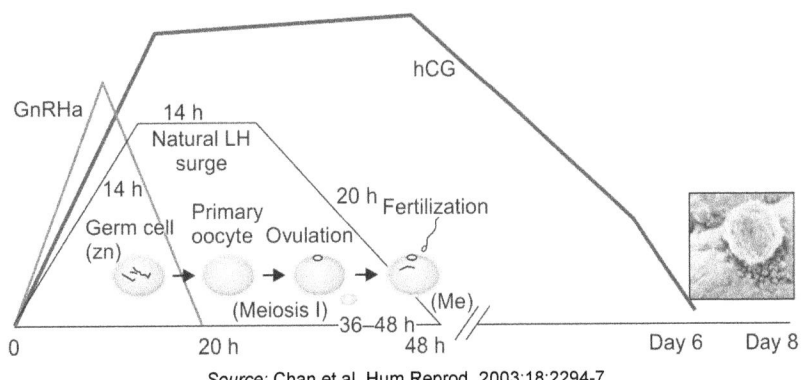

Source: Chan et al. Hum Reprod. 2003;18:2294-7

CHAPTER 58

10 Steps to Successful IUI

Apoorva Pallam Reddy, Rajeev Agarwal

Intrauterine insemination (IUI) is a simple, noninvasive, economical procedure of transferring a processed semen sample into the uterine cavity to increase the density of spermatozoa near the oocyte. There is significant increase in the number of IUI cycles over the years as the main advantage is lack of serious complications and increased cumulative pregnancy over months. However, the success of an IUI ranges between 7 and 20%. The key to success depends on various factors.

A. Choosing the ideal couple for an IUI is the most important factor for the success of an IUI. Women younger than 35 years with <4 years of infertility have higher probability of getting pregnant than older women. The success of IUI significantly decreases with increase in female partner age and the duration of infertility. It is also imperative that there should be confirmation of at least one functioning tube before performing IUI. Women with mild endometriosis and unexplained infertility have higher chances of conception with an IUI as compared to trying naturally.

B. Sperm parameters are the key factor for success from the male partner. Total motile sperm count (TMSC) of >1 million/mL in a post-wash sample is the minimum for performing an IUI. Total motile sperm count >5–10 million/mL significantly increases the chances of pregnancy. The main function of the sperm is fertilize the oocyte by penetrating the oolemma physically and deliver the genetic material. Men with abnormal morphology (<4%) fail to fertilize the oocyte and those with damaged DNA (DFI > 30%) carry higher risk of miscarriage. Hence, they are not ideal for considering IUI.

C. Ovulation induction specially with gonadotropins (GT) increases the success rates as compared to ovulogens or natural cycle. GT-IUI (17–20%) > CC+GT-IUI (13–15%) > CC-IUI (8–10%) > Natural cycle-IUI (3–5%). Achieving multifollicular genesis (2–3 follicles) although increases the chances of successful IUI, also increases incidence of multiple pregnancy. Hence using progressive increasing dose of ovulogens/GT to achieve 2–3 dominant follicles may be considered.

D. A premature luteinizing hormone (LH) surge is defined as a premature rise of LH (>10 IU/L) accompanied by a concomitant rise in P (>1 mg/L–3.2 nM/L). In stimulated IUI cycles the incidence is < 20%. This results in premature ovulation of an immature oocyte. Downregulation of an IUI cycle with gonadotropin-releasing hormone (GnRH) agonist or antagonist is not recommended on a routine basis as it does not increase the chances of pregnancy. Downregulation is considered only in cases of repeated cycles of premature ovulation or in case of persistent elevated day LH where one cycle of oral contraceptive pill (OCP) can be used to reduce basal LH.

E. Follicular monitoring is done routinely to assess the follicular and endometrial growth and determine the timing of IUI. The chances of pregnancy are higher if the endogenous LH surge coincides with that of exogenous ovulation trigger. Follicular maturity is assessed using both structural parameters of size as well as Doppler parameters. Once dominance is confirmed ovulation trigger is administered in such a way that IUI is scheduled at 36–38 hours. At our center we prefer performing the IUI in the morning hours as the clients are less stressed and the men have higher chances of giving a better sample.

F. Human chorionic gonadotropin (HCG) trigger, either recombinant or urinary, is routinely for ovulation trigger in IUI. Use of GnRH agonist trigger is associated with a defective luteal phase and poor pregnancy rates. Hence, routine use of GnRH agonist trigger is no advised for IUI cycles. If GnRH agonist trigger is given then aggressive luteal phase support in the form progesterone supplementation and single shot of 1,500–2,000 IU of HCG in the mid luteal phase is administered for rescuing luteolysis.

G. If the endometrial lining is thin (< 7 mm), estrogen supplementation may be given either in gel form for application or oral form. It is important to note that estrogen supplementation can be started only after the follicle reaches dominance. If estrogen is given prematurely, it can effect follicular growth and causes follicular arrest.

H. A second IUI is useful only if there are multiple follicles and if all of them have not ruptured at the time of first IUI. The second IUI is usually performed 12–24 hours from the first IUI.

I. Time of preparation to time of insemination should be <90 minutes to achieve best results.

J. Ultrasound guidance for IUI is helpful only when there is difficulty in negotiating through the cervical canal. Routine use does not add any benefit.

10 Steps to Successful IUI

Step 1 — Choosing ideal couple

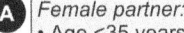 *Female partner:*
- Age <35 years
- Duration of infertility <4 years
- Unexplained/mild endometriosis
- Basal FSH <7 IU/mL
- At least one patent tube

 Male partner:
- Total motile sperm count 5–10 million/mL
- Morphology >4%
- DFI <30%

Step 2 — Ovulogens

 Use of *Gonadotropins* for ovulation induction has much higher pregnancy rate as compared oral ovulogens. When considered oral ovulogens letrozole is the first line of stimulation for PCOS women

Step 3 — No. of follicles

Cycles that result in *2–3 follicles* have higher chance of pregnancy as compared to monofollicular genesis

Step 4 — Downregulation

 There is no evidence that downregulation of an IUI cycle results in improvement in success rate. Only cases that need to be converted into an IVF or cases that show premature LH surge benefit from downregulation

Step 5 — Timing of ovulation trigger

 Size: 17–18 mm for exclusive GT stimulated cycles
18–20 mm for oral ovulogens + GT stimulated cycles
20–22 mm for only oral ovulogens stimulated cycles
Doppler: > ¾ perifollicular flow PSV → 10 cm/s RI—0.4-0.5

Step 6 — Type of ovulation trigger

 Recombinant hCG and urinary hCG result in similar ovulation rates
Similar pregnancy rates

Step 7 — Endometrial thickness

 Endometrial thickness of >7 mm with good vascularity and texture results in higher pregnancy rates

Step 8 — Timing of insemination

 Performing a single IUI at 36 hours results in the best pregnancy rates

Step 9 — Semen preparation technique

 Duration of abstinence 2–3 days
Timing of prepararations:
- Semen collection to sperm wash (max 30 min)
- Sperm wash to IUI time (ideally immediately)
- Semen collection to (IUI time < 90 min)

Technique of preparation: Normal male factor-swim up/OAT factor-density gradient

Step 10 — IUI technique

 USG guided VS blind: No benefit of USG guidance except in difficult negotiation
Type of cannula: Soft cannula preferred
Position of patient: No difference

(GT: gonadotropins; hCG: human chorionic gonadotropin; IUI: intrauterine insemination; DFI: DNA fragmentation index; FSH: follicle-stimulating hormone; PCOS: polycystic ovary syndrome; IVF: in vitro fertilization; LH: luteinizing hormone; USG: ultrasonography; OAT: oligoasthenoteratozoospermia; RI; resistivity index)

CHAPTER 59

Artificial Insemination: Donor

Dorothy P Ghosh, Rakhi Singh

A. *Clinical indications for donor insemination*
   - Couple with severe male factor infertility, unable to opt for intracytoplasmic sperm injection (ICSI) due to cost constraints
   - Azoospermia or severe abnormalities of semen quality where donor semen insemination is needed
   - Inheritable genetic condition of the male partner
   - An infection such as human immunodeficiency virus (HIV) of the male partner
   - Severe rhesus incompatibility has been a problem because of the male partner's homozygous status
   - Consanguineous marriages leading to early miscarriages due to autosomal recessive disorders.
B. *Donor Screening:*
   - Healthy males between 21 years and 35 years of age
   - Minimum semen parameters [as per American Society for Reproductive Medicine (ASRM)]
     - Volume more than 2 mL/sperm motility more than 50% moving activity
     - Sperm concentration more than 20 million/mL/sperm morphology normal range
   - Should not have injected drugs for nonmedical use
   - Screened negative for:
     - Chromosomal abnormalities
     - Autosomal recessive diseases like beta thalassaemia and Tay Sachs disease
     - HIV, Hepatitis B, Hepatitis C, syphilis, Cytomegalovirus
     - Hypertension, diabetes, sexually transmitted disease
     - Disseminated lymphadenopathy
     - Unexplained jaundice
C. *Donor profile:* Blood group and Rh status, height, weight, body color, eye color, and hair color recorded.
D. *Freezing technique:* Slow followed by rapid cooling
   - Consists of progressive sperm cooling over a period of 2–4 hours in two to three steps, either manually or automatically using a semi-programmable freezer.
   - The manual method is performed by simultaneously decreasing the temperature of the semen while adding a cryoprotectant in a stepwise manner and after plunging the sample in liquid nitrogen.
   - In spite of reports showing successful sperm freezing with manual techniques, the reproducibility of this procedure could pose some problems. For this reason, programmable freezers have been investigated.
   - Slow freezing, either manual or automated, causes extensive chemical-physical damage to the sperm probably because of ice crystallization.
E. *Thawing method of frozen semen sample:*
   - Thawing in a thermostat and water bath at 37°C for 10 minutes or
   - Thawing at room temperature for 15 minutes.
F. Donor semen samples are both recruited and stored by semen banks. An assisted reproductive technique (ART) clinic can't function as a semen bank.

ADVANTAGE AND DISADVANTAGES OF FROZEN DONOR SEMEN SAMPLE

Advantages

- Quarantine of donor semen till appropriate testing can be completed.
- Availability of consistent quality of sample.

Disadvantages

- The lifespan of the thawed specimen is only about 12 hours. So, timing of procedures has to be very precise.
- There was a significant decrease of sperm motility between fresh sperm and cryopreserved sperm due to impairment of mitochondrial activity.
- An alteration in mitochondrial membrane fluidity also leads to an alteration in mitochondrial membrane potential and release of reactive oxygen species (ROS).
- Cryopreservation has been shown to diminish the antioxidant activity of the spermatozoa making them more susceptible to ROS damage.

DETRIMENTAL EFFECTS OF CRYOPRESERVATION ON SPERM INTEGRITY

- Compared with other cell types, spermatozoa seem to be less sensitive to cryopreservation damage because of the high fluidity of the membrane and the low water content (about 50%).
- Several damaging processes could occur during freezing-thawing of human spermatozoa, such as thermal shock with formation of intracellular and extracellular ice crystals, cellular dehydration, and osmotic shock.
- Cryoinjury is not limited to the freezing process but may also occur during the thawing process as the ice melts or recrystallizes.

DNA Integrity in Relevance to Cryopreservation

- Freezing sperm in seminal plasma improves post thaw deoxyribonucleic acid (DNA) integrity: Sperm-frozen unprepared in seminal fluid seems to be more resistant to freezing damage than frozen prepared sperm.
- Further improvement can be achieved by preparing sperm and freezing after re-addition of seminal plasma. This may be due to the presence of abundant antioxidants in seminal plasma.
- Freezing-thawing procedure negatively affects DNA integrity.

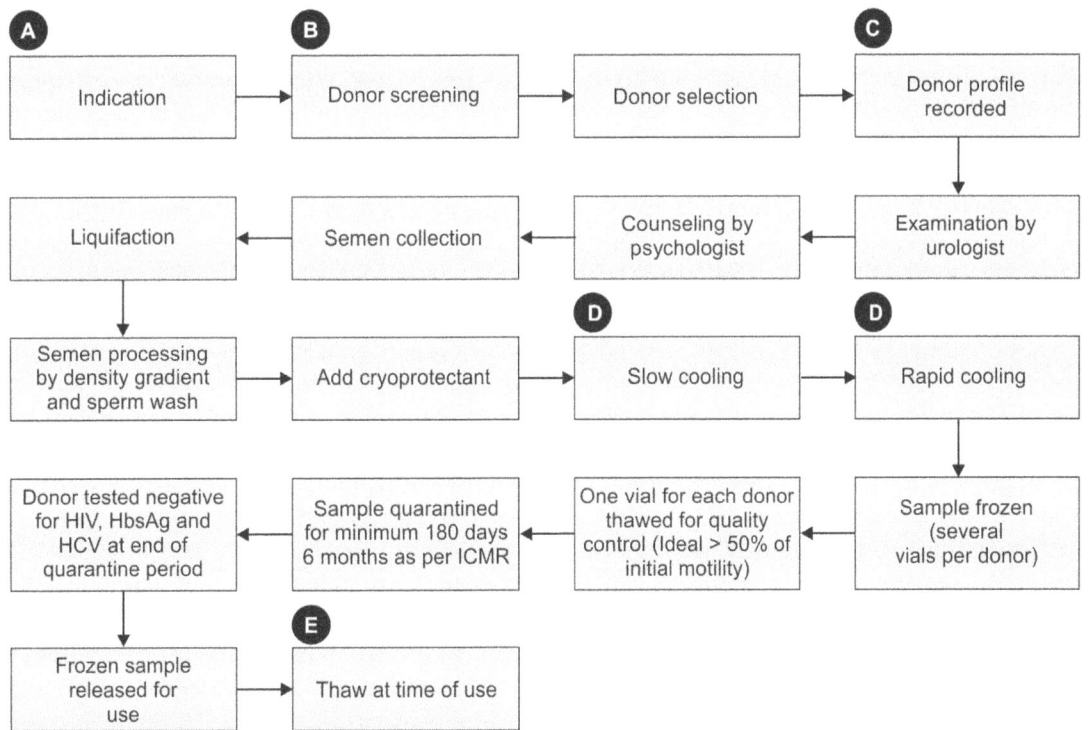

(HbsAg: hepatitis B surface antigen; HCV: hepatitis C virus; HIV: human immunodeficiency virus; ICMR: Indian Council of Medical Research)

CHAPTER 60

Luteal Phase Support in IUI

Apoorva Pallam Reddy, Rajeev Agarwal

A. Normal luteal function requires optimal preovulatory follicular development, proper luteinization of the granulosa cells to produce progesterone, continued tonic luteinizing hormone (LH) support, vascularization of the corpus luteum, and estrogen to induce progesterone receptors (PR) in the endometrium. Medicines and Healthcare Products Regulatory Agency (MHRA) recommends serum progesterone levels more than or equal to 14 ng/mL in the mid-luteal phase for maintaining pregnancy. Luteal phase defect (LPD) is defined as luteal phase duration less than 10 days and/or measurements of peak luteal progesterone less than or equal to 10 ng/mL. Women with impaired luteal function in an intrauterine insemination (IUI) require luteal phase support (LPS).

B. History of short menstrual cycles premenstrual spotting, elderly women and low body weight are considered risk factors for LPD.

C. Conditions associated with ovulatory dysfunction like hyperandrogenism, polycystic ovary syndrome (PCOS), endometriosis, hyperprolactinemia, and thyroid disorders are associated with low progesterone levels during the luteal phase and benefit from LPS during an IUI.

D. In gonodotropins (GT) stimulated cycles and cycles that have multifollicular genesis (>2 dominant follicles/>4 intermediate follicles), supraphysiological serum estradiol (E2) exerts negative feedback on LH secretion from the pituitary and cause premature luteolysis. The luteal phase in gonadotropin-stimulated cycles is 20% shorter (an average luteal phase lasts 11 days). LPS significantly increases clinical pregnancy rates (CPR) and live birth rates (LBR) in GT-stimulated cycles.

E. In clomiphene-stimulated cycles, the E2 receptor on pituitary axis is blocked by clomiphene citrate (CC). Hence supraphysiological E2 does not have a negative impact on LH secretion. The endogenous rise of LH is sufficient to maintain luteal support. No additional LPS is needed when the stimulation is done with CC alone in the absence of other risk factors for LPD. LPS does not impact CPR or LBR in CC-stimulated cycles. In letrozole-stimulated cycles, the E2 receptors on pituitary axis are not blocked like in CC. Hence supraphysiological E2 might still have a negative impact on LH secretion. If multifollicular genesis is achieved, LPS might improve CPR or LBR in letrozole-stimulated cycles. LPS significantly increases CPR and LBR in ovulogens + GT-stimulated cycles.

F. Starting LPS as early as on the day of ovulation is bound to be beneficial on uterine contractions. On the other hand, early exposure of high doses progesterone might be detrimental to the tubal peristalisis and impair embryo transport. There is no evidence regarding the best time to start progesterone supplementation. Startng either on the day of ovulation or the next day will yield similar pregnancy rates.

G. Oral micronized P4: The sustained release (SR) tablet contains P4 in a methylcellulose base which hydrates in the gastrointestinal tract providing a slow release matrix for a gradual release of progesterone. Sustained release pattern over 24 hours. Long elimination half-life of 18 hours with high protein binding of 90–99% leads to once a dosage convenience. The "smooth" release pattern avoids sudden drug release or "dose dumping" and therefore loss of drug due to hepatic metabolism minimizes dose-related central side effects, i.e. drowsiness.

H. Dydrogesterone is a stereoisomer of progesterone that is a highly selective synthetic progestin that binds almost exclusively to progesterone receptor. In contrast to natural progesterone, dydrogesterone has good oral bioavailability (28%).

I. Vaginal micronized progesterone has the benefit of ease of administration when compared with intramuscular (IM) injections of progesterone, lesser side effect profile, and higher bioavailability. No difference between gel/capsules with respect to LBR, miscarriage rate (MR), rate of early pregnancy bleeding, 8% gel/400–600 mg daily.

J. Parenteral progesterone is not routinely recommended for LPS in IUI.

K. Single dose of human chorionic gonadotropin (hCG) 7 days post-ovulation is shown to rescue corpus luteum from premature luteolysis. Secondly, hCG plays a role in biochemical cross-talking between the embryo and the decidua and promotes implantation. 2,000 IU IM increases the endogenous levels of both estrogen and progesterone.

L. Progesterone (P4) is needed to support early pregnancy and implantation. E2 is responsible for the induction of P4 receptors over the endometrium. Low serum E2 levels in luteal phase might impact PR. Supplementing estradiol valerate is not routinely recommended in IUI.

M. Endogenous FSH and LH surge induced by gonadotropin-releasing hormone agonist (GnRHa) is a physiological event with luteal phase steroid concentration near to those of normal cycles. GnRHa receptors have been described in the corpus luteum (CL) and human endometrium. Tesarik et al. reported that injection of a single dose of GnRHa in the luteal phase was shown to increase pregnancy, implantation, and birth rates suggesting a possible direct effect of GnRHa on the embryo.

N. All forms of LPS can be stopped by 7 weeks once the fetal note is established without compromising the LBR or increasing the miscarriage rate.

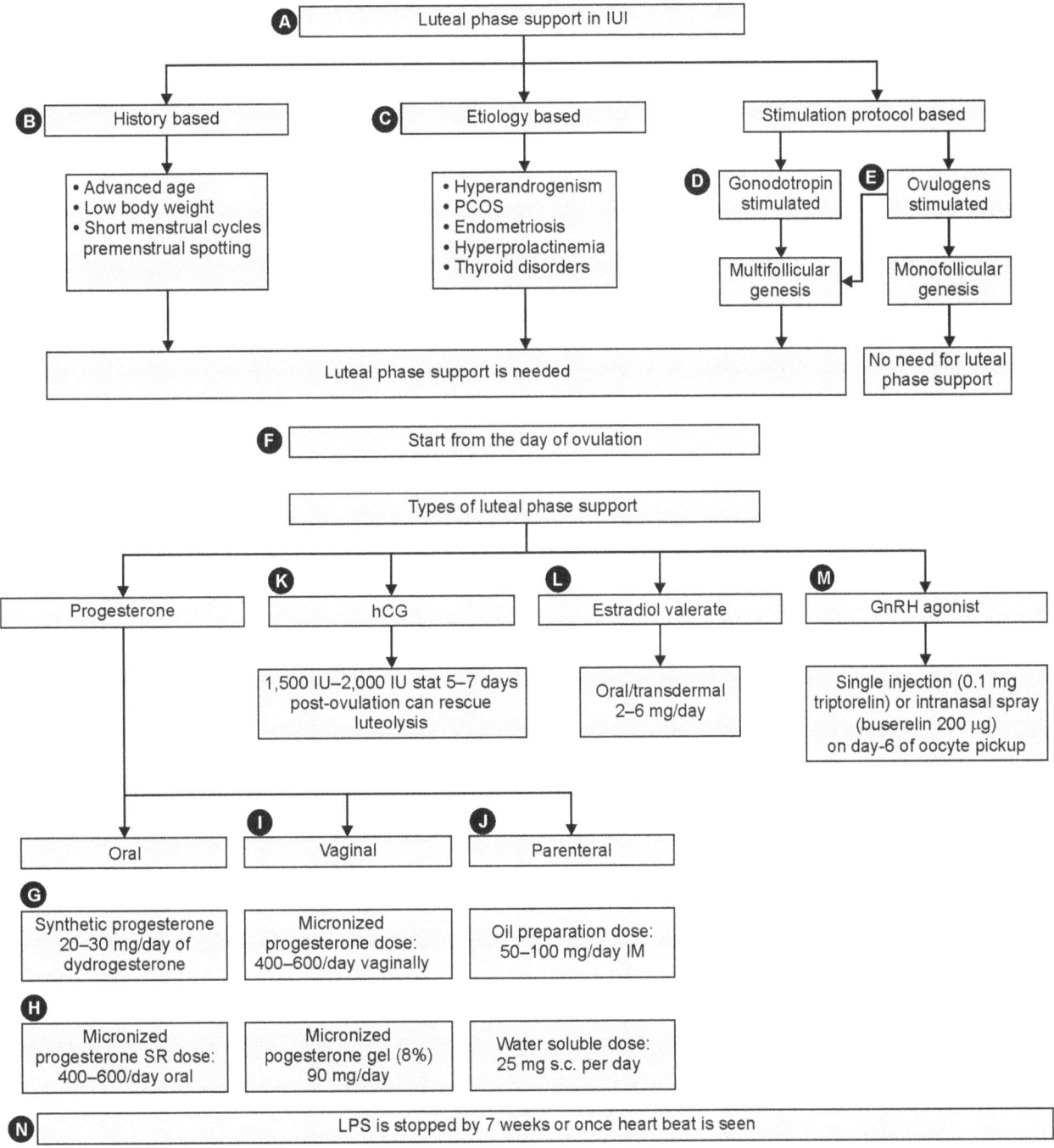

(GnRH: gonadotropin-releasing hormone; hCG: human chorionic gonadotropin; IUI: intrauterine insemination; LPS: luteal phase support; PCOS: polycystic ovary syndrome; IM: intramuscular; SR: sustained release; s.c. subcutaneous)

SECTION 15

In Vitro Fertilization

- Indications for In Vitro Fertilization-Male Factor
- Indications for In Vitro Fertilization-Female Factor
- Indications for ART—Unexplained and Emerging Factors
- Pre-IVF Evaluation
- Individualized Controlled Ovarian Stimulation
- Ovulation Induction in Assisted Reproductive Technique: Agonist Protocols
- Ovulation Induction in Assisted Reproductive Technique: Antagonist Protocols
- Controlled Ovarian Stimulation in Assisted Reproductive Technique
- Mild Ovarian Stimulation
- Role of LH in Controlled Ovarian Stimulation
- Triggers for Ovarian Stimulation: IVF
- Oocyte Pickup
- Embryo Transfer
- Luteal Phase Support in IVF
- Diagnosis of Ovarian Hyperstimulation Syndrome
- Management of Ovarian Hyperstimulation Syndrome
- Batch In Vitro Fertilization
- Cycle Preparation for Batching Embryo Transfer
- Endometrial Preparation for FET: Natural Cycle
- Endometrial Preparation for FET: Hormonal Replacement Therapy
- Oocyte Donor Recruitment Protocol
- Oocyte Donor Controlled Ovarian Stimulation

CHAPTER 61

Indications for In Vitro Fertilization-Male Factor

Venu Gopal M, Simi Fabian

INTRODUCTION

The indications for assisted reproductive technique (ART) can be broadly divided into male, female, unexplained, and emerging factors.

Male infertility contributes to 20–30% cases of infertility. Medicines have a limited role in most of the cases. Intrauterine insemination (IUI) seldom succeeds if post-wash inseminate has less than 1 million motile sperms. Over the years, intracytoplasmic sperm injection (ICSI) has overtaken as procedure of choice for men with severe oligoasthenozoospermia, obstructive azoospermia, and in some cases of nonobstructive cases of azoospermia with the count threshold for ICSI being different in different laboratories.

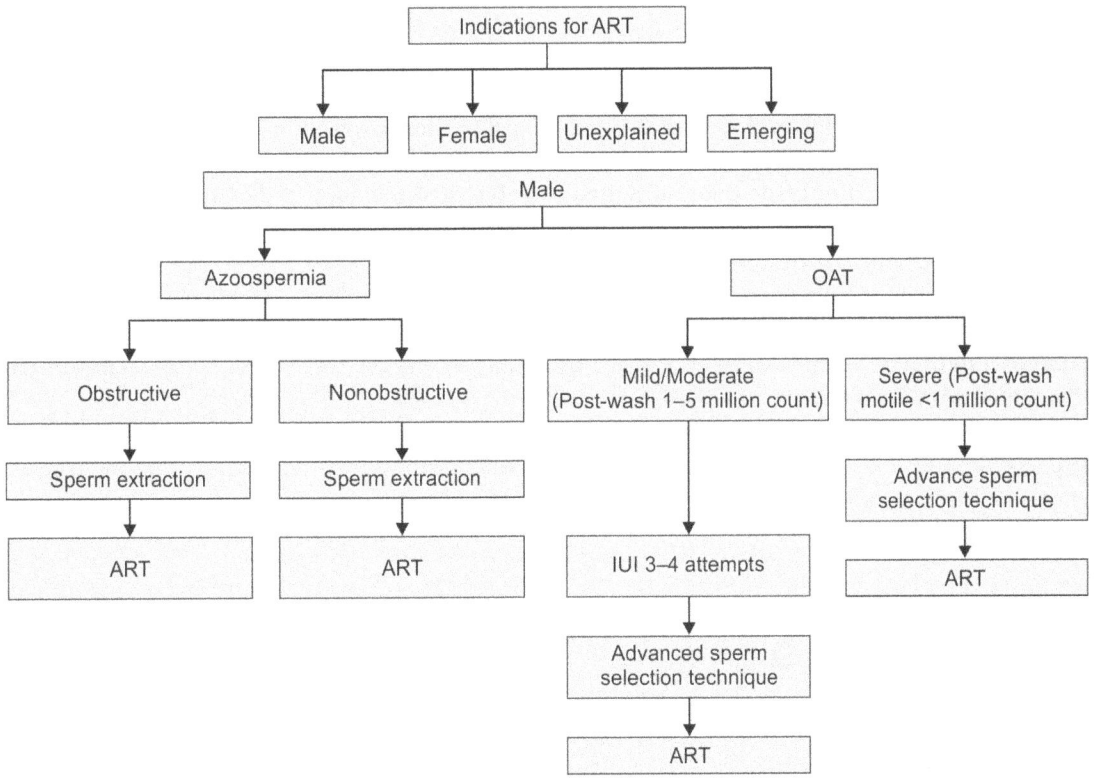

(ART: assisted reproductive technique; IUI: intrauterine insemination; OAT: oligoasthenoteratozoospermia)

CHAPTER 62

Indications for In Vitro Fertilization-Female Factor

Venu Gopal M, Simi Fabian

INTRODUCTION

Abnormality in the female partner with a normal male resulting in infertility is seen in 30% of the subfertile couple. About 10% of the infertile couples have, a coexisting, female and male partner abnormality resulting in infertility. The four main components assisting in female reproduction are (1) the ovary, (2) the uterus, (3) the fallopian tubes connecting both, and (4) the pelvis stationing all these organs. Any dysfunction in one or more of these factors results in infertility.

A. *Ovulatory dysfunction:* World Health Organization (WHO) group I and group III patients have well-defined management guidelines. WHO group II patients, majority of them have polycystic ovary syndrome (PCOS), constitute almost 70% of anovulatory patients. This group of patients are the most challenging considering the risk of ovarian hyperstimulation syndrome (OHSS), poor oocyte quality, and poor fertilization indices. For all women in group I and group II who fail to achieve pregnancy either through timed intercourse or intrauterine insemination (IUI), assisted reproductive technique (ART) becomes the final resort.

   Women with premature ovarian failure are categorized into WHO group III. Oocyte donation through ART is a realistic option of achieving pregnancy for these women.

B. *Tubal disorders* contribute roughly 25–30% of cases of infertility. The obstruction is proximal or distal. It is always a dilemma deciding whether to proceed with assisted reproduction or to advice tubal reconstructive surgeries for such patients. Endoscopic procedures have evolved significantly but quantification of damage to inner cilia and lining of fallopian tube remains a challenge. Hence, for women with advanced tubal disease or failed tubal re-anastomosis or those with tubal occlusion, ART becomes the mainstay of treatment.

C. *Uterine factors* have been associated with infertility. Patients with uterine agenesis and functional ovaries benefit from surrogacy. Similarly patients with refractory endometrium secondary to Asherman's, unexplained persistent thin endometrium, multiple recurrent cavity distorting fibroids, adenomyosis, etc. which cause recurrent implantation failure have surrogacy as an option.

D. *Pelvic/Peritoneal factors:* The pelvis harbours all the reproductive organs and a healthy reproductive environment is essential for their normal functioning as well as maintenance of tubo-ovarian relation. Endometriosis and pelvic inflammatory disease are the two major factors that effect pelvic factors.

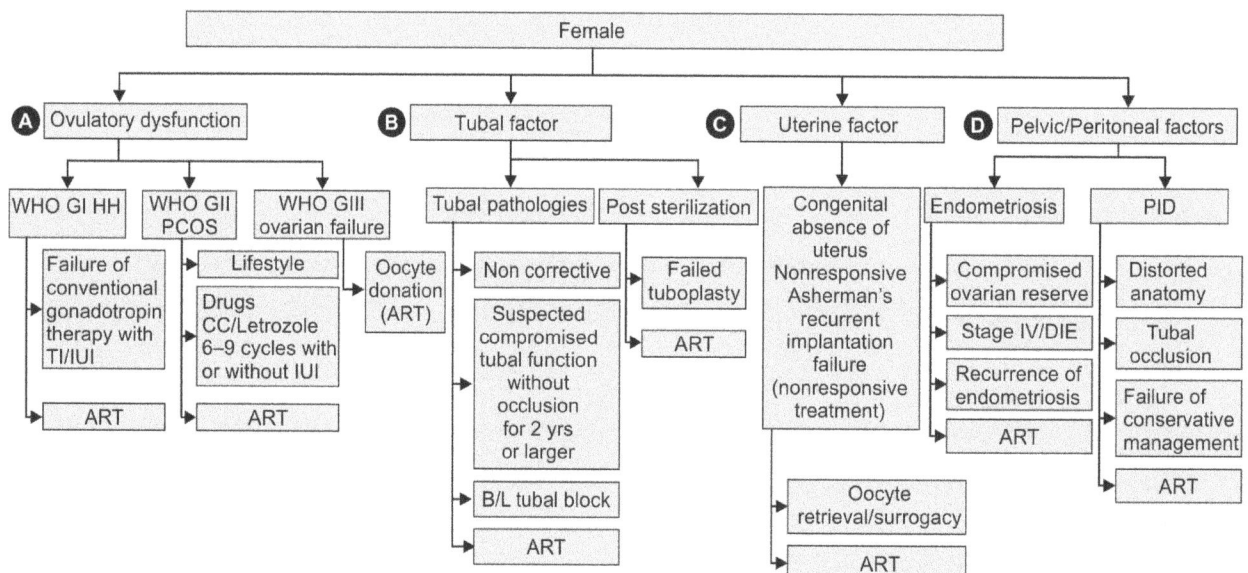

(ART: assisted reproductive technique; CC: clomiphene citrate; DIE: deep infiltrating endometriosis; HH: hypogonadotropic hypogonadism; IUI: intrauterine insemination; PCOS: polycystic ovary syndrome; PID: pelvic inflammatory disease; TI: timed intercourse; WHO: World Health Organization; B/L: bilateral)

CHAPTER 63

Indications for ART—Unexplained and Emerging Factors

Venu Gopal M, Simi Fabian

A. Unexplained infertility is one area where the waiting game may yield results. It is difficult to prognosticate which patient will benefit from which intervention. There are many empiric therapies available but assisted reproduction shortens time to pregnancy and hence age is an important factor while deciding upon the same. In women with unexplained infertility the age of the female partner and duration of infertility plays a key role in the deciding further management.

B. In younger women (<35 years) with >5 years of married life, failure of a minimum of 2 years expectant management, failed multiple intrauterine inseminations (IUIs) (3-6 attempts), assisted reproductive technique (ART) is indicated to increase the chance of pregnancy.

C. In older women (>35 years) waiting too long might drastically reduce the possibility of pregnancy even with ART. Hence, failure to get pregnant after 6 months of spontaneous attempt should be followed by three attempts of gonadotropins (GT) stimulated IUI. Moving to ART should be considered in cases of failed IUI.

D. All women older than 40 years should be offered ART directly.

E. *Emerging indications for assisted reproduction* are the most exciting and include fertility preservation, preimplantation genetic diagnosis and screening and gestational surrogacy.

Various options are available to young women for fertility preservation before commencement of radiotherapy or chemotherapy for fertility preservation. Similarly sperm freezing should always be considered in males. Many women in late reproductive years who are single may wish to preserve oocytes for the future as reproductive insurance.

Preimplantation genetic diagnosis (PGD) has established its place in patients who are at high risk of transmitting genetic abnormalities to their offspring. Preimplantation genetic screening (PGS) though a debatable issue is now being widely offered for embryo selection in assisted reproduction in a wide array of cases.

Women with no functional uterus or markedly abnormal uterus or those suffering from serious medical disorders are now able to create a family using a gestational carrier.

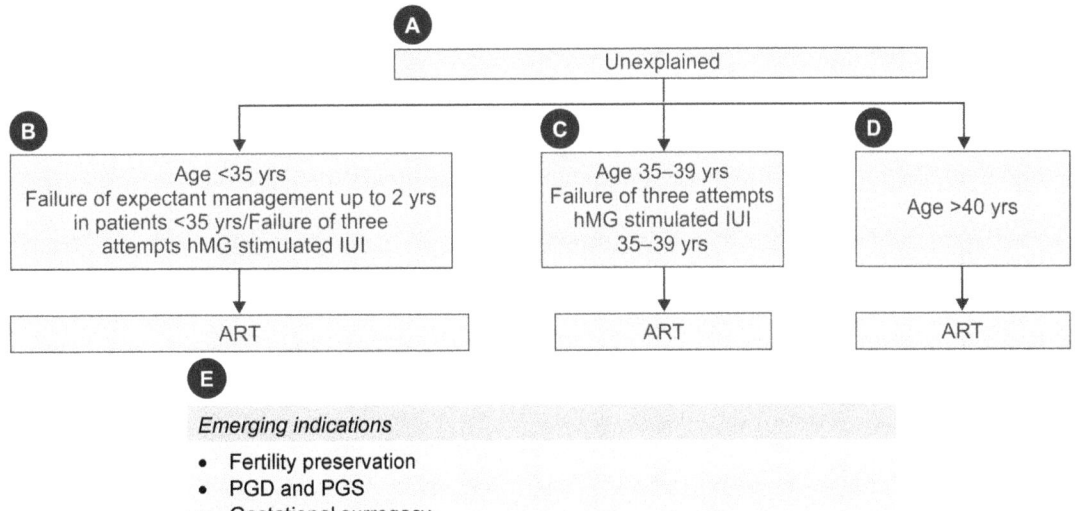

(ART: assisted reproductive technique; hMG: human menopausal gonadotropin; IUI: intrauterine insemination; PGD: preimplantation genetic diagnosis; PGS: preimplantation genetic screening)

CHAPTER 64

Pre-IVF Evaluation

Venu Gopal M, Simi Fabian

MALE PARTNER EVALUATION

Semen analysis remains the cornerstone of male partner investigation. Ultrasound is done only for confirmation of clinically suspected pathologies. Genetic testing identifies patients with genetic anomalies and facilitates genetic counseling prior to assisted reproduction. Y deletions are done in cases of severe oligoasthenoteratozoospermia and in azoospermia for prognostication. Cystic fibrosis transmembrane conductance regulator (CFTR) screening is a mandatory part of investigation in cases of obstructive azoospermia. In the Indian context, screening in both partners is also a routine for human immunodeficiency virus (HIV), venereal disease research laboratory (VDRL), hepatitis B surface antigen (HBsAg), and HCV (hepatitis C virus).

FEMALE PARTNER EVALUATION

Antral follicle count (AFC) and anti-Müllerian hormone (AMH) are preferred over follicle-stimulating hormone (FSH), inhibin or estradiol levels for predicting the ovarian response as poor normal or high. However, they cannot predict probability of live birth. Ovarian reserve tests can also be used to decide a dosage of gonadotropin to be used for stimulation.

Intracycle monitoring is useful in assisted reproductive technique (ART) to confirm downregulation, adjust dose of gonadotropins, determine time of trigger, and to identify time of transfer of embryos. A combination of ultrasound and biochemical markers is used to follow-up in ART cycles. Serum estradiol (E2) is primarily correlated to follicle dynamics while the role of progesterone measurement at start and end of cycles remains a matter of debate. Serum progesterone levels are important at start of cycle as elevated progesterone levels during start are due to incomplete luteolysis and consistent with decreased pregnancy. Similarly, elevated progesterone on the day of trigger shows premature progesterone exposure to the endometrium, alteration in implantation window and thus is associated with reduced pregnancy.

Two-dimensional (2D) ultrasound is invaluable in assessing both follicular growth and endometrium while use of three-dimensional (3D) ultrasonography (USG) with Doppler is an additive option if available.

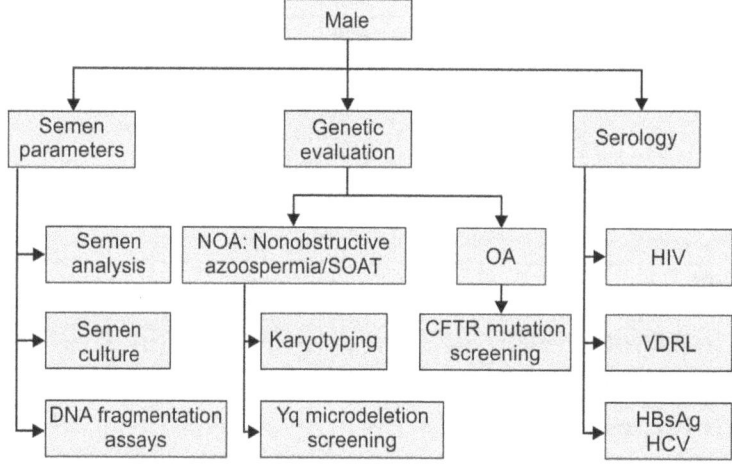

Pre-IVF Evaluation

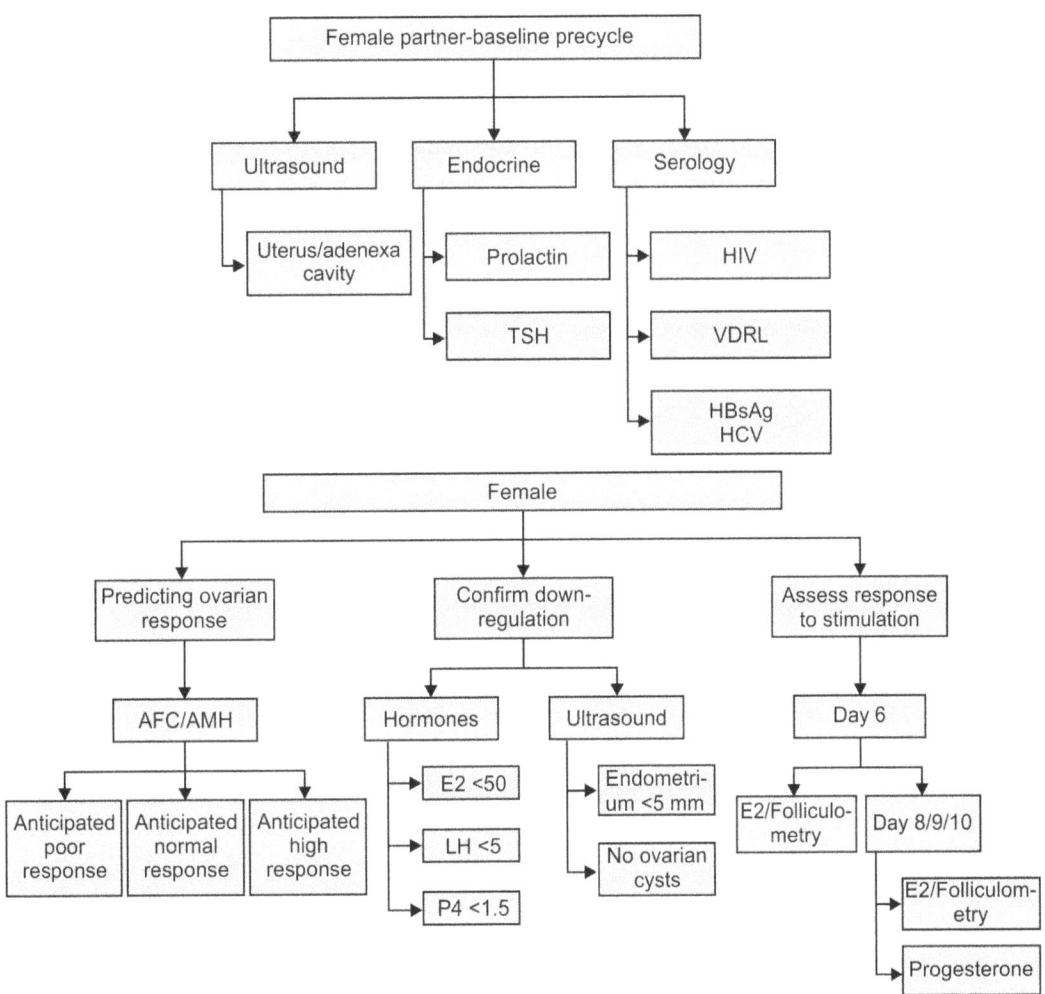

(AFC: antral follicle count; AMH: anti-Müllerian hormone; CFTR: cystic fibrosis transmembrane conductance regulator; DNA: deoxyribonucleic acid; HBsAg: hepatitis B surface antigen; HCV: hepatitis C virus; HIV: human immunodeficiency virus; LH: luteinizing hormone; OA: obstructive azoospermia; SOAT: severe oligo-astheno-teratozoospermia; TSH: thyroid-stimulating hormone; VDRL: venereal disease research laboratory; E2: estradiol; P4: progesterone)

CHAPTER 65

Individualized Controlled Ovarian Stimulation

Apoorva Pallam Reddy, Nandita Palshetkar

INTRODUCTION

The three major components of an assisted reproductive technique (ART) cycle include:
1. Initiation of multifollicular genesis with the administration of exogenous gonadotropins (GT) and/or oral ovulogens—starting dose
2. Prevention of endogenous luteinizing hormone (LH) surge using gonadotropin-releasing hormone (GnRH) analogs (antagonists/agonists)—downregulation and finally
3. Inducing an endogenous LH surge or mimicking it with exogenous human chorionic gonadotropin (HCG) to initiate final oocyte maturation—ovulation trigger. It cannot be emphasized enough that there is no single protocol that suits the needs of all the patient profiles. Identifying the best protocol for each individual increases the reproductive outcome of ART over all.

Prior to start of stimulation, all the patients must be assessed for their antral follicle count (AFC) and anti-Müllerian hormone (AMH) in order to predict the response at the end of stimulation. Based on this prediction, all the patients for controlled ovarian stimulation (COS) can be categorized into either high responder, normal responder, or poor responder. The stimulation protocol differs according to the category of the patient. The aim of controlled ovarian stimulation in ART is to achieve a reasonable number of oocytes that can cumulatively result in a live birth. Studies have shown that obtaining 8–12 oocytes significantly improved the probability of ART resulting in a live birth. All stimulation protocols should ideally aim at resulting in 8–12 number of oocytes when feasible.

HIGH RESPONDERS

Presence of more than 19 follicles more than or equal to 11 mm in size on day of oocyte maturation trigger and/or more than 19 oocytes collected post-oocyte pickup (OPU) characterize a high response (Griesinger et al. 2016). They have an inherent increased risk of ovarian hyperstimulation syndrome (OHSS). Hence, the stimulation protocol should aim at reducing the risk of OHSS. GnRH antagonist stimulation is the recommended protocol for women with polycystic ovary syndrome (PCOS) and women with predicted high response. The antagonist stimulation reduces the risk of OHSS, improves safety profile without compromising the efficacy. It is not recommended to use agonist protocol, mild stimulation with clomiphene citrate (CC) or a natural cycle. Although there is a mild reduction in the OHSS levels with the use of letrozole in mild stimulation and choosing lower starting doses (<150 IU) as compared to conventional (150–225 IU), this is not proven to be beneficial, hence not recommended. Use of agonist trigger during an antagonist cycle significantly reduces the risk of OHSS.

POOR RESPONDERS

A poor responder has a diminished response to conventional ovarian stimulation characterized by generally less than or equal to 3 follicles on day of oocyte maturation trigger and/or less than or equal to 3 oocytes obtained after OPU. Both antagonist and agonist cycles are equally effective in poor responders. When an agonist cycle is opted for, choosing the short protocol is preferred as compared to the long protocol. Mild ovarian stimulation with CC seems to improve reproductive outcome. Use of higher doses of GT (>400 IU) is not recommended as it is not associated with proportionate increase in the number of oocytes obtained or increase in the live birth rate. Although evidence is weak, a dual trigger is considered to increase the number of mature oocytes obtained.

Ovarian reserve tests	Poor	Normal	High
AFC	<7	7–14	>14
AMH	<1.1 ng/mL	1.1–0.5 ng/mL	>3.5 ng/mL
Starting dose of GT (IU)	300–450	225–300	150–225
Protocol	–	–	–
Antagonist	Recommended	Strongly recommended	Strongly recommended
Agonist	Recommended	Strongly not recommended	Strongly not recommended
Mild stimulation with CC	Recommended	No evidence	Not recommended
Mild stimulation with letrozole	Not recommended	Not recommended	Might reduce OHSS chance. But not recommended
Mild stimulation with low dose GT	No evidence	Not recommended	Recommended
High dose GT	Not recommended	No evidence	Strongly not recommended
Natural cycle IVF or modified natural cycle	Not recommended	Not recommended	Not recommended
Trigger	Dual trigger/HCG trigger	HCG trigger/agonist trigger	Agonist trigger

(AFC: antral follicle count; AMH: anti-Müllerian hormone; CC: clomiphene citrate; HCG: human chorionic gonadotropin; IVF: in vitro fertilization; OHSS: ovarian hyperstimulation syndrome; GT: gonadotropins)

NORMAL RESPONDERS

Any response other than high or poor is called a normal response. Although the risk of OHSS is slightly lower as compared to high responders, antagonist protocol is still recommended in normal responders. Mild stimulation is not recommended in normal responders. A HCG trigger is appropriate routinely. However, in the rare event of a predicted normal responder, hyperresponding during stimulation, a GnRH agonist trigger should be given.

It should be kept in mind that there is no single protocol that is suitable for patients of all categories. Customized and individualized controlled ovulation stimulation protocols should be tailor made according to the patient's profile. The starting dose of GT is divided between recombinant follicle-stimulating hormone (rFSH) and human menopausal gonadotropin (HMG) or rLH in a 2:1 ratio also keeping in mind the basal FSH and LH ration. For example if a decision to start a dose of 300 IU is taken, this can be divided into:
a. 150 IU of rFSH + 150 IU of HMG if the basal LH levels are normal or
b. 300 IU of rFSH if the basal LH levels are elevated.

It is noteworthy that 150 IU of HMG has both 150 IU of FSH and 150 IU of LH component. Using exclusive HMG results in a 1:1 exposure of FSH and LH. The debate pertaining to the superiority of rFSH over HMG or vice versa is never ending. However, most studies have failed to shown any difference in the pregnancy rates between rFSH and HMG.

Ovulation Induction in Assisted Reproductive Technique: Agonist Protocols

Rohan Palshetkar, Biswanath Ghosh Dastidar, Nandita Palshetkar

Prevention of endogenous luteinizing hormone (LH) surge is an important component in any assisted reproductive technique (ART) cycle. This not only helps in scheduling the oocyte pickup but also averts the premature luteinization of follicles. The synthesis and release of LH is under the control of hypothalamic gonadotropin-releasing hormone (GnRH). Downregulating the GnRH receptors (agonist protocol) or blocking the GnRH receptors (antagonist protocol) prevents the endogenous release of LH.

This also ensures that the physician has the cycle under strict control of exogenous gonadotropins and is sure of the circulating levels of gonadotropins. Controlled ovarian stimulation with gonadotropins is started from day 2/3 of the menstrual cycle. Monitoring of the follicles should be done by ultrasonography (USG). The dose of gonadotropins should be altered according to response. The granulosa cells lining the growing graafian follicles, secrete the hormone estradiol into the blood stream. Hence serum estradiol levels also can be used in combination with follicular monitoring for evaluation of response to ovarian stimulation.

Gonadotropin-releasing hormone agonists have been widely used in infertility. GnRH agonists are decapeptide molecules that have a structure similar to endogenous GnRH but have altered amino acids at 6th and 10th position. This alteration in their structure significantly increases their affinity towards the GnRH receptors and increases their biological activity compared to the endogenous GnRH. Once the GnRH agonist attach to the receptors, they cause an initial flare response, that results in an initial increase in the serum follicle-stimulation hormone (FSH) and LH levels (Flare response). This can result in cyst formation in certain protocols. Once the initial flare settles, desensitization of receptors is achieved and downregulation is established. Pituitary desensitization usually occurs within 5 days of starting therapy with GnRH agonist and, therefore, prevents premature LH surge.

There are various agonist protocols that can be used. They are listed here in Table 1.

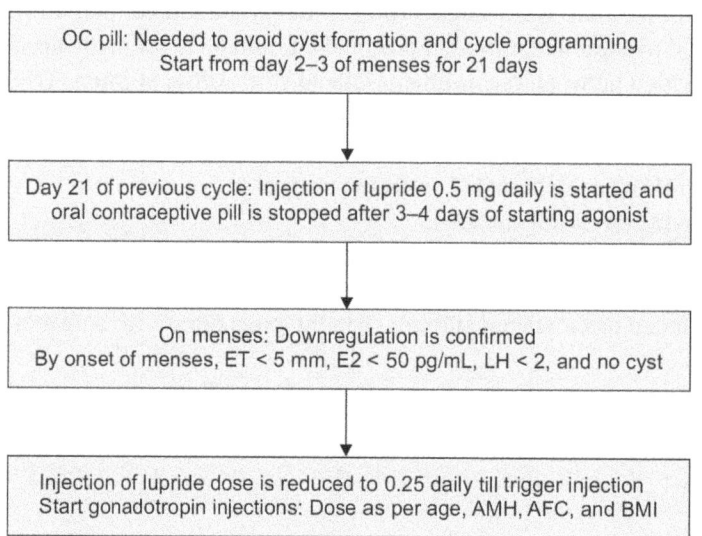

(AFC: antral follicle count; AMH: anti-Müllerian hormone; BMI: body mass index; ET: embryo transfer; LH: luteinizing hormone; OC: oral contraceptive; E2: estradiol)

TABLE 1: Various types of agonist protocols.

Protocols	Duration of administration	Route of administration	Starting day of GnRH agonist	Stopping day of GnRH agonist
Ultrashort	3 days	SC	D2 of cycle	D4
Short	8–12 days	SC	D2 of cycle	Day of trigger
Long follicular	28–35 days	SC	D2 of previous cycle	Day of trigger
Long luteal	21–28 days	SC	D21 of previous cycle	Day of trigger
Long follicular depot	Once	Depot	Single dose on D2 of previous cycle	
Long luteal depot	Once	Depot	Single dose on D21 of previous cycle	
Ultralong	8–12 weeks/Depot 2–3 times	SC/Depot		

(GnRH: gonadotropin-releasing hormone; SC: subcutaneous)

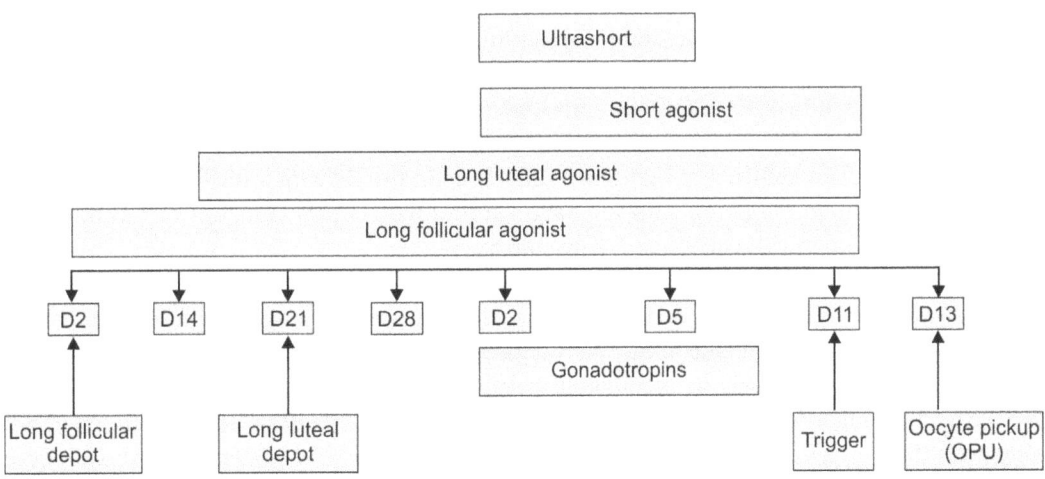

CHAPTER 67
Ovulation Induction in Assisted Reproductive Technique: Antagonist Protocols

Rohan Palshetkar, Biswanath Ghosh Dastidar

One of the most important advances in the clinical aspect of reproductive medicine was the introduction of gonadotropin-releasing hormone (GnRH) antagonists. Cetrorelix acetate is currently the most commonly used antagonist. GnRH antagonist are medications that have high affinity towards GnRH receptors and act by blocking the receptors completely once bound. They have a competitive inhibitory effect over the GnRH receptors that is rapidly reversible in the presence of higher levels of GnRH. The main advantage of the antagonist over agonist is that it creates immediate dose dependant suppression of the pituitary without any flare effect. Secondly, when a higher bolus of GnRH agonist is administered externally, the GnRH molecules can displace the antagonist from the receptor site and cause stimulation of the GnRH receptor releasing endogenous luteinizing hormone (LH). The same principle is applied for using GnRH agonists for ovulation trigger (release of endogenous LH causes the ovulation trigger.) The competitive blockage facilitates the prevention of premature luteinization besides enabling the physician to proceed with controlled stimulation of the ovaries by means of exogenous gonadotropins.

As the antagonist preparations cause immediate blockage of pituitary gonadotropin secretion, number of injections, which are administered, are lesser than agonist, thus improving patient compliance. These protocols are particularly favored for polycystic ovary syndrome (PCOS) patients and are superior in prevention of ovarian hyperstimulation syndrome (OHSS). Although there have been concerns over the impact of antagonists on the endometrium and eventual pregnancy rates, studies have not shown any significant difference in results with antagonists, if used appropriately. A Cochrane review concluded that compared with long-agonist protocol, GnRH antagonists substantially reduces the incidence of OHSS without reducing the likelihood of live birth.

There are many antagonist preparations available. The third generation antagonists have the least risk of anaphylaxis and edema making them safe and tolerable. There has been no documented teratogenic effects or impact on the quality of the oocyte even at higher dose. Minor side effects like headache, fatigue, nausea and malaise, etc. have noted that get settled once the medication is withdrawn. In an antagonist cycle, gonadotropin stimulation is started from day 2 or day 3 of menstrual cycle and antagonist (cetrorelix acetate, 0.25 mg daily) started either from day 6/7 of cycle or based on response [rising estradiol (E2) levels, usually above 500–600 or lead follicle > 14–15.9 mm]. It was observed that there was a decreased pregnancy rate when antagonist was started at E2 levels less than 300 or above more than 1,100. Correct timing for starting antagonists is crucial to in vitro fertilization (IVF) success as early or late initiation is likely to result in inadequate ovarian stimulation or premature luteinization, respectively.

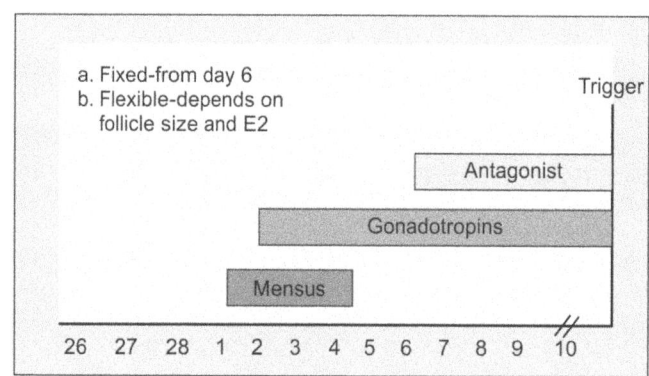

```
                    GnRH agonist
         1   2   3   4   5  [6]  7   8   9  [10]
         pyro(Glu)–His–Trp–Ser–Tyr–Gly–Leu–Arg–Pro–Gly–NH₂
         Activation of the    Increased GnRH      Biologic activity
          GnRH receptor    receptor affinity ~20x    increased
```

Generic names	Trade name	Half-life	Relative potency	Admin route	Recommended dose
Native GnRH			1	IV, s.c.	
Nonapeptides					
Leuprolide	Lupron lupride	90 min	50–80 20–30	S.c. IM depot	500–1,000 mg/d 3.75–7.5 mg/month
Buserelin	Superfact, supercure	80 min	20–40	S.c., nasal spray	200–500 mg/day 300–400 3 to 4 times/day
Histrelin	Supprelin	<60 min	100	S.c.	100 mg/day
Goserelin	Zoladex	4.5	100 50–100	S.c. S.c. implant	100 mg/day 3.6 mg/month
Decapeptides					
Nafarelin	Nasral synarel	3–4 hrs	200	Nasal	200–400 twice daily
Triptorelin	Decapeptyl	3–4.2 hrs	36–144	S.c. im depot	100–500 mg/day 3.75 mg/day

(GnRH: gonadotropin-releasing hormone; s.c.: subcutaneous; IV: intravenous; IM: intramuscular)

CHAPTER 68

Controlled Ovarian Stimulation in Assisted Reproductive Technique

Apoorva Pallam Reddy, Kathyaini VS

Evaluating FSH, LH, and E2 on the day 2 of cycle helps us in determining if the current cycle is capable of resulting in an optimal response and if yes what is the best stimulation regimen.

On the other hand, a good ultrasound examination sometimes may over power the need for performing a hormonal profile. Absence of any ovarian cysts or an endometrium thinner than 6 mm confirms a downregulated cycle and is sufficient to start stimulation. The hormonal profile, although preferred, is not mandatory before starting every stimulation.

A. *Role of FSH in controlled ovarian stimulation (COS):* Follicle-stimulating hormone (FSH) and luetinizing hormone (LH) both, in appropritate levels, are required for development of a healthy oocyte. In controlled ovarian stimulation, the ovaries are exposed to significantly higher doses of gonadotropins (GT) for longer duration of time resulting in an increased FSH window, thus stimulating multiple follicle growth. FSH stimulates the antral follicles to produce estrogen and increase the size of the follicle. Each follicle has an estrogen rich microenviroment that is required for a healthy mature oocyte. The dominance of estradiol (E2) and FSH in follicular fluid is essential for sustained accumulation in granulosa cells, continued follicular growth, and E2 production. Elevated levels of FSH on D2 of cycle is an indication of poor recruit of antral follicles and increased chances of poor response. Hence incase of elevated FSH administering one cycle of oral contraceptive pill (OCP) or waiting for a cycle with low FSH levels might be a better approach.

B. *Role of estradiol in COS:* The early appearance of estrogen within the follicle allows the follicle to respond to relatively low concentrations of FSH. Severe downregulated cycle with low E2 levels (<30 mg/mL) might result in suboptimal response. Estrogen priming for 1–2 days might increase the response.

C. *Role of LH in COS:* Role of LH in COS is a like a double edged sword. Neither too much nor too less is good for the COS. If the levels of LH are more than the FSH, there is more production of androgen from the theca cells compared to the conversion into estradiol in granulosa cells under FSH effect. This causes a androgen dominant milieu in the follicle leading poor oocyte quality or oocyte atresia (LH ceiling effect). If the LH levels are less than the threshold levels, then sufficient androgen is not produced which is a precursor for the estradiol synthesis resulting in failed follicular growth. Higher levels of LH as compared to FSH results in more number of immature oocytes [e.g. polycystic ovary syndrome (PCOS) patients having high basal LH levels, have higher chances of obtaining more number of immature oocyte specially if stimulated with human menopausal gonadotropin alone (HMG) instead of recombinant follicle-stimulating hormone (rFSH)]. Hence based on the basal LH levels the decision to add LH component in the form of either rLH or HMG is decided. LH component should be added from the beginning of the stimulation if the basal LH is <1 IU/mL. There is emerging evidence that adding LH component from the beginning of the cycle instead of in the middle of the cycle has higher reproductive outcomes even if the basal LH is in normal range. In women with elevated LH, stimulation is either started with rFSH alone or plan B can be followed.

D. *Role of P4 in COS:* The role of assessing progesterone (P4) value on d2 remains dubious. A recent meta-anlysis has concluded that patients who have P4 more than 1.5 ng/mL have less pregnancy rates as compared to the ones with P4 less than 1.5 ng/mL. The diagnostic value is questionable cause and there is no definitive change in treatment strategy. Elevated P4 values in day 2 are associated with poor pregnancy rates.

E. *Plan B*: When day 2 FSH, LH, E2, and P4 are elevated, two to three doses of 0.25–0.5 mg of gonadotropin-releasing hormone (GnRH) antagonist/day sc helps in normalizing the endocrine profile. This also helps in syncronizing the cycle partly. Any functional cyst noted can be aspirated, followed-up with GnRH antagonist and continue assisted reproductive technique (ART) stimulation.

F. The decision for total starting dose of GT is dependant on factors like age, body mass index (BMI), previous response, antral follicle count (AFC), and anti-Müllerian hormone (AMH).

G. It is advised to take the GT at the same time everyday maintaining strict cold chain.

H. The response to controlled ovarian stimulation is monitored by follicular study. The routine use of serum E2, LH, and P4 is not advised for evaluating response. If an adequate response is observed, no change in the dose is made. In case of a suboptimal response, consider increasing the dose and/or adding LH if not done. After a size of 12 mm, a healthy follicle grows at the rate of 1–2 mm/day.

I. In the initial GnRH antagonist dose finding studies, it was proposed that endogenous LH rise happens on day 6 of stimulation; however, recent studies suggest starting antagonist on day 5 of stimulation is suggested.
J. Ovulation trigger is given after documenting more than or equal to three dominant follicles of more than 17 mm.

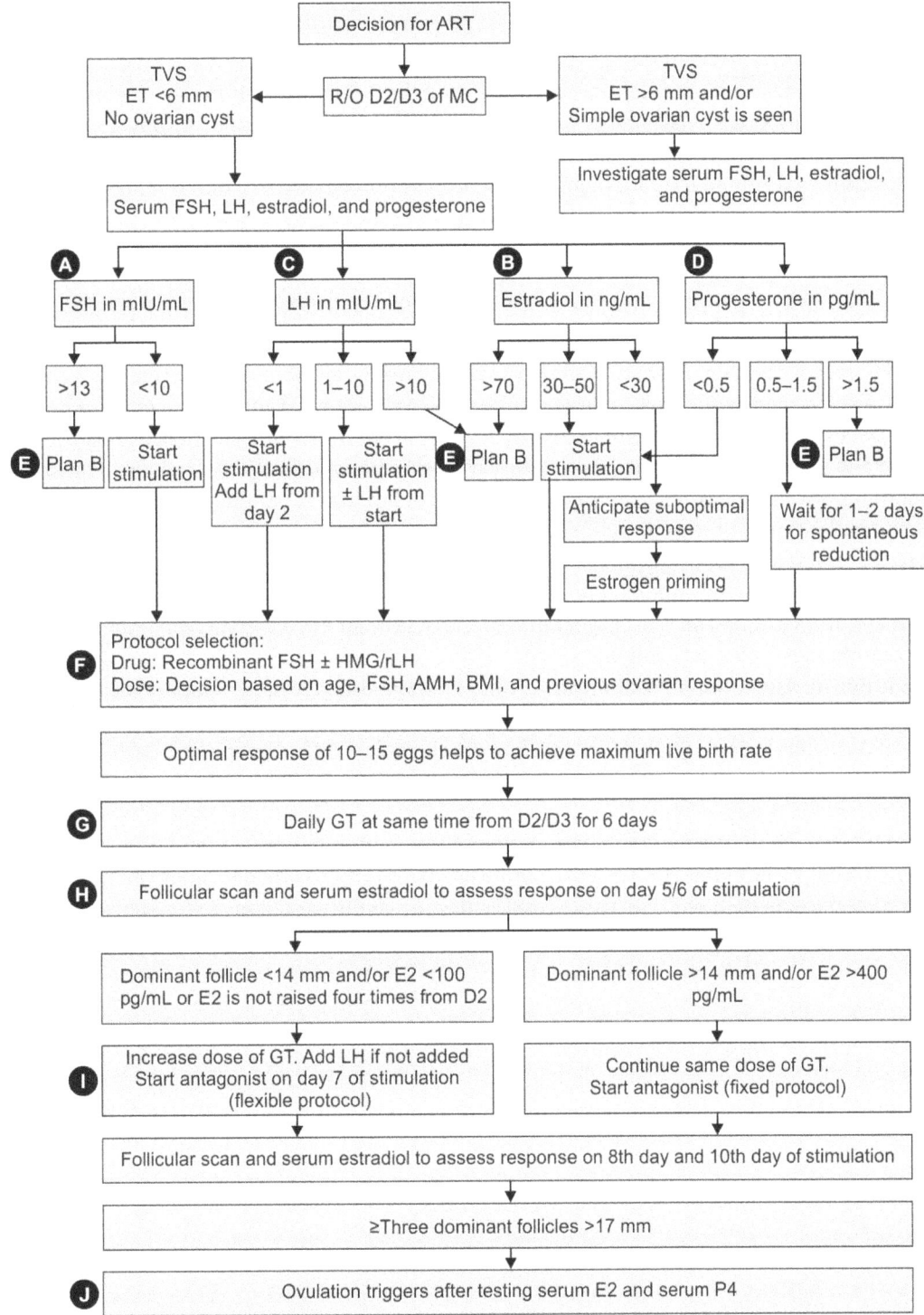

(AMH: anti-Müllerian hormone; ART: assisted reproductive technique; BMI: body mass index; E2: estradiol; ET: embryo transfer; FSH: follicle-stimulating hormone; HMG: human menopausal gonadotropin; LH: luteinizing hormone; rLH: recombinant luteinizing hormone; P4: progesterone; TVS: transvaginal sonography; MC: menstrual cycle; GT: gonadotropins; D2: day 2 of MC; D3: day 3 of MC)

CHAPTER 69

Mild Ovarian Stimulation

Aswathy Kumaran, Pratap Kumar

A. The idea of a mild ovarian stimulation is to produce better quality oocytes as compared to the conventional or high-dose stimulation that aim at obtaining maximum number of oocytes at one go. It consists of using either: (1) gonadotropins at lower than usual dose or for a shorter period of time with or without antagonist use; (2) oral agents are used alone or in combination with gonadotropins and antagonists.
B. Mild ovarian stimulation can be tried for high, normal, and poor responders. Proposed arguments favoring use of mild stimulation are:
   - *Poor responders*: It is suggested that higher cost of high-dose gonadotropins does not add value in poor responders.
   - Reducing cost and time commitment in normal responders.
   - Reducing risk of ovarian hyperstimulation syndrome (OHSS) in both high and normal responders.
   - Increasing gonadotropin stimulation may increase risk of chromosomal abnormalities in a dose-dependent manner. However, it has been shown that even in unstimulated cycles, about 36.4% of embryos can be aneuploidy.
   - *Controlled ovarian stimulation harms endometrium*: With the coming of vitrification many centers have adopted the free all policy to circumvent the problem of asynchrony of endometrium with high estrogen levels. Also, it may be ideal for a woman to maximize oocyte recovery from one stimulation so as to ensure a favorable cumulative pregnancy rate. Such a process may increase OHSS chances but with expanding options to avoiding OHSS, many doctors and patients may prefer this option.
C. Due to the lack of standardization in protocol there is deficiency of strong evidence supporting the efficacy of mild stimulation as compared to conventional protocol (basic dose of 225 IU/day). The anticipated response in a mild stimulation is 2–8 oocytes based on the category of responder. Presence of less than two dominant follicles is usually taken as the criterion for cycle cancellation.
D. The use of only oral ovulogens for mild stimulation is not recommended in view of higher incidence of cancellation.
E. Follicle-stimulating hormone (FSH) and human menopausal gonadotropin (hMG) can be used in combination or alone at a total dose not exceeding 150 IU starting early in the cycle (D4) or later in the cycle (D5). Use of exclusive gonadotropins mandates the use of gonadotropin-releasing hormone (GnRH) antagonist for preventing premature luteinizing hormone (LH) surge.
F. Use of both oral ovulogens and gonadotropins has the benefit of using endogenous gonadotropins as well as exogenous gonadotropins. Clomiphene citrate (CC) or letrozole are used from D2–6. Gonadotropins can be started concurrently from D4–5 or started sequentially on D7–8. Use of GnRH antagonist is not mandatory in this protocol. Some studies have shown clinical pregnancy rates to be better in cycles not using antagonist as compared to the cycles using antagonist.

Mild Ovarian Stimulation

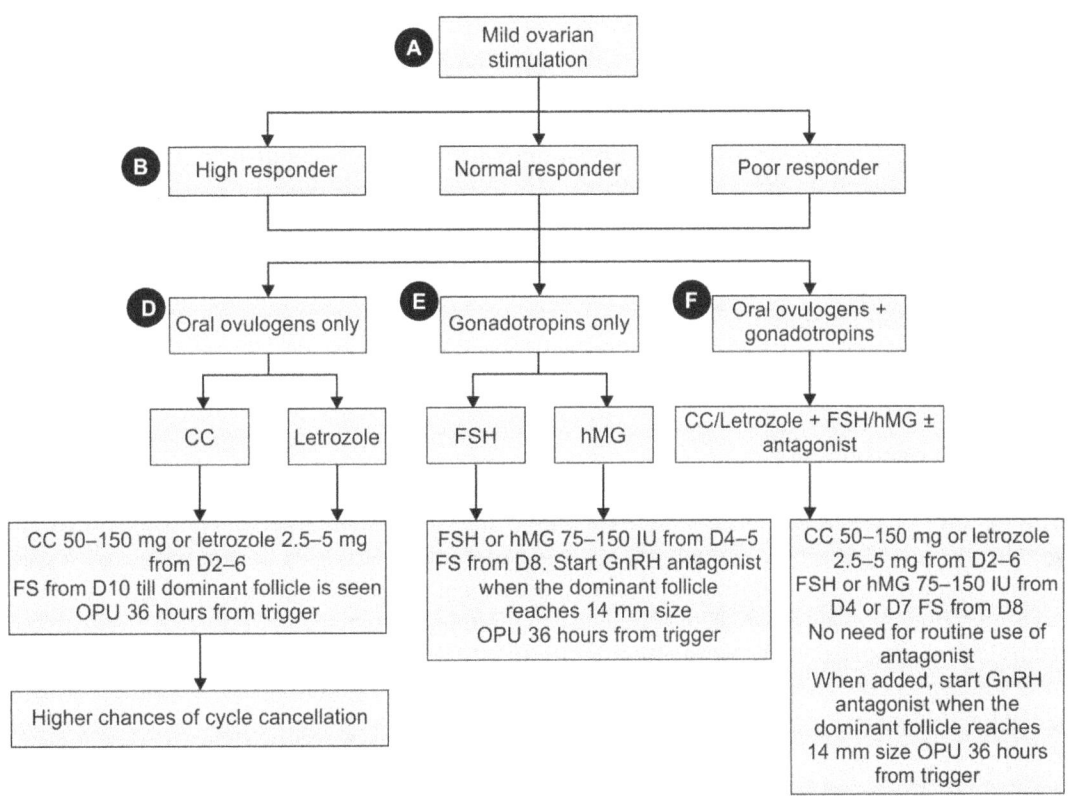

(FS: follicle size; CC: clomiphene citrate; FSH: follicle-stimulating hormone; GnRH: gonadotropin-releasing hormone; hMG: human menopausal gonadotropin; OPU: oocyte pickup)

CHAPTER 70

Role of LH in Controlled Ovarian Stimulation

Sankalp Singh, Vandana Ramanathan

INTRODUCTION

Although exogenous follicle-stimulating hormone (FSH) is the main regulator of follicular growth in stimulated cycles, luteinizing hormone (LH) plays a key role in promoting steroidogenesis and follicle development. As per the 2 cell 2 gonadotropin theory, in the early follicular phase, the theca cells have predominant LH receptors and the granulosa cells have mainly FSH receptors. Stimulation of LH receptors results in the synthesis of androgens from the theca cells. The androgens cant be converted into estradiol in theca cells due to lack of the enzyme aromatase. These androgens act as a substrate to the aromatization happening in granulosa cells under stimulation of FSH receptors. The granulosa cells cannot synthesize androgens from cholesterol due to lack of the enzyme P450 CYP 17. Thus, granulosa cells are dependant on the theca cells for the synthesis of androgens and theca cells are dependent on granulosa cells for the aromatization of androgens. Absence of adequate LH activity in the beginning of the cycle, results in low androgen production from the theca cells, low estradiol production in the granulosa cells, ultimately leading to failure in follicular growth. On the other hand in women with LH activity higher than the FSH activity in the beginning of the cycle (e.g. polycystic ovary syndrome (PCOS) pts have reversal in the FSH:LH ratio) there is more androgen that is being produced by the theca cells under the influence of LH compared to the aromatization happening in the granulosa cells under FSH influence. This results in an androgen predominant milieu in the follicle leading to follicular atresia.

A. *LH preparations available include*:
   - Recombinant LH (r-LH)—with only LH activity driven by pure LH
   - Human menopausal gonadotropin (HMG) 1:1 ratio of FSH/LH in which LH activity is driven by human chorionic gonadotropin (hCG)
   - Human chorionic gonadotropin
   - Combination of recombinant FSH and recombinant LH, with 2:1 ratio of pure FSH/LH activity.

   All these preparations have equal efficacy and there is no conclusive evidence yet for choosing one over the other.

B. *Hypogonadotropic hypogonadism*: Women of this subgroup (WHO Group I) do not have the threshold level of endogenous LH required to achieve optimal follicular development and steroidogenesis during therapy with FSH alone. They need a combination of FSH and LH to stimulate proper follicular growth and estradiol production. The follicles stimulated by FSH alone also do not consistently rupture after hCG administration, luteinize poorly, and oocytes may have a lower fertilization rate. A daily dose of 75 IU r-LH is sufficient for promoting optimal follicular development.

C. *Hyporesponders:* This condition is clinically evident in the form of an "initial slow response" or "stagnation" in follicle growth after 4-5 days of FSH administration in a normoresponder woman. The options in such a situation include either stepping up the dose of FSH or adding 75 IU of a LH containing preparation. The latter has been shown to be of considerable benefit in improving the in vitro fertilization (IVF) outcome.

D. *Advanced age*: Rationale for the use of LH in women with age more than 35 years: with increasing age, there is— (1) reduced function of LH receptors; (2) reduced androgen receptors; (3) reduced bioactive LH; and (4) reduced intraovarian paracrine activity. Some studies have shown that there is no significant benefit of adding LH in this subgroup of patients with respect to improvement in the live birth rate. But, there are also studies which have shown that addition for LH improves clinical pregnancy rate. Again, there is no consensus regarding the day from which the LH preparation has to be added, with some studies suggesting to start from day 1, and others from day 6 of controlled ovarian stimulation (COS). In clinical practice, since the addition of LH is unlikely to have any detrimental effect, we can consider starting LH from day 1 of COS.

E. *Poor responders:* There is biased opinion regarding the addition of LH in poor responders as few studies have shown benefit of adding LH in poor responders, and some have shown that it does not improve pregnancy rate. Due to heterogeneous nature of study designs, there is, as of now, no strong evidence backing the use of LH in this subgroup. Till such time, addition of LH from day 1 of COS should be considered.

F. Many authors have tried to suggest a cutoff for defining an LH threshold level in long agonist protocol needed for optimal follicular growth, but there is no single value which has proven to be of clinical benefit. Arguments against the need of LH in normogonadotropic women in long agonist protocol are: (1) normal LH level prior to downregulation is able to prime small follicles (LH>1 IU/mL); (2) Spare Receptor Hypothesis—less than 1% receptors need to be occupied for the action of LH; (3) suprapraphysiological levels of FSH may balance the lack of LH by inducing compensatory paracrine activity in granulosa cells. Studies have shown that there is no detrimental effect of low LH on cycle outcome in antagonist protocol. However, in clinical practice, it might be acceptable to add LH once the midfollicular LH level drops to less than 1 IU/L.

G. Rationale for LH priming in GnRH downregulated cycles, where LH supplementation is started 1 week prior to starting rFSH is—(1) LH receptor can be found on theca cells of preantral and antral follicles; (2) LH priming will increase the androgen levels and thereby increase the FSH sensitivity of the follicles. The studies done till date have failed to prove any benefit of LH priming in IVF.

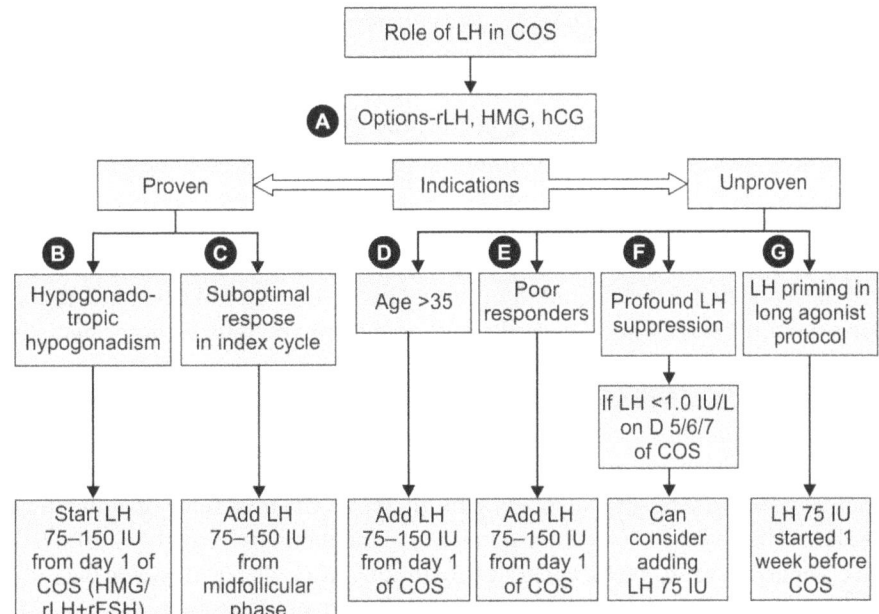

(COS: controlled ovarian stimulation; HMG: human menopausal gonadotropin; LH: luteinizing hormone; rLH: recombinant luteinizing hormone; rFSH: recombinant follicle-stimulating hormone)

2 Cell 2 Gonadotropin theory

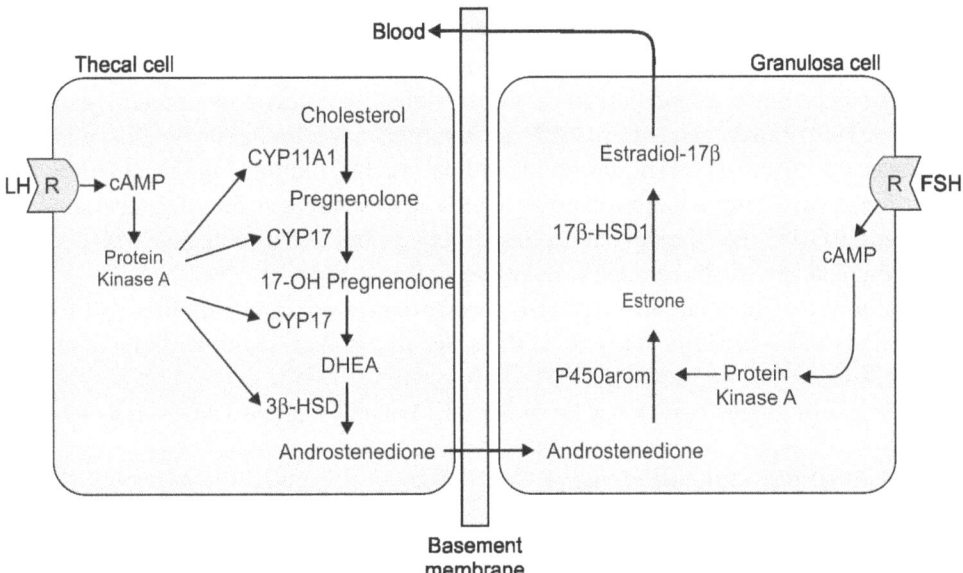

(LH: luteinizing hormone; cAMP: cyclic adenosine monophosphate; CYP17: cytochrome P450 17α-hydroxylase/17,20-lyase; 3β-HSD: 3β-Hydroxysteroid dehydrogenase; FSH: follicle-stimulating hormone; DHEA: dehydroepiandrosterone; OH: hydroxy; R: receptor; 17β-HSD: 17β-Hydroxysteroid dehydrogenases; P450arom: aromatase)

CHAPTER 71

Triggers for Ovarian Stimulation: IVF

Meenu Handa

Ovulation trigger in controlled ovarian stimulation ensures the final oocyte maturation, resumption of meiosis and separation of cumulus oocyte complex from the follicular wall into the follicular fluid. It is also imperative to choose the optimum time and type of the trigger to minimize complications of ovarian hyperstimulation and also maximize the yield of mature oocyte. Preovulatory luteinizing hormone (LH) surge plays a very important role in the resumption of meiotic arrest and leading to final maturity of metaphase II (MII) oocyte now ready for fertilization.

A. It is imperative to classify the patient based on their age, antral follicular count, anti-Müllerian hormone (AMH), and body mass index (BMI) as normoresponder, expected poor responder or hyper-responder before starting the stimulation. Type of anticipated trigger can determine the preferred stimulation protocol in some patients. In hyper-responders, antagonist protocols are preferred so that an agonist trigger can be given to avoid ovarian hyperstimulation syndrome (OHSS).

Human chorionic gonadotropin (hCG) shares a striking resemblance to the structural as well as biological molecule of LH and hence used as standard LH surrogate for triggering. An important difference is prolonged half-life of hCG (>24 hours, LH 60 min) due to delayed degradation caused by the presence of distinct C-terminal sequence.

B. Intensive ultrasound monitoring is a must. The total number of dominant follicles, intermediate follicles, and serum estradiol levels determine the type of trigger as well as timing.

C. Optimum time of trigger in assisted reproductive technique (ART) cycle is when mean diameter of 2–3 leading follicles of more than 17–20 mm is achieved.

D. When the total serum estradiol level is less than 3,000 pg/mL or the number of dominant follicles is less than 15, a conventional trigger using hCG is considered ideal as this increases the possibility of performing a fresh transfer.

E. Urinary hCG dose should be 5,000–10,000 IU intramuscular/subcutaneous for highly purified preparations. Studies have shown that in comparison to 10,000 IU, lower dose of urinary hCG of 5,000 IU yields the same number of meiotic II and similar ongoing pregnancy rates and minimizes risk of OHSS significantly.

F. Recombinant hCG dose of 250 μg is equivalent to 6,500 IU of urinary hCG. Similar ovulation rates (92% vs 86%) and clinical pregnancy rates are observed with recombinant hCG 250 μg and urinary hCG 5,000 IU administration. Also less local reactions are observed with recombinant hCG.

G. If more than 20 growing follicles are observed (>14 mm in size) and if serum estradiol levels >3,000 pg/mL, gonadotropin-releasing hormone (GnRH) agonist is preferred trigger to avoid risk of OHSS.

H. Gonadotropin-releasing hormone agonist can also be used as a trigger in vitro fertilization (IVF) cycles when using GnRH antagonist protocol. Some researchers have observed that he induced natural endogenous LH and follicle-stimulating hormone (FSH) surge, created by GnRH agonist trigger, is found to be beneficial for oocyte quality and maturity. It also takes the advantage of shorter half-life of natural LH, minimizing risk of OHSS. Doses used can be 0.2 mg triptorelin, buserelin 0.5 mg or leuprolide 1 mg. GnRH agonist has been found to have similar yield of MII with a significant decrease in OHSS risk. Though luteal phase has been found to be defective with GnRH agonist trigger, it can be well supplemented and can be rescued with aggressive luteal support.

I. If the patient hyperstimulates when stimulated with an agonist protocol, coasting technique (withholding gonadotropin stimulation) is applied or hCG is withheld to avoid OHSS. Significant drop in implantation rate is seen if coasting is done for more than 4 days.

J. Dual trigger (GnRH agonist trigger followed by low dose hCG 1,500 IU) can be also given to achieve adequate luteal phase.

K. Ovum retrieval is planned at 35–36 hours of trigger.

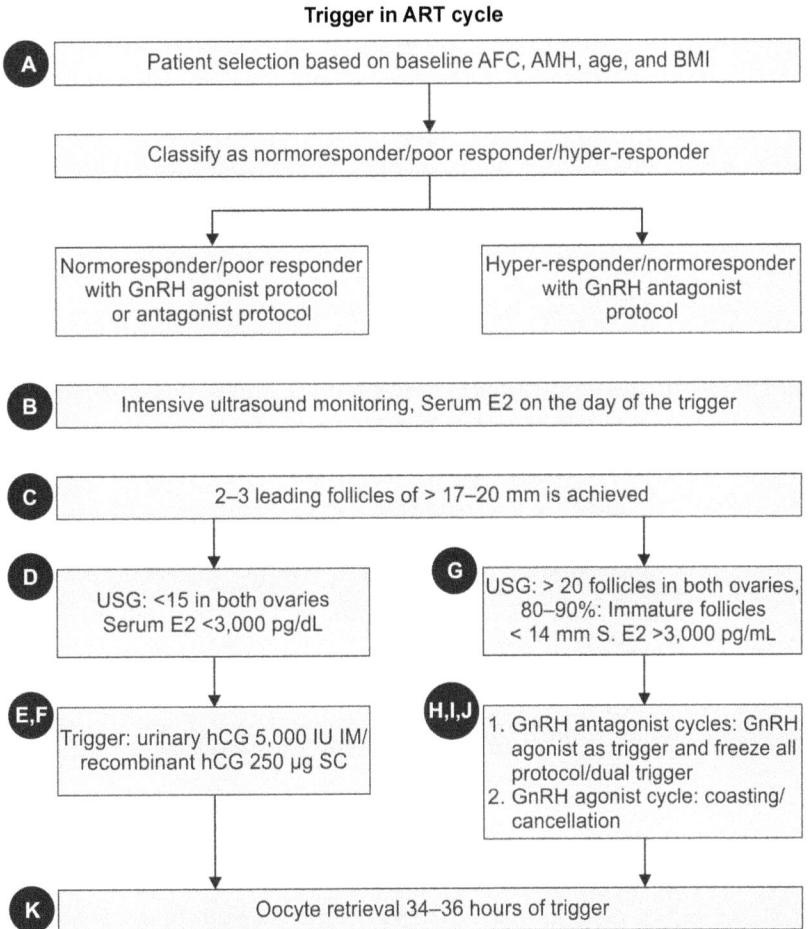

(AFC: antral follicle count; AMH: anti-Müllerian hormone; BMI: body mass index; E2: estradiol; GnRH: gonadotropin-releasing hormone; hCG: human chorionic gonadotropin; USG: ultrasonography; SC: subcutaneous)

Section 15: In Vitro Fertilization

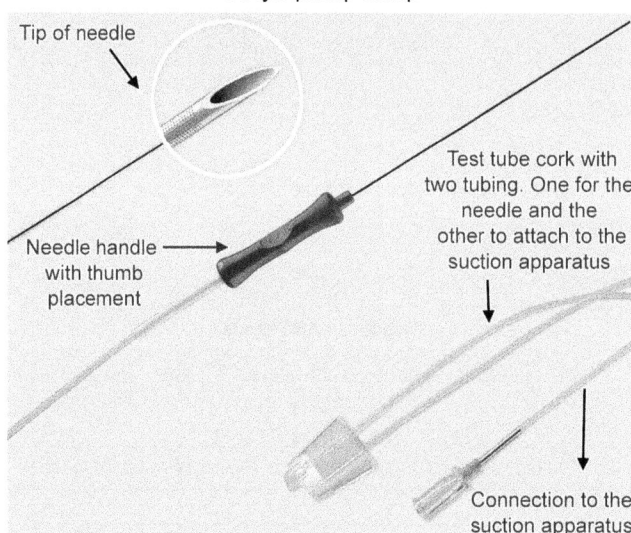

Oocyte pickup set up

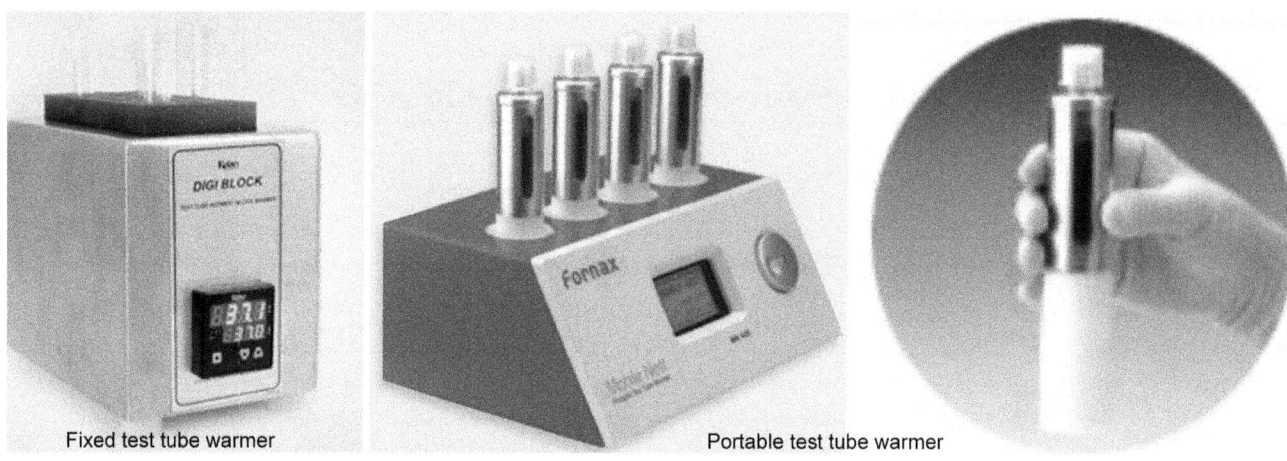

Fixed test tube warmer · Portable test tube warmer

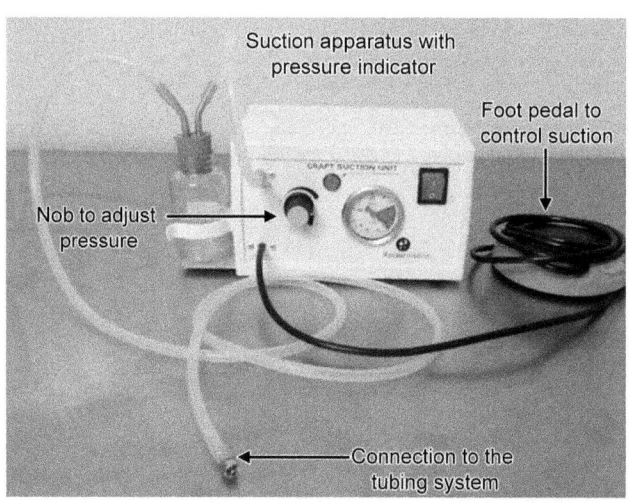

CHAPTER 72

Oocyte Pickup

Aditya Khurd, Vandana Khurd

A. Oocyte pickup (OPU) is one of the most important processes of assisted reproductive technique (ART) where the cumulus-oocyte complex (COC) are aspirated from the follicles. When first introduced all pickups were done laparoscopically which has progressed to doing in a much noninvasive technique like ultrasound guided aspiration. Timing the egg pickup from the trigger is crucial as the percentage of mature oocytes obtained can be increased by prolonging the interval between ovulation trigger and oocyte retrieval. Most pickups are scheduled at 35–36 hours from the trigger. In a meta-analysis by Wang et al. the fertilization rate, implantation rate, and pregnancy rate did not differ significantly between oocyte retrieval less than 36 hours after ovulation trigger and oocyte retrieval more than 36 hours after ovulation trigger. Waiting for longer than 36 hours increases the chances of follicular rupture thus effecting the final number of oocytes. There is no difference in determining the time of OPU based of the type of stimulation protocol used or the type of final ovulation trigger.

B. *Preoperative checklist*:
   - *Patient check*: Identity, consent, latest ultrasound report and hormone levels (if done), emptying bladder, and preoperative antibiotic prophylaxis.
   - *Equipment check*: Ultrasound machine, connection of tubing with needle and suction pump, aspiration of culture media with oocyte pickup needle, and suction and pressure check test tube warmer with temperature at 37°C.

C. Anesthesia for the procedure is usually with the help of intravenous (IV) propofol as it has antiemetic property and fast recovery. Other methods like acupuncture, nitrous oxide, and even local anesthesia have been used. Prolactin rise due to stress during OPU has in some reports been suggested to cause poor embryo development. The vaginal is cleansed using plain saline multiple times to remove any vaginal discharge. Use of antiseptic solutions like povidone iodine or savlon is strictly prohibited.

D. *Some practice tips to minimize complications*: Avoid multiple punctures to the vagina or the ovarian capsule. To avoid puncturing the great vessels, use color Doppler freely. Also, increase the gain of the machine to brighten the capsule of the ovary. When in doubt, see the cross-section and the longitudinal section of the entity. The follicle will remain oval or ovoid whereas vessel will take long tunnel-like picture.

E. Ovaries which are adherent to the uterus posteriorly may require the transcervical approach and when ovaries are posterior and adherent to the uterine fundus, a transmyometrial approach may have to be taken.

   E1 In a rare situation, ovaries which are high placed in the pelvis or near the abdominal wall, a transabdominal aspiration is easier and safer technique as compared to transvaginal pickup. Sufficient pressure with the ultrasound probe should be applied transabdominally to go as close to the ovary as possible to prevent inadvertent visceral injury.

   E2 Follicles should be aspirated in a sequential and systematic way to avoid missing out on any follicle from the ovary. Needle should be kept within the ovary as much as possible and maximum follicles should be aspirated in minimum pricks, to minimize the amount of trauma to the ovarian capsule. When follicles within one ovary are aspirated, the needle is withdrawn from the vagina and the needle is flushed with culture media to clear any blood. The other ovary is then aspirated.

F. Oocyte pickup needle should be thin enough to cause less pain but thick enough to recover maximum oocytes. One study compared 15 gauge, 17 gauge, and 18 gauge needles and found less pain with 18 gauge without compromising oocyte numbers. The diameter of the needle does not have any effect on the quality of the oocyte but may impact the time of procedure. Maintaining the right suction pressure is critical because if the pressure is too low the oocyte might not be aspirated and if the pressure is too high then the oocyte might be damaged. 100–110 mm of Hg is an ideal pressure. Before starting the actual procedure, aspirate in vitro fertilization (IVF) media into the needle and the tubing system. This helps in checking pressure as well as the dead space of 1–2 mL in the collecting system is filled. Thus preventing any damage to the oocyte in the process of collection. If pressure is not achieved, check for any cracks in the tube, if the aspiration system is attached tightly to the test tube or not, any kinking of the pipes and rotate the needle in the follicle to make sure that walls are not collapsed on the needle tip. The suction should be initiated only after the follicle is punctured. If started before entering the follicle there is a possibility of air being sucked in that might result in damage to oocyte—cappuccino effect. The suction should be maintained till the follicle is completely aspirated and the needle is out—this prevents the back flow of the oocyte or loosing the oocyte in pelvis due to fall in pressure. Each 20 mm size follicle has about 3-4 mL follicular fluid. Once the follicle is completely aspirated, the test tube collecting it should be changed. The change of the test tubes should ideally happen between each follicular aspiration and not between.

G. Aspirate the follicles that are in the periphery first and most accessible before moving on to others. The tip of the needle should be visible at all times to prevent any inadvertent damage to other pelvic structures. Once both ovaries are aspirated, a final check is done to see for the presence of any missed follicles. Intermediate follicles also may be aspirated to reduce the risk of OHSS. A Cochrane review looked at flushing versus simple aspiration for oocyte retrieval and found no difference in oocyte numbers or other clinical outcomes, but the operative time was significantly increased by flushing. The test tubes with follicular aspirates should be transferred to the laminar air flow for the embryologist to screen. All the COC are pipetted and transferred into the incubator to await IVF/ICSI.

H. *Complications*: Although the risk of serious complications due to OPU is quite low, various complications related to the procedure have been reported, including infection; bladder, bowel, appendix, and ureteral injuries; vaginal bleeding at the entrance of the needle; and minimal to massive bleeding due to needle injuries to pelvic veins. Other complications may result from the administration of IV sedation or general anesthesia.

I. Based on the number of cumulous-oocyte complexes picked, the response can be categorized as normal, suboptimal, poor, or hyper.

TIPS FROM EDITORS DESK

1. Before giving the trigger, always check for the availability of anesthetist and embryologist at the anticipated time of pickup.
2. Ask the patient to arrive 1-2 hours prior the pickup to avoid any last minute hiccups.
3. Ask the patient to empty bladder before entering the theater. This reduces the chances if inadvertent bladder injury during OPU as well prevents the need to empty bladder during the OPU.
4. Place the patient in low lithotomy position. This facilitates easy access to both vaginal and abdominal routes of OPU. Mild pressure from the abdominal region may be given to fix the ovaries.
5. The collection test tubes should be placed in the test tube warmer minimum 20 minutes prior to the actual pickup to maintain the optimum temperature for oocytes. Variation in the temperature can result in damage to the meiotic spindles and thus increasing the possibility of biochemical pregnancies and early pregnancy loss. Note that the part of the test tube inside the warmer is the only part maintaining temperature of 37°, hence follicular fluid should be collected only till that level and not to be filled till the brim. Once collected the test tubes should be immediately transferred in a temperature maintained test tube carrier or by hold in hand to the embryology lab for oocyte screening.
6. Once the follicle is punctured with the needle tip, make sure that the tip remains in the center of the follicle at all times. If the tips goes too close to the wall of the follicle, the collapsing wall can block the tip of the needle and prevent the aspiration of the follicle. When more than 75% of the follicle is emptied, the needle is rotated multiple times repeatedly to prevent the collapsing of the follicle wall over it and create a churn kind of movement that increases the chance of aspirating the COC.
7. At the end of procedure ensure complete hemostasis at the vault. Mild oozing can be controlled with pressure with gauze for 5-10 minutes. If active bleeding is seen, a couple of stitches with no. 1 vicryl may be needed.

Oocyte Pickup

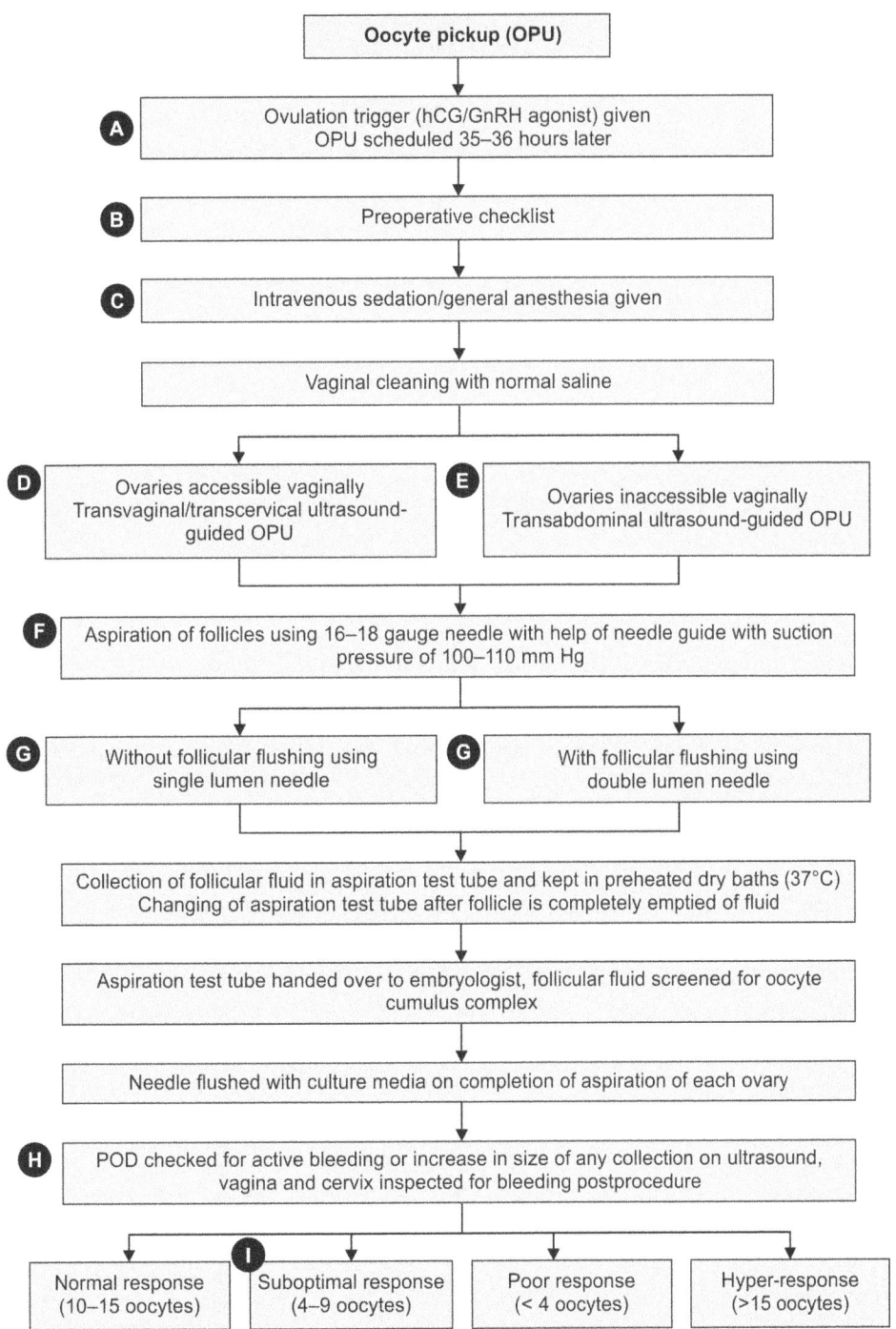

(GnRH: gonadotropin-releasing hormone; hCG: human chorionic gonadotropin; POD: pouch of doughlas)

CHAPTER 73

Embryo Transfer

Parasuram Gopinath, Kartika D Kumar

A. Embryo transfer (ET) is the process of depositing embryos in the uterus of a female with the intent to establish a pregnancy. Even though a simple procedure, it is considered as one of the most crucial steps in vitro fertilization (IVF).
B. The morphological assessment of the embryo is carried out on the day of transfer (i.e. day 2/3/5) and are graded according to the number, regularity of blastomeres, and percentage of fragmentation seen.
C. Endometrial receptivity is altered if the serum progesterone levels are elevated or in cases of thin endometrium with poor vascularity. The cutoff for serum progesterone beyond which an ET is canceled varies. In a fresh cycle 1–1.25 ng/dL is taken as cutoff. Whereas in a FET cycle 0.5 ng/dL is taken as the cutoff beyond which the probability of embryo implantation is reduced. The serum progesterone levels should be tested before giving the trigger in a fresh cycle or before starting progesterone supplementation in a FET cycle. Hence, a decision for transferring embryos is taken only if the desired levels of progesterone are noted are noted on the day of trigger or before starting progesterone supplementation.
D. The good quality embryos selected for transfer are transferred into a center well dish containing the transfer media and placed in the incubator until the transfer is performed and the remaining embryos are either cryopreserved or discarded after discussing with the patient and her partner. The poor quality embryos and unfertilized oocytes are discarded.
E. After identification and matching of patient and embryo(s), the patient is placed in lithotomy position with partially filled bladder which facilitates visualization of the uterus using transabdominal ultrasound (TAS). If the bladder is not adequately full, wait for another 15–20 minutes to improve the visualization. If the bladder is over distended, a catheter can be used to drain the bladder partially to ensure adequate visualization. A sterile cusco's speculum is used to visualize the cervix. Some clinicians have suggested the use of a warm speculum to reduce the discomfort for the client thus reducing the probability of uterine contractions. However, there is no evidence backing the same. Cleansing the vagina is usually done using normal saline. This is performed 2–4 times gently to clear any vaginal and cervical secretions or discharge. Use of bactericidal agents like povidone iodine is strictly prohibited as they are embryotoxic.
F. Prior to inserting the outer sheath of ET catheter, the cervix is cleansed with cotton swab to remove mucus from the endocervical canal. Presence of excess cervical mucous results in higher chances of retained embryos in the catheter post transfer. A sterile cotton swab, tuberculin syringe sans the needle or even a simple cotton swab can be used to remove the excessive cervical mucous. There is no added advantage of one agent over the other. The cervical canal may be flushed gently with IVF media making sure the median does not enter the uterine cavity. The outer sheath of catheter is guided through the cervical canal and placed at the level or just beyond the internal under ultrasound guidance.
G. Once the outer sheath has negotiated the internal os, the inner soft catheter is loaded with the embryos (after load technique). The inner catheter is irrigated with transfer media and aspirated in the following in sequence. First an air bubble, then medium containing embryo(s), and then again an air bubble (total volume of the earlier not exceeding 20–30 μL).
H. The loaded inner catheter is threaded through the outer sheath of the ET catheter into the endometrial cavity. Place the tip of the catheter in the upper or middle third of the endometrial cavity (i.e. the thickest part), no closer than 1 cm to the fundus.
I. Expel the embryo(s) with the microliter syringe, just enough to see both the air bubbles fall into the cavity along with the intermediate medium containing embryos. The catheter is withdrawn gently with a rotatory movement so as to prevent the re-aspiration of the expelled embryos. Maintain pressure on plunger to prevent backflow of embryos.
J. Check the catheter for retained embryos, if present reload and immediately retransfer embryos.
K. The patient can get up and leave immediately without routinely being provided any period of bed rest.
Symptoms such as slight cramping and spotting are rare, but may occur. The routine use of tocolytics before embryo transfer to reduce uterine contractions is not recommended. However, in case of recurrent implantation failure or

presence of myometrial waves on the ultrasound before transfer, use of atosiban (Atosiban is a receptor antagonist for oxytocin) can be considered. (Dose: 6.75 mg of intravenous bolus preparation over 1 minute, 30 minutes before the transfer followed by a infusion—18 mg in the 1st hour after ET followed by 12 mg in next 2 hours).

L. In cases of difficult transfer—(1) The cervical canal can be negotiated by using catheter with stylet or cervical dilator or (2) The catheter is introduced by gently pulling the cervix with a vulsellum.

M. In case of frozen thawed embryo cycles, the embryos are incubated for a period of 2 hours prior to transfer.

N. The use of analgesics and other techniques are used as needed for patient comfort but not for improving pregnancy rates.

The ASRM guidelines for number of embryos (fresh or frozen) to transfer

Characteristics	Number of cleavage stage embryos to transfer	Number of blastocysts to transfer
<35 years old, most favorable prognosis*	1–2 (1 recommended)	1
Other women < 35 years old	≤2	≤2
35–37 years old, more favorable prognosis*	≤2	≤2
Other women 35–37 years old	≤3	≤2
38–40 years old, more favorable prognosis*	≤3	≤2
Other women 38–40 years old	≤4	≤3
41–42 years old, favorable prognosis and all others	≤5	≤3

*(1) First IVF cycle, good quality embryos, and sufficient excess embryos for cryopreservation or (2) Previous IVF success. In donor oocyte cycles, the age of the donor is used to determine the number of embryos to transfer.

(ASRM: American Society for Reproductive Medicine; IVF: in vitro fertilization)

Effect of various interventions over the improving reproductive outcome

Interventions	Effect	Level of evidence (grade)
Ultrasound guidance	Recommended	A
Soft embryo catheter	Recommended	A
Bed rest	Not recommended	A
Acupuncture	Not recommended	B
Transcutaneous electrical acupoint stimulation	Equivocal	B
Routine antibiotic prophylaxis	Not recommended	B
Specific type of glove usage	Not recommended	B
Removal of cervical mucus	Recommended	B
Correct embryo transfer (ET) catheter placement in the upper or middle area of uterine cavity > 1 cm from fundus	Recommended	B
Immediate withdrawal of embryo catheter	Recommended	B
Mucus on catheter tip after ET	Does not affect pregnancy rates	B
Retained embryos and retransfer	Does not affect pregnancy rates	B
Use of analgesics	Equivocal	C
Routine anesthesia	Not recommended	C
Blood on catheter tip after ET	Does not affect pregnancy rates	C
Injection speed of the catheter at time of ET	Insufficient evidence	C
Chinese medicine	Equivocal	C

Embryo Transfer

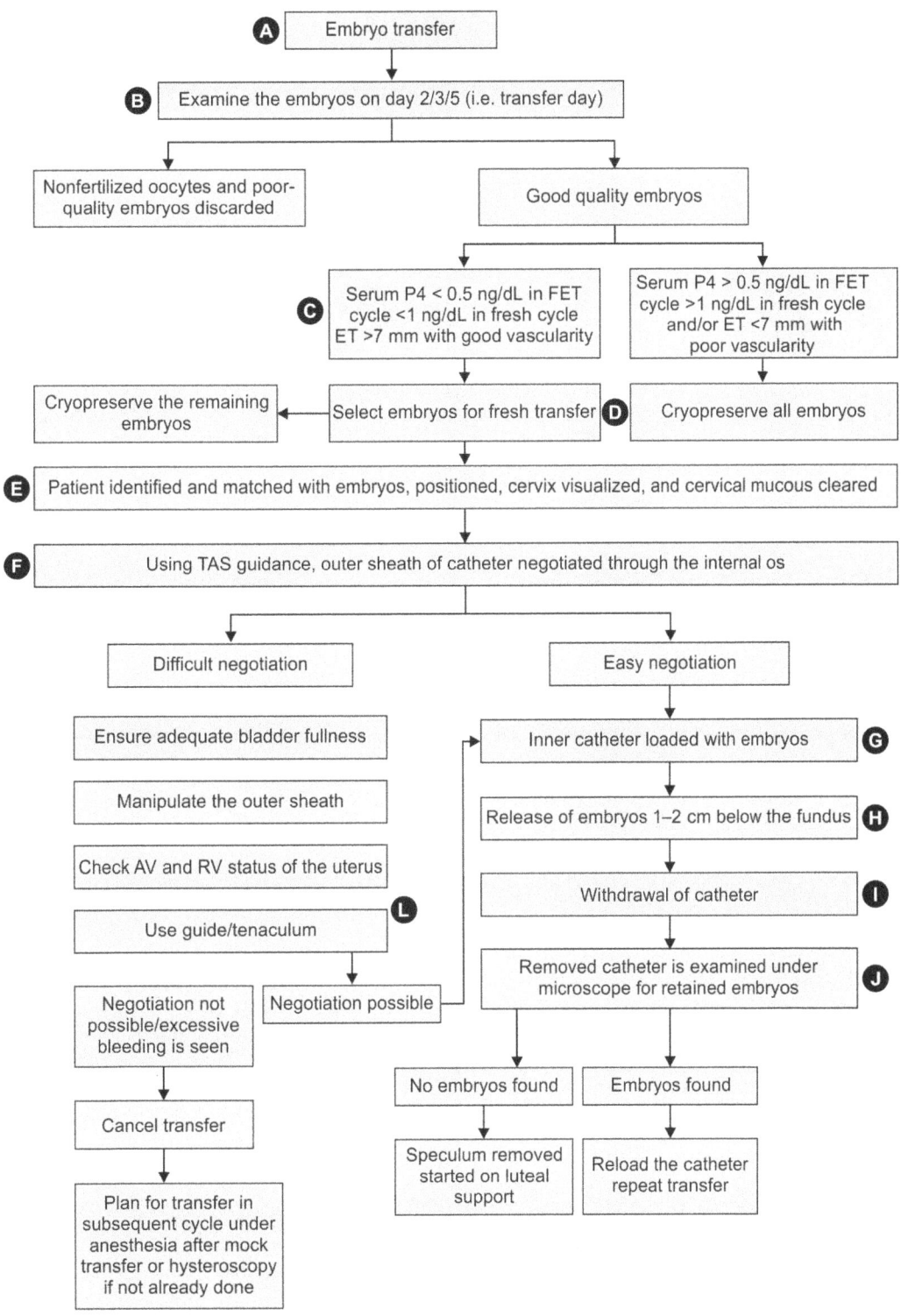

(ET: embryo transfer; P4: progesterone; TAS: transabdominal ultrasound; AV: anteverted; RV: retroverted)

Section 15: In Vitro Fertilization

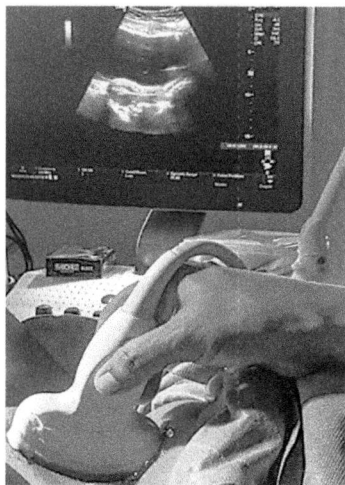

Ultrasound guidance significantly improves the pregnancy rates

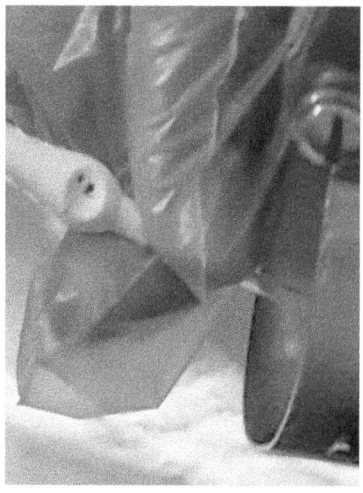

Thumb rest on the embryo transfer catheter is in sync with the direction of catheter tip.
If the direction of the tip is not maintained there is increased chances of ectopic pregnancy

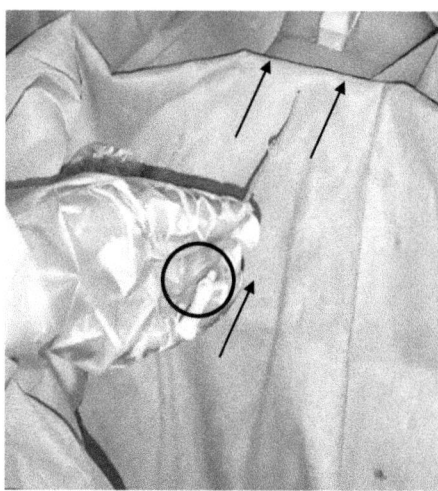

With Thumb rest in the center, the direction of release of embryos is forward

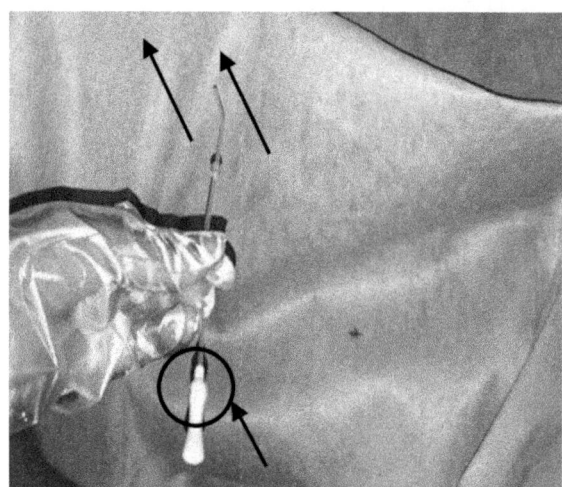

With Thumb rest to left side, the direction of release of embryos is towards left cornu

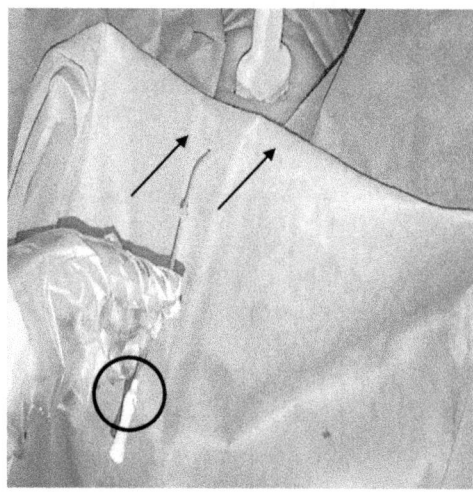

With Thumb rest to right side, the direction of release of embryos is towards right cornu

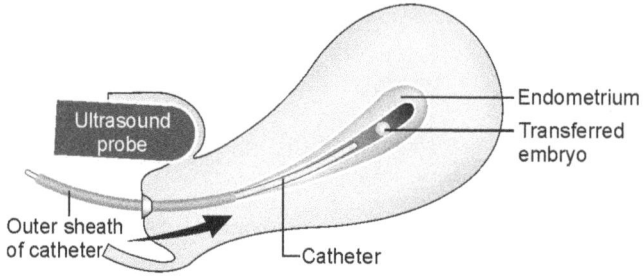

Placing the embryos 1–2 cm below the fundus increases conception rates

CHAPTER 74

Luteal Phase Support in IVF

Aarti Deendayal, Hema Desai

LUTEAL PHASE SUPPORT

Luteal phase deficiency (LPD) is insufficient endogenous progesterone required to manage the predecidual changes in endometrium to support the implantation and growth of the normal embryo. Research suggested LPD as a clinical entity and an etiological factor for subfertility, implantation failure, and recurrent miscarriages. The exogenous supplementation of progesterone (Luteal phase support: LPS) is capable of supporting the pregnancy and minimizes the pregnancy loss.

A. The disruption of corpus luteum and eventual LPD in a fresh cycle assisted reproductive technique (ART) occurs due to the supraphysiological levels of serum estradiol causing the premature luteolysis. This interferes with normal corpus luteum function, necessitating LPS.

B. In frozen embryo transfer (FET) cycles, due to absence of physiological corpus luteum, external progesterone needs to be supplemented till the embryonic placentation is self-sufficient (8–12 weeks). Apart from these, low follicle-stimulating hormone (FSH), altered luteinizing hormone (LH): FSH ratio, progesterone receptor resistance, thyroid and prolactin disorders, polycystic ovarian disease (PCOD), obesity, and endometriosis also manifest LPD.

C. Time of initiation is debatable. The general consensus is for the onset of administration immediately after the oocyte pickup (OPU). Lower implantation and pregnancy rates have been observed when intramuscular (IM) progesterone is started a day before oocyte retrieval. This might be due to advancement in the secretory transformation of the endometrium with an early closure of the window of receptivity. In FET cycles, after adequate endometrial preparation, progesterone is started 3 and 5 days prior to the day of embryo transfer (e.g. for a day 3 embryo transfer on Saturday, progesterone is started on Wednesday; for day 5, progesterone supplementation is started on Monday).

D. Luteal phase support is the administration of progesterone externally to maintain the normal secretory endometrium necessary for the implantation and growth of embryo. There is no evidence to support the use of progesterone in natural cycles. Progesterone use for LPD has shown to improve the implantation rate, ongoing pregnancy rate, and live birth rate (LBR).

There are various routes of progesterone administration, each with its own agreement and disagreements.

D1 *Progesterone intramuscular preparation* is oil-based, which is painful with local inflammatory reaction and sometimes leads to abscess formation. This route is found to be effective with high bioavailability. Minimal dose of 25 mg/day to 50 mg daily is needed to achieve predecidualization.

D2 *Oral administration of micronized progesterone* is generally not preferred because of its rapid liver interaction and systemic side effects. Excessive drowsiness and gastrointestinal upset are common side effects. Oral dydrogesterone 20 mg/day is the preferred form of synthetic progesterone commonly used.

D3 *Vaginal route of administration* is well-accepted and found to be effective. It is very effective due to its direct transport across the vaginal endothelium. The micronized progesterone is available as pessaries and hydrophilic gel. Its effect is short-term and has poor bioavailability. The pessaries need to be used 2–3 times a day with a dosage of 200–800 mg in divided doses. The gel is used only once daily in a 90 mg prefilled syringe in slow release form.

Of late much attention is focused on subcutaneous (SC) administration of progesterone, a *water-soluble preparation* in cyclodextrin. The progesterone is encapsulated in cyclodextrin, with high polarity. In the body, cyclodextrin gets digested and liberates the free progesterone into the circulation. This has become a new therapeutic effective alternative to IM and vaginal administration. The use of a daily dose of 25 mg SC progesterone is calculated to be effective to achieve good predecidual changes.

E. Gonadotropin-releasing hormone agonist (GnRH-a) are also tried as LPS. It acts as a luteotrophic agent, stimulating endogenous secretion of FSH and LH from the pituitary. It enables early diagnosis of pregnancy, improves LBR, and clinical pregnancy rate. GnRH-a is given as a single injection (0.1 mg triptorelin) or intranasal spray (buserelin 200 µg) on day-6 of oocyte pickup.

F. Oral estrogen administration for LPS is controversial. Both estrogen and progesterone affect the quality of endometrium and thereby the implantation of embryo. Sufficient estrogen levels are important in inducing progesterone receptors in the endometrium. Serum estrogen may be depleted post-OPU due to aspiration of granulosa cells in oocyte retrieval stimulation. Oral estradiol valerate 2–4 mg/day is used along with progesterone. Oral administration is better avoided in women with high risk of venous thromboembolism. Transdermal patch of estrogen provides better bioavailability and is safe due to its hepatic bypass.

G. Luteal phase support with human chorionic gonadotropin (hCG) administration stimulates the corpus luteum to increase the endogenous synthesis of estrogen and progesterone in ART cycles. It may also enhance implantation rates. However, the potential risk factor here is of moderate to severe ovarian hyperstimulation syndrome (OHSS). The risk of OHSS is found to be twice as higher with hCG than with progesterone. hCG is essential in luteal phase of women with hypogonadotropic hypogonadism undergoing ovulation induction. The rate of miscarriages, multiple pregnancies, and live birth rates are found to be similar between hCG and progesterone groups. There is no advantage of combining both the regimes.

H. Adjuvants like glucocorticoids showed better pregnancy rates, however, there is no evidence to support its usage. Aspirin is empirically used as LPS and is thought to improve blood flow to the endometrium. Its use inhibits cyclooxygenase (COX), which is essential for implantation. However, due to lack of robust evidence, it is not routinely recommended. Low molecular weight heparin (LMWH) is thought to improve the pregnancy outcomes, in a subgroup of patients with antiphospholipid antibody (APLA) syndrome. The injudicious use of aspirin or heparin should not be practiced. The endometrium or uterine lining—was considered a sterile environment for a very long time. We now know that there is a unique community of bacteria that reside in the uterus, like almost everywhere else in the body. Studies have shown that *Lactobacillus*-dominance in the endometrium led to a significant increase in success rates of IVF implantation, pregnancy, and live birth. Taking a high-quality probiotic containing *Lactobacillus* spp. and *Bifidobacterium* spp. daily helps to promote colonization of the vagina.

I. Luteal phase support can be stopped after 8 weeks once fetal heart rate (FHR) is detected in fresh cycles and by 12 week in FET cycles. However, LPS duration may be tailored to individual preference.

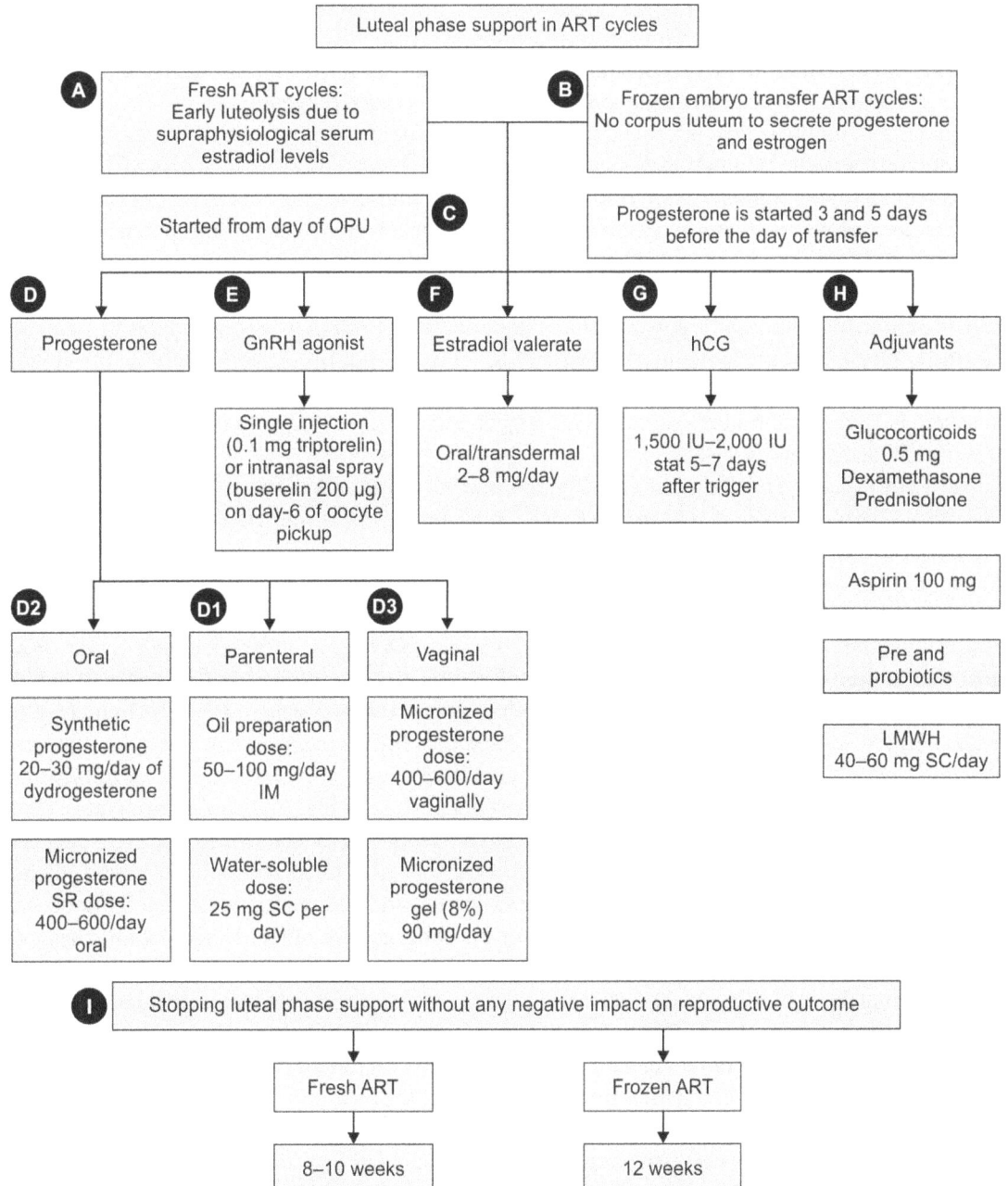

(ART: assisted reproductive technique; GnRH: gonadotropin-releasing hormone; hCG: human chorionic gonadotropin; LMWH: low molecular weight heparin; OPU: oocyte pickup; IM: intramuscular; SR: sustained release; SC: subcutaneous)

CHAPTER 75A

Diagnosis of Ovarian Hyperstimulation Syndrome

Kavitha Gautham

A. Ovarian hyperstimulation is a serious yet rare complication as a result of controlled ovarian stimulation as a part of assisted reproductive technique (ART) procedures. Mild and moderate hyperstimulation is more commonly seen as compared to severe grades which can be life threatening if not managed diligently.

B. Understanding the pathophysiology is crucial in the management of ovarian hyperstimulation syndrome (OHSS). Vascular endothelial growth factor (VEGF) and many other proangiogenic growth factors that are secreted by the granulosa cells of the dominant follicle are responsible for the pathophysiology of OHSS. These factors increase the global vascular permeability resulting in accumulation of fluid into extravascular or third spaces like peritoneal cavity, pleural cavity, pericardial cavity, and dependent edema. The shift causes hemoconcentration and reduced perfusion to the renal and hepatic tissues leading to low protein synthesis, elevated liver enzymes, oliguria, or anuria and higher probability of venous thrombosis. Human chorionic gonadotropin (HCG), which is commonly used for ovulation trigger, seems to play a central role in the pathophysiology of OHSS. It is proposed to increase the circulating levels of VEGF, messenger ribonucleic acid (RNA) and other angiogenic factors aggravating the symptoms. The symptoms are most severe 8–10 days after administering HCG trigger. Studies have shown that withholding HCG, completely eliminates the risk of developing OHSS.

C. All women must be evaluated for the risk of OHSS before starting ovarian stimulation. Younger women with low body mass index (BMI), high anti-Müllerian hormone (AMH), high antral follicle count (AFC), elevated serum estradiol on the day of trigger (>4,000 pg/mL), multiple dominant follicles, or higher intermediate follicles on the day of trigger are all considered risk factors for development of OHSS.

D. Evaluating the risk of OHSS before starting ovarian stimulation helps in determining the suitable stimulation protocol. The incidence of OHSS in ovulation induction with oral ovulogens, although extremely rare is not unheard of. Starting stimulation with lower doses of oral ovulogens and/or gonadotropins (least effective dose possible) should be considered for all cases of ovulation induction for intrauterine insemination. When considering for in vitro fertilization (IVF) stimulation, use of antagonist cycle for pituitary suppression gives the opportunity to use gonadotropin-releasing hormone (GnRH) agonist for ovulation trigger, thus avoiding the administration of HCG. Studies have shown that withholding HCG significantly reduces the risk of OHSS. In the same lines, clinicians have considered the use of recombinant luteinizing hormone (LH) for ovulation trigger instead of HCG to decrease the risk of OHSS. The main advantage of recombinant LH (rLH) is that it can be used for all types of ovarian stimulation including clomiphene citrate, letrozole, gonadotropins, GnRH agonist cycles, and GnRH antagonist cycle without compromising the possibility of pregnancy in the concurrent cycle. On the contrary, use of GnRH agonist for trigger significantly reduces the possibility of pregnancy in the concurrent cycle, hence advised to either opt for a freeze all protocol or consider use of small doses of HCG (1,500–2,000 IU) to salvage premature luteolysis (Humaidan protocol). Reducing or with holding the subsequent doses of gonadotropin (Coasting technique) although reduces the risk of OHSS, also is considered to reduce the total number of oocytes obtained. Medical therapy with metformin, cabergoline, aspirin, letrozole and sometimes even montelukast is proposed to reduce the incidence of onset as well as severity of disease. Letrozole is considered to reduce the synthesis of estradiol levels and thus reduce the chances of OHSS. Reducing the total number of embryos transferred decreases the incidence of late onset OHSS (OHSS in the 1st trimester of pregnancy as consequence of endogenous raise in HCG). Administering 1000 ml of 6% HES hydroxyethyl starch over 60 minutes within in 4 hours of oocyte pickup (OPU) significantly reduces the probability of OHSS.

E. Diagnosis of OHSS is made using signs and symptoms of hypovolemia and generalized edema. The severity is assessed by testing for complete blood count, serum electrolytes, liver function tests, and renal function tests.

F. Assessing the severity of the disease helps in planning the management ahead.

Diagnosis of Ovarian Hyperstimulation Syndrome

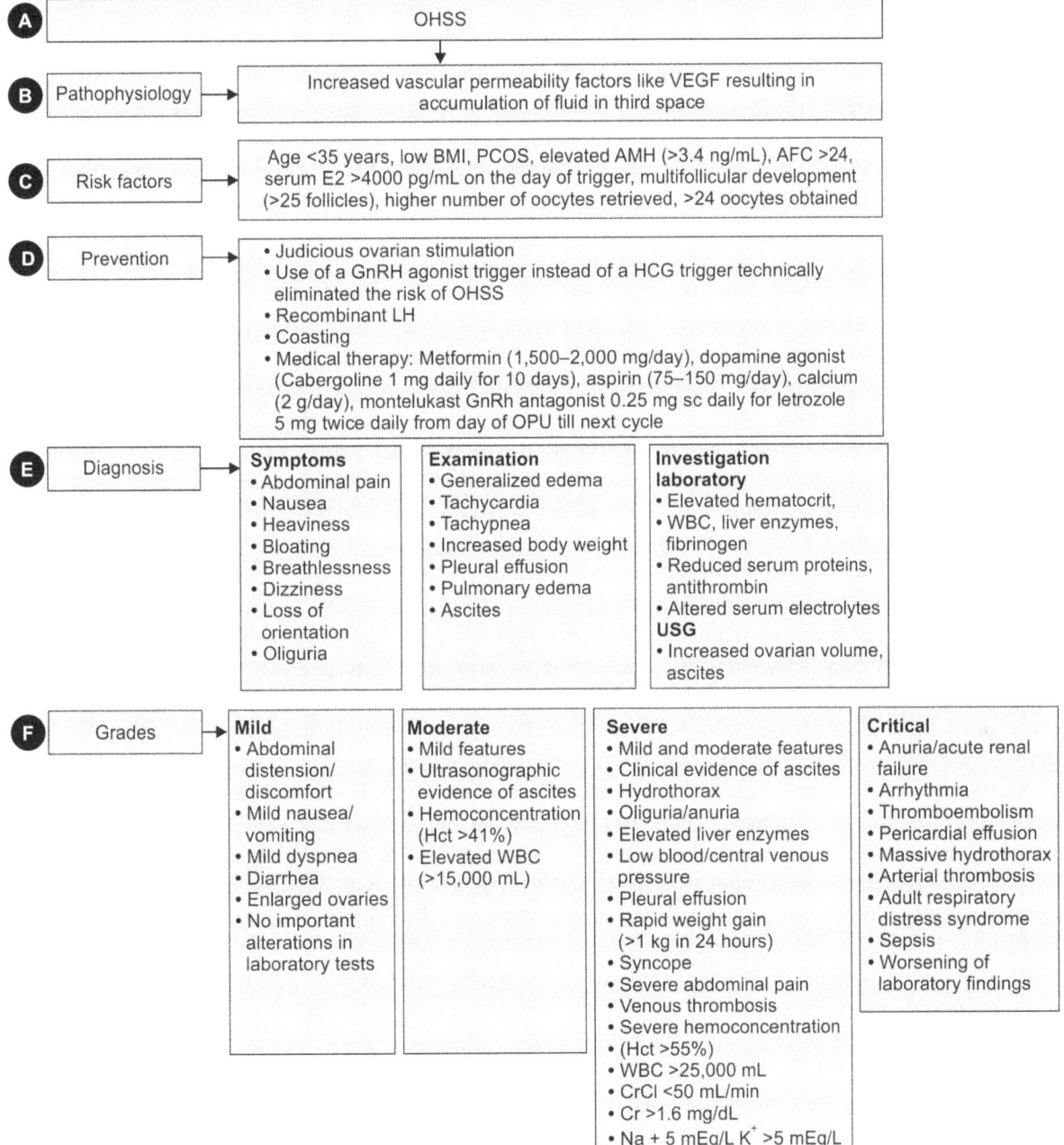

CHAPTER 75B

Management of Ovarian Hyperstimulation Syndrome

Apoorva Pallam Reddy, Rajeev Agarwal

A. Mild and moderate cases of OHSS can be managed on outpatient department (OPD) basis. Symptomatic management with analgesics and antiemetics with protein rich diet helps in improving symptoms. Close monitoring with hematocrit and white blood cell (WBC) count assessment helps in picking up severe cases early. Even a 2% raise in hematocrit (HCT) value from 45% to 47% can have deleterious effects, hence should be considered trigger for admission.

B. Use of crystalloid solutions in management of OHSS is a double-edged sword. It helps in maintaining the intravenous volume and thus improves renal perfusion. However, due to increased vascular permeability and loss of intravascular protein into third space, the fluid eventually shifts into third space. Hence, judicious use of isotonic solutions is warranted. When adequate fluid balance is not maintained, then colloid solutions should be administered to maintain adequate urine output and hematocrit less than 45%. 1.5–3 liters of fluid replacement might be required per day to maintain renal perfusion and urine output. Colloid preparations like albumin and starch increase the colloid oncotic pressure of the intravascular system thus reducing the shift of fluid into the third space. Use of GnRH antagonist also causes endogenous suppressions and reduces the severity of OHSS. 0.5 mg daily for 5–10 days depending on the symptoms reduces the severity.

C. Renal hypoperfusion causes reduced glomerular filtration, hyperkalemia, hypernatremia, oliguria, and finally anuria with renal failure. Hence, monitoring renal output using catheterization is useful. Less than 30 mL/hour of urine output is detrimental. Furosemide is a diuretic that reduces the total fluid volume in the body even from the third space and improves the urine output. However, furosemide should be always given in combination with colloid preparations that help in maintaining intravascular volume otherwise it can cause further rise in hemoconcentration. Dopamine infusion also improves renal perfusion.

D. Aspiration of ascitic fluid helps in reduction of the intra-abdominal pressure, improvement of symptoms of pressure, and increased renal output. Tense ascites, severe oliguria, anuria, and rising levels of serum creatinine are some indications for performing paracentesis. This can be done both abdominally or vaginally under ultrasound guidance. A maximum of 4 L of fluid can be aspirated at one go. Paracentesis is contraindicated in hemodynamically unstable patients or in cases of suspected hemoperitoneum. Even after paracentesis, there is continued shift of fluid from the intravascular spaces to peritoneal cavity. To overcome this, the technique of peritoneo-venous shunting was suggested where ascitic fluid that is rich in protein content is recirculated into the intravascular spaces.

E. Hemoconcentration increases the risk of venous thromboembolism. Hence use of heparin prophylaxis (prophylactic enoxaparin = 40 mg/day) is warranted in severe and critical cases of OHSS. In the presence of suspected deep venous thrombosis or pulmonary embolism, therapeutic doses of heparin (therapeutic enoxaparin = 1.5 mg/kg/day) should be initiated.

F. A multidisciplinary approach involving a hematologist and intensivist should be practiced for the management of severe and critical cases of OHSS.

Management of Ovarian Hyperstimulation Syndrome

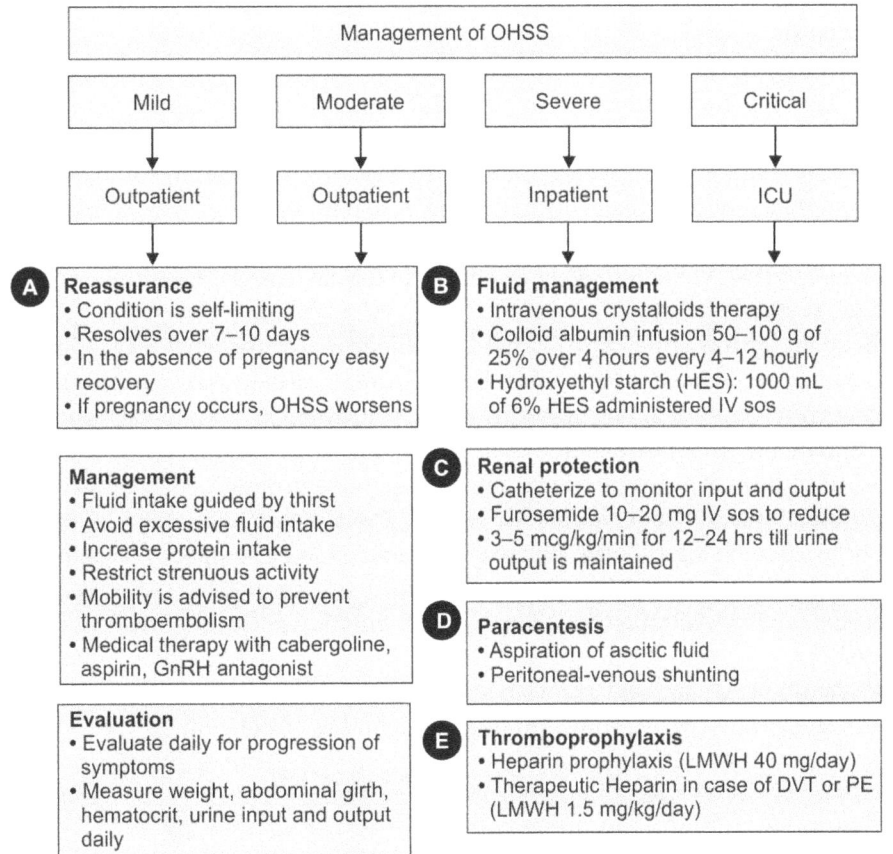

(DVT: deep vein thrombosis; GnRH: gonadotropin-releasing hormone; ICU: intensive care unit; LMWH: low molecular weight heparin; OHSS: ovarian hyperstimulation syndrome; PE: pulmonary embolism)

CHAPTER 76A

Batch In Vitro Fertilization

Parikshit Tank, Jaydeep Tank

A. Batch in vitro fertilization (IVF) is required in practice for centers which do not have a full-time embryologist capable of handling all the aspects of assisted reproduction. It is also a desirable practice for centers where a full-time embryologist is available for reasons such as maximizing efficiency of utilizing medium, manpower, medical tourism, and even avoiding weekends. The first step to making an IVF batch schedule is to fix the date of the embryo transfer (ET).

B. The oocyte pickup (OPU) should be done 2–3 days before the ET. There is flexibility here for 2–3 days between OPU and ET depending on center's preference, travel schedule of the visiting embryologist/assisted reproductive technique (ART) team, and workload.

C. As per standard practice, the trigger time is calculated as 35 hours before the OPU is scheduled. The choice of trigger is based on risk of ovarian hyperstimulation. The time schedule is same whether human chorionic gonadotropin (hCG) or gonadotropin-releasing hormone (GnRH) agonist trigger is used.

D. Considering an average responder, the average number of days of gonadotropin stimulation needed is 9–10 days. The day of starting stimulation is calculated by deducting 9–10 days before the day of trigger. We prefer antagonist cycles for the sake of safety, flexibility of trigger choice, and universal applicability without compromising the results. Stimulation is with menopausal gonadotropin or recombinant follicle-stimulating hormone (FSH) and the antagonist is added on day 6 of the stimulation.

E. Our choice for scheduling the menstrual cycle is a 30-μg combined oral contraceptive (COC) pills. It should be stopped 7 days before stimulation is scheduled to begin. This allows a withdrawal bleed to occur and gives enough time for COC washout. The concept of a 7-day washout is derived from the standard pill-free interval, which should suffice ovarian and endometrial restoration. Alternative protocols for scheduling such as luteal phase estradiol, varying the day of trigger, and the use of antagonist before starting stimulation have been described. They all have the same efficacy in scheduling and pregnancy rates are not affected.

F. The COC should be given for at least 15 days before it is scheduled to be stopped. This allows the withdrawal bleed to be predictable. The COC can be given for any length of time. It is suggested to keep this to less than 45 days so that there are fewer episodes of breakthrough bleeding. A longer duration of COC use does not affect stimulation since there is a 7-day washout.

G. As depicted in the algorithm, to plan a OPU on 13th June, the patient should get her cycle by 1st June and she should be given oral contraceptive pills (OCPs) for withdrawal based on this calculation.

Batch IVF—How to schedule cycles?

- A. E.g. 16th June (D3 embryo transfer)
- B. E.g. 13th June (Day of OPU) at 9 am
- C. E.g. 11th June (Date of trigger) at 10 pm
- D. E.g. 2nd June-date of starting stimulation/preferably day 2 of cycle
- E. Last pill on 24th May
- F. Start pills at-least from 10th May

(IVF: in vitro fertilization; OPU: oocyte pickup)

CHAPTER 76B
Cycle Preparation for Batching Embryo Transfer

Apoorva Pallam Reddy, Rajeev Agarwal

A. Apart from scheduling oocyte pickup (OPU), scheduling an embryo transfer also is equally important. With the improvement in technique of vitrification, the number of frozen embryo transfer (FET) cycles are on the rise. In addition, there is significant increase in the total number of oocyte donation cycles happening that require the synchronizing both recipient and donor cycles. The recipient embryo transfer date is synchronized with that of the pickup date of an oocyte donor. In order to schedule a FET on a particular day, the following algorithm may be followed. First, the date of transfer is decided (June 16th and the calculation are done backward).

B. Most clinicians transfer the embryos on 6th day of progesterone supplementation for a Day 5 embryo and 4th day of progesterone supplementation for a Day 3 embryo (accepted and practiced widely). However, there is a different school of thought that promotes the transfer of Day 5 embryo on 7th day and Day 3 embryo on 5th day of progesterone supplementation. Studies have failed to establish any added benefit by increasing the duration of progesterone priming.

C. The cycle is anticipated 5–7 days after stopping the oral contraceptive pill (OCP). If the cycle occurs prematurely before the anticipated date, 0.25 mg of gonadotropin-releasing hormone (GnRH) antagonists is administered subcutaneously from the Day 2 daily till the day before we intend to start medications either for endometrial priming in FET or for controlled ovarian stimulation in assisted reproductive technique (ART).

D. Giving GnRH antagonist, although helps in synchronizing the cycles of all women undergoing a batch, it also slightly increases the duration and dose of gonadotropins required for achieved dominant follicles.

E. The main disadvantage of batching is that, on occasions, the trigger may be given too early (16–17 mm or less) in order to synchronize the pickup with that of a batch resulting in lesser number of mature or the lining might not be ready due to fixed number of estrogen stimulated days..

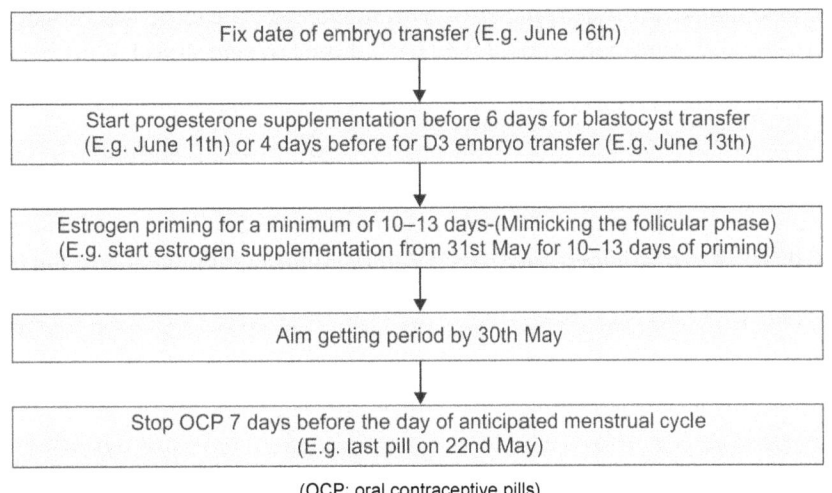

(OCP: oral contraceptive pills)

CHAPTER 77

Endometrial Preparation for FET: Natural Cycle

Apoorva Pallam Reddy, Mithila Mahesh

With the advent of better embryo freezing techniques, many clinics have moved to an "all freeze" protocol where the embryos are frozen in a fresh cycle and transferred later in another month. Thus, the focus has now shifted to methods of preparing the endometrial lining for receiving this embryo. For implantation there has to be synchrony between the growing endometrium and the embryo development stage.

The various regimes used to prepare the lining are:
- *Natural cycle*: Frozen embryo transfer is carried out in a natural cycle after spontaneous ovulation. The hypothesis has been that the window of implantation is widest in this method of embryo transfer.
- *Modified natural cycle*: In this cycle, the ovulation is artificially triggered by a human chorionic gonadotropin (hCG) injection given to mimic the luteinizing hormone (LH) surge.
- *Hormone replacement therapy (HRT) cycle*: HRT or hormone replacement cycle is one where estrogen hormone is given in varying doses to artificially create the endometrial lining without folliculogenesis.

Various studies have shown that no matter which method of lining preparation is undertaken, the success rates are the same.

A. For those with regular cycles and those who ovulate regularly, natural cycle without any ovulogens can be employed. For those who do not ovulate spontaneously, clomiphene citrate or aromatase inhibitors, with or without gonadotropins are used for ovulation induction.
B. The patient is called back around day 9 and follicular study initiated both for monitoring the growth of the dominant follicle as well as the thickness of the endometrium. The patient is called back again the next day or day after depending on the growth of the follicle and the clinic protocol.
C. Different authors have defined LH surge differently. Measuring a LH value by follicle size 13 mm helps in establishing a baseline LH level. Most clinics will measure the value daily thereafter. Frydman (1981) has defined LH surge as 180% rise of a previous LH value and more than or equal to 18 IU/L. A more recent study has further refined the criteria and suggested that a cutoff of 17 IU/L be taken, but a lot of focus be given on the additional drop in estradiol value which happens a day after the surge thus making the diagnosis more robust.
D. In a modified natural cycle, once the follicle is 18 mm size and the corresponding endometrial lining looks good, an hCG trigger (5,000 IU or 10,000 IU) can be given to artificially create an LH surge without waiting for the natural one.
E. From the day of LH surge or ovulation trigger, D3 embryo is transferred after 5 days and D5 embryo is transferred after 7 days. For example, if LH surge is noted on June 1st, D3 embryo transfer is done on June 6th and D5 embryo transfer is done on June 8th.

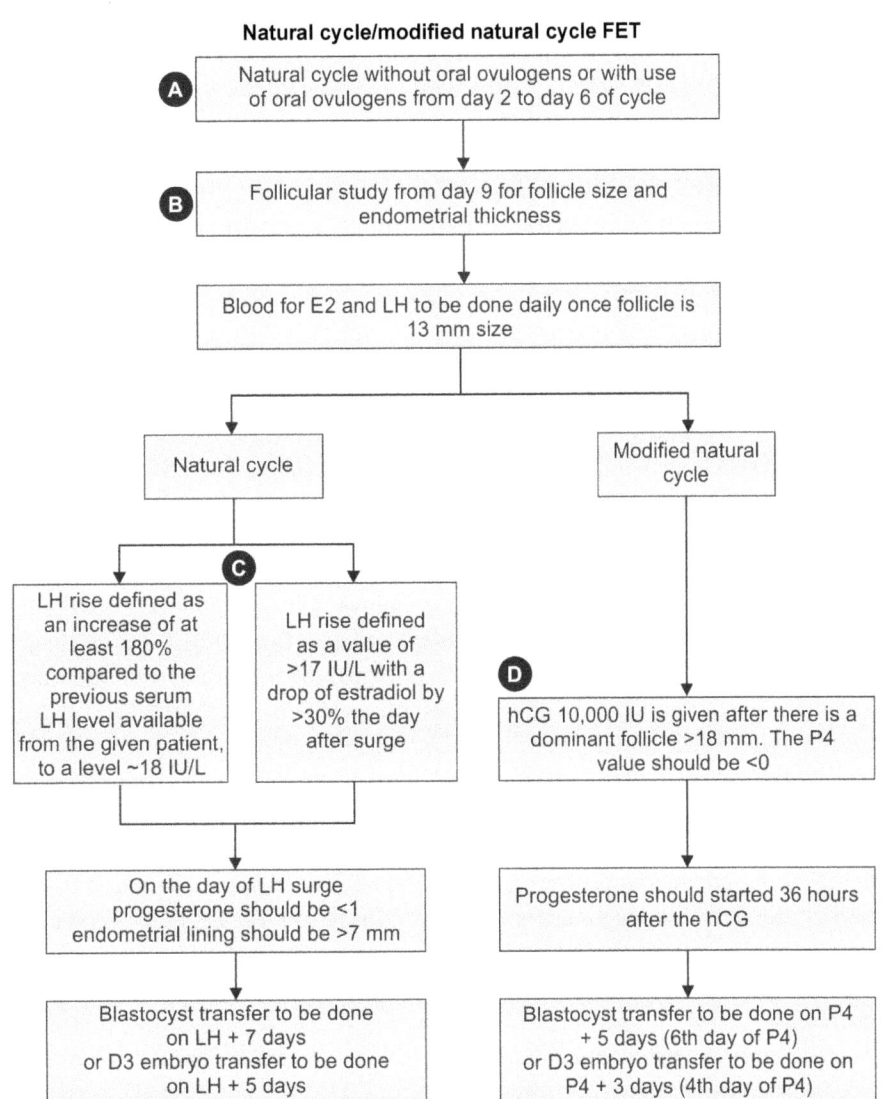
(FET: frozen embryo transfer; hCG: human chorionic gonadotropin; LH: luteinizing hormone; E2: estradiol; P4: progesterone)

CHAPTER 78
Endometrial Preparation for FET: Hormonal Replacement Therapy

Ritu Hinduja, Nikita Banerjee

Freezing is an important aspect of assisted reproductive technique (ART). It gives the ability to store the extra embryos formed in an ART cycle for future use and thus adding to the cumulative pregnancy rates. With the advent of vitrification and increase in the post thaw survival rates of embryos, the incidence of frozen embryo transfer (FET) has increased. FET cycles not only allow the flexibility in deciding the date of transfer but also are proposed to increase the pregnancy rates due to the lack of supraphysiological estradiol impact on the endometrium. Hormone replacement therapy using estradiol valerate and progesterone for the follicular phase and luteal phase is the most common method of endometrial preparation for FET cycles. The estradiol supplemented simultaneously downregulates the pituitary. Hence, the risk of spontaneous luteinizing hormone (LH) elevation is negligible.

A. In order to mimic the endocrine conditions of the endometrium of a normal cycle in an artificial cycle, estrogen and progesterone are administered consecutively. Baseline ultrasonography (USG) is done to rule out ovarian cyst and ensure a thin endometrium before starting hormonal replacement for preparation of endometrium for freeze-thaw embryo transfer.

B. The earlier estradiol is commenced, the lesser is the risk of unwanted follicular development and ovulation. Estradiol is introduced before the 4th day of the cycle. Estrogen can be administered as an oral tablet, transdermal plaster, or estrogen gel. The most widely used form is estradiol valerate oral tablet which can be given in progressively increasing doses beginning with 2 mg reaching a daily dose of 8 mg or using a constant and fixed dose (6–12 mg/day).

C. After 7–11 days, a transvaginal evaluation of endometrium is done to see the effect of estrogen. By this time, endometrium should grow and achieve trilaminar pattern.

D. If the endometrium is more than 7 mm, trilaminar, and there is absence of dominant follicle, the endometrium is prepared and progesterone is added to initiate the secretory changes. Thus, an attempt is made to mimic the physiologic midcycle estrogen–progesterone transition.

E. Before starting the luteal support, serum progesterone is done to rule out premature luteinization. Various studies point toward different cutoffs but in general if the progesterone value is less than 0.5 ng/mL in a freeze-thaw cycle, premature luteinization is less likely and the patient can be started with luteal support.

F. Progesterone can be administered vaginally, intramuscularly, or orally. Vaginal micronized progesterone can be given at doses of 600–1,200 mg daily as two to three divided doses. After the Lotus trial, oral dydrogesterone may replace micronized vaginal progesterone as the standard of care for luteal phase support in in vitro fertilization (IVF), owing to the oral route being more patient-friendly than intravaginal administration, as well as it being a well-tolerated and efficacious treatment. Intramuscular progesterone is given at dose of 50–100 mg daily. Aqueous preparation can also be administered at 25 mg subcutaneously daily dose.

G. Optimal time for embryo transfer lies between luteal days +3 and +5, where luteal day +1 is the second day of exogenous progesterone treatment.
According to the stage of embryo vitrification P + 5 for day 5 blastocyst transfer and P + 3 for day 3 embryo transfer.

H. After embryo transfer, serum beta human chorionic gonadotropin (bHCG) is done, to confirm pregnancy 10 days after blastocyst transfer or 12 days after day 3 embryo transfer.

I. If the endometrium, on the other hand, is less than 7 mm on first scan after commencing estrogen treatment then the dose of oral estrogen can be increased, e.g. from 12 mg/d to 16 mg/d. Alternatively, vaginal estrogen or estrogel can be added. Various adjuvant treatments have been advocated by many. These include addition of sildenafil, intrauterine granulocyte-colony stimulation factor (G-CSF), and use of platelet-rich plasma (PRP). These adjuvants are of doubtful efficacy and need further research.

J. If the endometrium does not improve despite increasing the dose, then intrauterine adhesions may be suspected which can be confirmed and removed hysteroscopically followed by E+P (estrogen + progesterone) supplementation.

Endometrial Preparation for FET: Hormonal Replacement Therapy

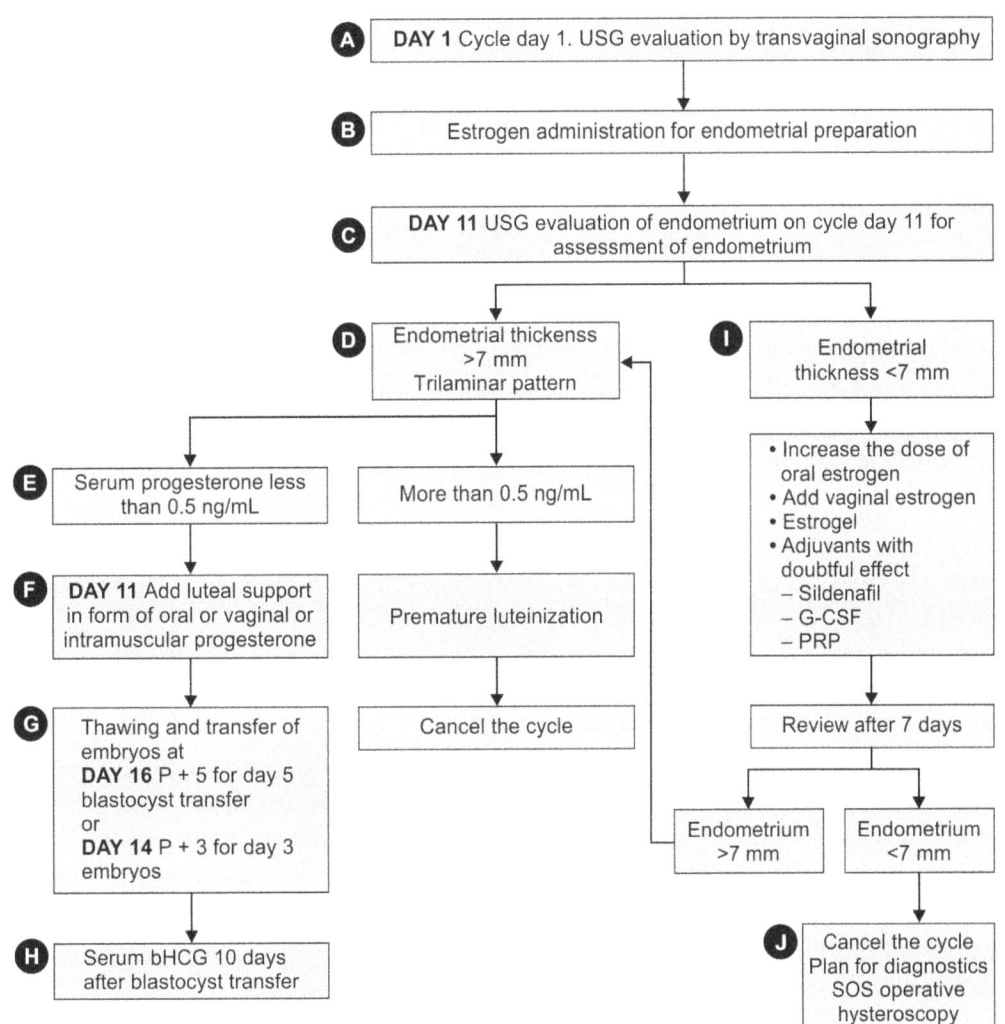

(bHCG: beta human chorionic gonadotropin; G-CSF: granulocyte-colony stimulation factor; PRP: platelet-rich plasma; SOS: if necessary; USG: ultrasonography)

CHAPTER 79

Oocyte Donor Recruitment Protocol

Neelam Bhise, Sushma Mandava

Anonymous oocytes donation as opposed to sperm donation is an invasive procedure covering controlled-ovarian stimulation, oocytes retrieval, and anesthesia. Psychological counseling and appropriate consents are mandatory part of the procedure.

SOURCING OF DONOR

The donor can be sourced through the assisted reproductive technique (ART) bank and she can be compensated financially by the bank.

The parties involved in process of consenting:
- In vitro fertilization (IVF) clinic
- ART bank
- Donor
- Recipients.

The consents and agreements involved between ART bank and donor, ART bank and recipient to be taken by ART bank.

Form: S	Form: R1	Form: K
Contract between the ART bank and the patient	Contract between the ART bank and the oocytes donor	Consent form for the donor of egg

Criteria for donor selection:
- Age between 21 years and 35 years. If age of donor is more than 34 years, the age should be revealed to the recipient as a part of informed consent.
- If donor is Rh negative, report should be informed to the recipient. Blood group matching between donor and recipient although desired is not mandatory.
- Proven fertility of the donor is desirable but not mandatory.

Concerns about repetitive oocytes donors: The risks assessed include risk ovarian hyperstimulation syndrome (OHSS; 1–2%), serious acute complications (0.5%), risk of future cancers, and risk of affecting donors egg reserve. Although existing data cannot permit conclusive recommendations, a concern for the issues of the safety and well-being of oocytes donors' warrants consideration. It is prudent to limit the number of stimulated cycles for a given oocytes donor to 6.

Oocyte sharing from indigent infertile patient: Indian Council of Medical Research (ICMR) guidelines 2017 have accepted oocytes sharing from indigent infertile patient with well-informed consent, in order to compensate the expenses toward indigent infertile patient.

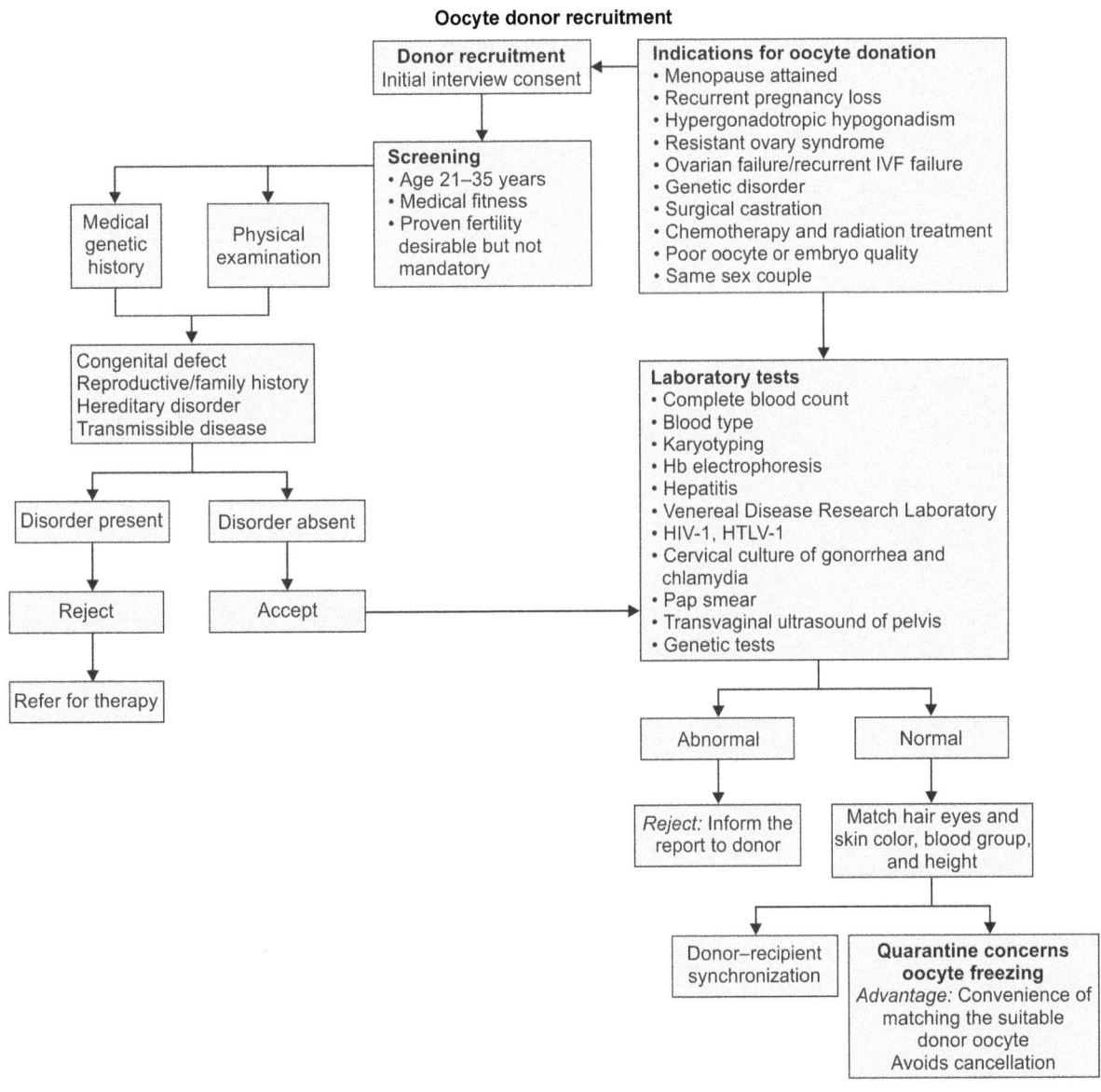
(HTLV: Human T-cell lymphotropic virus)

CHAPTER 80

Oocyte Donor Controlled Ovarian Stimulation

Neelam Bhise, Sushma Mandava

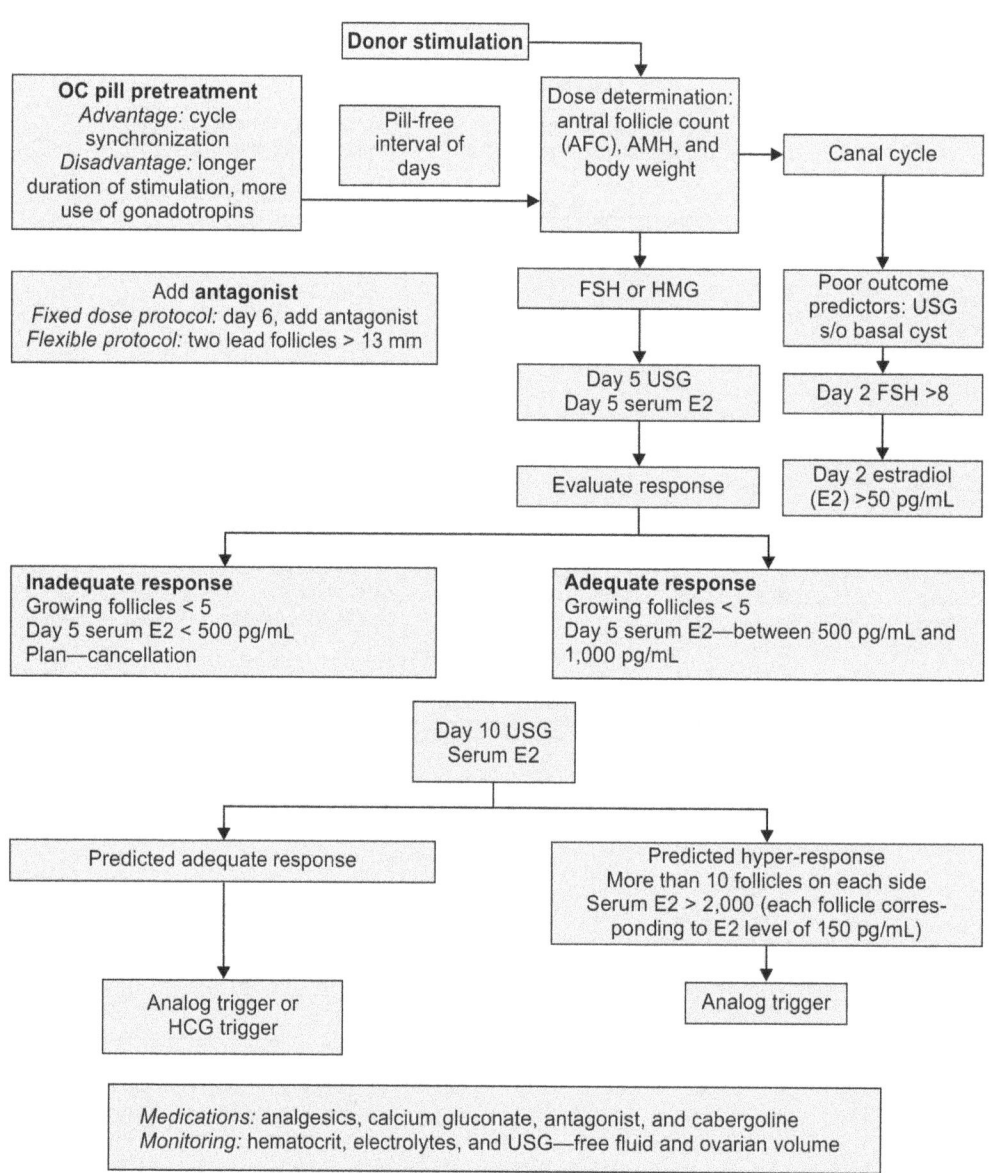

(AMH: anti-Müllerian hormone; FSH: follicle-stimulating hormone; HCG: human chorionic gonadotropin; HMG: human menopausal gonadotropin; OC: oral contraceptive; USG: ultrasonography; s/o: suggestive of)

SECTION 16

Sperm Preparation Techniques

- Sperm Preparation for Assisted Reproduction Techniques
- Advanced Sperm Preparation
- Sperm Retrieval Techniques

CHAPTER 81

Sperm Preparation for Assisted Reproduction Techniques

Saroj Agarwal, Rajeev Agarwal

Sperm preparation is essential prior to either artificial insemination (AI), in vitro fertilization (IVF), or intracytoplasmic sperm injection (ICSI). This constitutes not only separation of sperms from the seminal contents, but also enables the selection of the ejaculated spermatozoa before the performance of the treatment. This also helps in removal of the certain components of the seminal fluid that may act hostile for fertilization. Methods like the swim-up or the density-gradient centrifugation are the most commonly used technique for sperm preparation.

SEMEN COLLECTION

The first fraction of the ejaculate, mainly from the prostate, is rich in spermatozoa. Hence, during ejaculation, it is of paramount importance to collect the entire volume of the sample. The last fraction of the semen consists of vesicular fraction, less rich in spermatozoa. Loss of this initial fraction may lead to erroneous assessment of the semen features. In case of the AI, the semen sample will not contain the best portion of the spermatozoa. It is strongly recommended to collect the semen following an abstinence period of 2–3 days to maximize the conception rate.

After sample collection and liquefaction, it is recommended to perform the evaluation of semen volume, viscosity, appearance, and pH measurement. Next step involves motility, concentration, and morphology assessments.

SPERM PREPARATION TECHNIQUES

There are a range of techniques like simple wash, swim-up, and density gradient which can be used to prepare sperm and the technique used will depend upon the type of assisted reproductive technique procedure and the quality of the semen sample. Newer technologies, such as magnetic-activated cell sorting (MACS), microfluidics, electrophoresis, motile sperm organelle morphology examination (MSOME), and birefringence eliminate the centrifugation steps and can improve the selection of sperm with higher deoxyribonucleic acid (DNA) integrity, normal morphology, and motility as well as improved AI outcomes.

CONVENTIONAL SPERM PREPARATION TECHNIQUES

A. *Simple washing*: This technique is the easiest and quick to fulfill, no filter is used to select spermatozoa as it is performed by mixing the semen sample with a washing medium and centrifuging the mixture twice at 300–500 g for 5–10 minutes. The supernatant is discarded and the pellet is resuspended. Simple washing procedure normally is used with semen samples with a good concentration of highly motile sperm.

B. *Swim-up*: First described by Mahadevan and Baker in 1984, it is still mainly adopted by IVF laboratories worldwide. Normal sperm parameters and high sperm motility are prerequisite to adopt this method, based on the ability of sperm to swim actively from the prewashed pellet into a placed over medium. This is very easy and cheap procedure allows for the recovery of a clean fraction of highly motile sperm. On the other hand, during the centrifugation steps, leukocytes and other pellet components may induce oxidative stress. The portion of culture medium recovered, enriched with sperm, can be analyzed to estimate final motility and concentration of the processed sample.

C. *Density-gradient centrifugation*: Two types of density gradients, continuous or discontinuous, can be prepared. While in continuous gradients, a gradual increase in density is created in the conical test tube, in a discontinuous gradient, a clear boundary between the two phases is present. Nowadays, a discontinuous gradient, the most widely used, contains colloidal silica coated with silane having different densities, 40% (v/v) and 80% (v/v). Semen sample is placed on the top of density media. During centrifugation, cells stratify in different layer of the gradient, according to their density. Motile and morphologically competent sperm have higher density (1.10 g/mL) compared to immature or abnormal sperm (1.06–1.09 g/mL), thus they form a pellet at the bottom of the tube. This is the ideal procedure when the sample has scarce parameters, thus it is mainly used for oligozoospermic, asthenozoospermic, and teratozoospermic patients.

Sperm Preparation for Assisted Reproduction Techniques

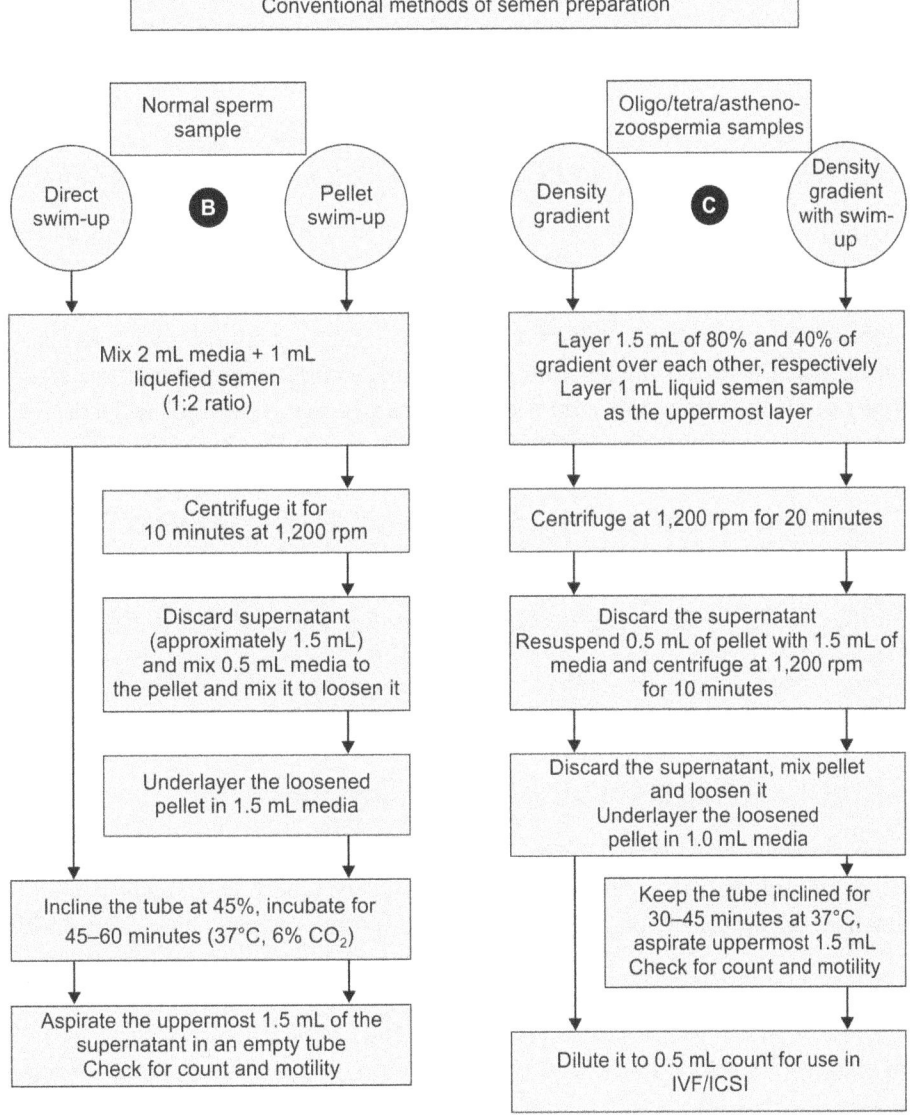

(IVF: in vitro fertilization; ICSI: intracytoplasmic sperm injection)

CHAPTER 82

Advanced Sperm Preparation

Saroj Agarwal, Rajeev Agarwal

INTRODUCTION

Advanced sperm preparation techniques for intracytoplasmic injection (ICSI) assists the embryologist in choosing structurally intact and mature sperm with high deoxyribonucleic acid (DNA) integrity for fertilization. Different modalities utilize various parameters of sperm structure, physiology, or function to allow selection of the genetically and functionally superior sperm.

SELECTION BY DIFFERENTIAL NET ELECTRIC CHARGE ON SPERM SURFACE

A. *Electrophoretic system:* The electrophoresis-based technology segregates the sperms using an electric field based on size and electronegative charge. Expression of CD52 protein on the sperm membrane correlates positively with normal sperm morphology. Presence of CD52 increases the electro negativity of the sperm thus making selection easy.
B. *Zeta potential method:* Mature sperms with intact chromatin have high negative surface electrical charge, called "Zeta potential". Advanced sperm selection can be done using this negative zeta electrokinetic potential. When the sperm are suspended in a positively charged tube, the negatively charged mature sperms will adhere to the tube used for ICSI while nonmature sperm will not adhere and are discarded.

SELECTION OF NONAPOPTOTIC SPERM FROM APOPTOTIC SPERMS

C. *Magnetic-activated cell sorting (MACS):* MACS uses Annexin V antibody conjugated super paramagnetic microbeads that bind to spermatozoa whose plasma membranes have externalized phosphatidylserine which is a marker for signs of early apoptosis.
D. *Annexin V glass wool filtration:* Glass wool filtration separates motile sperm cells from other contents of semen by filtration through densely packed glass wool fibers.

SELECTION OF HIGHLY MOTILE SPERM FROM IMMOTILE ONES

Microfluidics: Spermatozoa are sorted depending on their ability to swim across the semen stream into the medium stream. Studies have shown that the motility of the sperm sample increased significantly by almost 100% with use of microfluidic device with the added benefit that the morphology of the isolated sperm was better after microfluidic sorting.

SELECTION BASED ON SPERM MEMBRANE MATURITY

Hyaluronic acid (HA) binding sites: Hyaluronic acid binding sites on the sperm plasma membrane are an indicator of sperm maturity.
E. *PICSI (Physiological intracytoplasmic sperm injection):* In PICSI, HA is added to a sterile Petri dish, and then a washed or centrifuged sperm sample is placed onto the HA areas.
F. *Sperm slow:* A droplet of treated sperm [density gradient centrifugation (DGC), direct swim up (DSW), conventional swim up (CSW)] is connected to a droplet of fresh culture medium via a pipette tip, while on the other side of the clean culture droplet, a sperm slow solution, which contains HA, is also connected by a pipette tip. Sperm that bind with HA become slowed and are collected from the middle medium to be used in ICSI.

SELECTION BASED ON ULTRAMORPHOLOGY

G. *Motile sperm organelle morphology examination (MSOME):* The sperms are selected based on the microscopic observation of their morphology. Sperm are analyzed with enhanced magnification of 6300 × using Nomarski optics. MSOME assesses the morphology of the acrosome, postacrosomal lamina, the midpiece, mitochondria, vacuoles, and the nucleus. Sperms with large vacuoles are associated with poor chromatin integrity. Vacuoles occupying >50% of the space of the head or >4% of the nuclear area are considered large.

Intracytoplasmic morphologically selected sperm injection (IMSI). IMSI is the technique of injecting a sperm selected through MSOME. Some studies suggest that selection of the sperms by MSOME and performing IMSI is associated with higher implantation rate, clinical pregnancy rate, and live birth rates. It is most beneficial for men with severe teratozoospermia. However, incubation of the sperms for 2 hours prior to IMSI has raised concerns over the added length of the procedure.

H. *Sperm birefringence by using polar microscopy:* Sperm birefringence can be evaluated using an inverted microscope equipped with polarizing and analyzing lenses, which allows the selection of birefringent acrosome reacted spermatozoa during ICSI without negatively impacting sperm motility or viability.

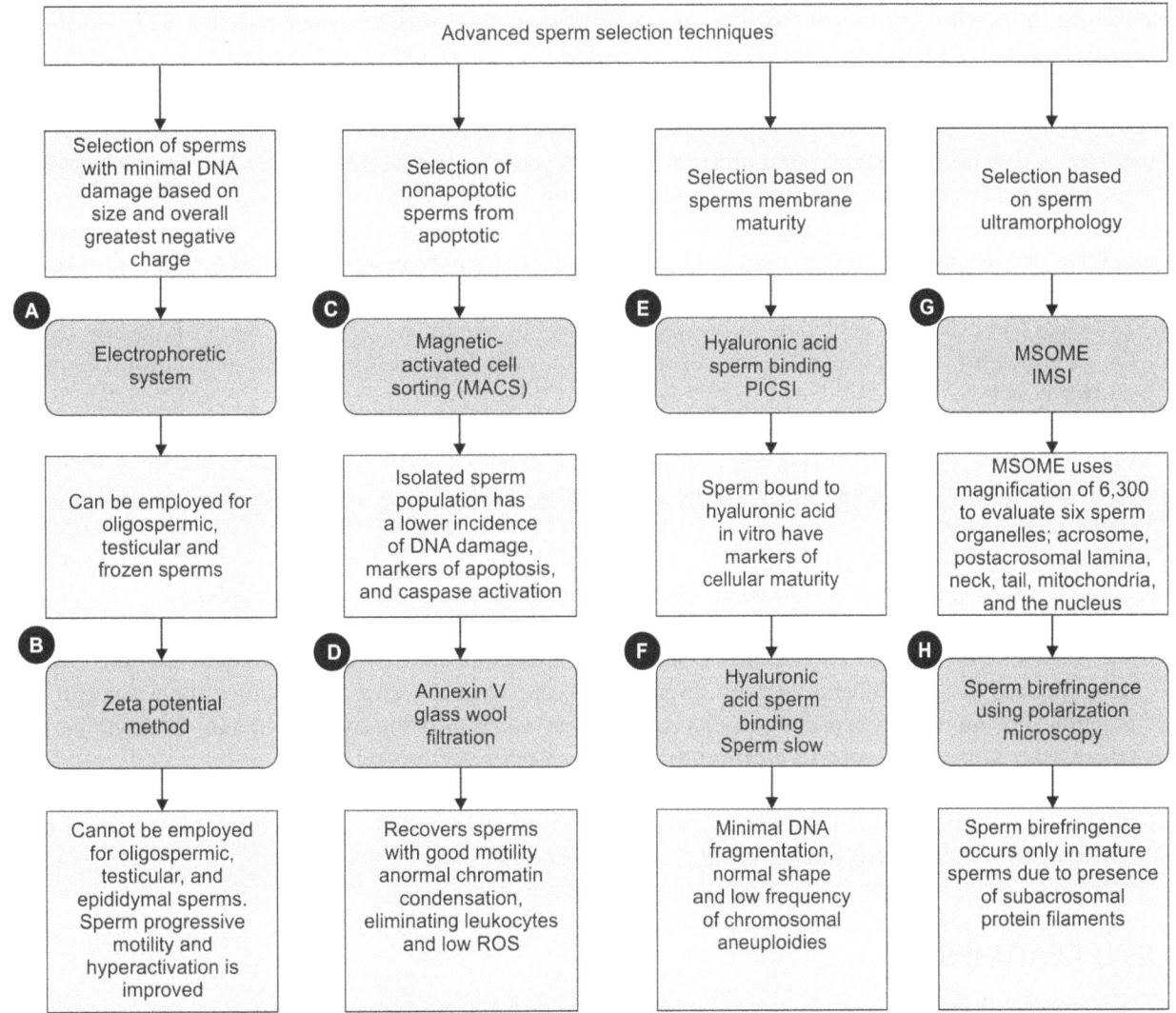

(PICSI: physiological intracytoplasmic sperm injection; MSOME: motile sperm organelle morphology examination; IMSI: intracytoplasmic morphologically selected sperm injection; DNA: deoxyribonucleic acid; ROS: reactive oxidative species)

CHAPTER 83

Sperm Retrieval Techniques

Dorothy P Ghosh, Apoorva Pallam Reddy, Rajeev Agarwal

In case of absence of sperms in an ejaculated sample, an attempt is made to retrieve the sperms directly from the male genitals to achieve a genetically similar offspring using intracytoplasmic sperm injection (ICSI) technique. Azoospermia (obstructive and nonobstructive), elevated DFI, total astheno/necrozoospermia, failure to ejaculate sperm on the day of procedure, etc. are some of the indications for performing sperm retrieval.

A. In men with obstructive azoospermia, sperm may be retrieved from the epididymis and/or the testis, while in men with nonobstructive azoospermia only testicular sperm retrieval techniques are useful.

Procedure type	Open	Percutaneous
Epididymal	MESA; OFNA	PESA
Testicular	Conventional, MD-TESE, SST	TESA; NAB; Tru-cut

MESA: microsurgical epididymal sperm aspiration; OFNA: open fine needle aspiration; PESA: percutaneous epididymal sperm aspiration; MD-TESE: microdissection testicular sperm extraction; SST: single seminiferous tubule biopsy; TESA: testicular sperm aspiration; NAB: needle aspiration biopsy

The choice of technique should be least invasive with maximum possibility of obtaining normal spermatozoa.

B. *Percutaneous epididymal sperm aspiration (PESA):* PESA is done for either diagnostic purposes to confirm the presence of viable spermatozoa prior to ICSI or therapeutic indications carried out at the same day of oocyte pickup.

   Procedure: A fine needle attached to tuberculin syringe is inserted through the scrotal skin into the epididymis. PESA is repeated at a different site (from cauda to caput epididymis). The amount of fluid aspirated is often minimal (0.1 mL). Men with obstructive azoospermia have distended epididymis and have higher chances of sperm retrieval using PESA. This is the most noninvasive form of sperm extractions and can be done under local anesthesia.

C. *Testicular sperm aspiration*
   - Testicular parenchyma is percutaneously aspirated using fine needle (e.g. 18 gauge). Needle is usually inserted at the anteromedial or anterolateral portion of the superior testicular pole, in an oblique angle toward the medium and lower poles.
   - The tip of the needle is moved in and out the testis in an oblique plane to disrupt the seminiferous tubules and sample different areas. Testicular sperm aspiration (TESA) or testicular sperm extraction (TESE) may be performed at the contralateral testis, if insufficient or no sperm are obtained.

D. *Testicular sperm extraction*
   - Testis is not exteriorized
   - Multiple biopsy specimens can be collected from upper, middle, and lower testicular poles.

E. *Microsurgical testicular sperm extraction (Micro-TESE)*
   - The procedure is performed under microscopic magnification to increase the precision of the procedure: 6–8X magnification for a single large midportion incision in the avascular area of the tunica albuginea and 16–25X magnification for dissection of the testicular parenchyma searching of the enlarged islets of seminiferous tubules (more likely to contain germ cells and eventually normal sperm production).
   - Enlarged tubules are removed using microsurgical forceps. If all tubules are similar in appearance, random microbiopsies are performed at each testicular pole. Specimens are then washed grossly to remove blood clots and are sent to the laboratory for processing and search for sperms.
   - Extensive teasing may help in releasing more sperm from tissue.

SALIENT FEATURES

- Presence of significantly elevated follicle-stimulated hormone (FSH) associated with small bilateral testes and low inhibin B levels is indicative of nonobstructive azoospermia (NOA) and is associated with reduced chances of obtaining

sperms even in one of the sperm retrieval technique. However, a biopsy may be considered to determine the likelihood of sperm retrieval in ICSI candidates with NOA.
- The presence of either spermatozoa on a wet preparation or hypospermatogenesis on testicular histopathology is highly predictive of successful sperm retrieval in future retrieval attempts.
- Closed procedures such as PESA and TESA may result in better yield of sperm in obstructive cases whereas open surgeries is superior to needle aspirations in nonobstructive patients.
- Epididymal retrievals are only indicated in cases of obstructive azoospermia; whereas, testicular extractions can be used in both obstructive and nonobstructive cases.
- Microsurgical epididymal sperm aspiration (MESA) is indicated for obstructive azoospermia (OA) cases, whereas Micro-TESE is recommended for the most severe NOA cases.
- Intracytoplasmic sperm injection outcomes using motile fresh or frozen epididymal sperms seems not to differ.
- Immotile spermatozoa through the method of sperm tail flexibility test is selected as viable sperm for ICSI.
- Post thaw testicular sperm are often found to be immotile or exhibit only a twitching motility. ICSI results in such cases are found to be lower than fresh ones.
- Success of sperm retrieval in case NOA is mainly dependent on the technique used. Hence, choosing the right technique is of paramount importance. Successful percutaneous testicular aspiration retrieval rates range from 10% to 30% and is significantly lower than the 50% success rate reported for testicular sperm extractions.
- Overall 30–60% of men with NOA have focal areas of sperm production within the testis leading to successful sperm retrievals.

DNA FRAGMENTATION TEST IN RELEVANCE TO SPERM RETRIEVAL TECHNIQUES

- DNA fragmentation is mainly a post-testicular event, during which the sperm chromatin is damaged while being stored and transported through the seminiferous tubules and epididymis. The double helical chromatin undergoes breakage at one or more places resulting in DNA fragmentation. DNA fragmentation levels were significantly lower in testicular sperm than those found in ejaculated sperm (4.8 ± 3.6 vs $23.6 \pm 5.1\%$, $P < 0.001$). ICSI cycles with ejaculated sperm that have DNA fragmentation >15% had significantly lower pregnancy rates as compared to those obtained from testicular sperm (5.6% vs 44.4%, $P < 0.05$).

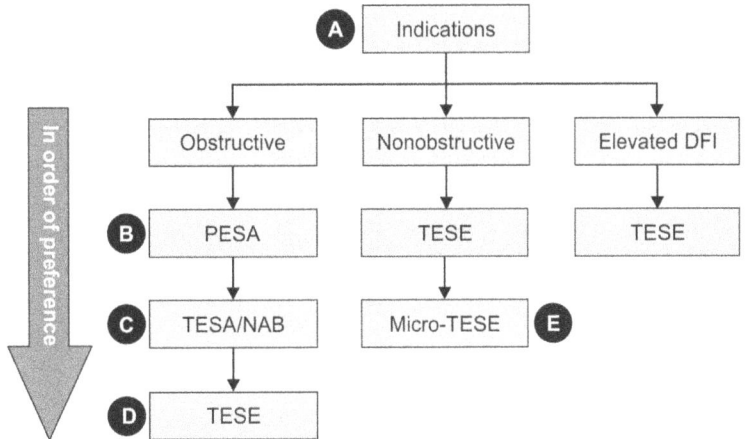

(DFI: DNA fragmentation index; PESA: percutaneous epididymal sperm aspiration; TESA: testicular sperm aspiration; TESE: testicular sperm extraction; NAB: needle aspiration biopsy)

Type of procedure	Technique	Tip	Advantage	Disadvantage
PESA (PERCUTANEOUS)	Head of epididymis is punctured and aspirated using a 22–26 G tuberculin syringe or butterfly needle	Maintain gap between the rubber of the plunger and the media in the syringe to prevent direct contact of the sperms with the rubber	Most noninvasive	As epididymis is only palpated and not visualized precision may be effected
TESA (PERCUTANEOUS)	Testicular body is aspirated with a 18–22 G butterfly needle attached to a 20 cc syringe that creates suction	Color Doppler ultrasonography has been used to guide the aspiration so as to avoid blood vessels and reduce hematoma formation	Simple, non-surgical procedure that can be performed under LA	
Needle aspiration biopsy (PERCUTANEOUS)	A 18-G scalp vein needle is using to aspirate and cut testicular tissues to obtain seminiferous tubules	Color Doppler ultrasonography has been used to guide the aspiration so as to avoid blood vessels and reduce hematoma formation	Both the testicular fluid and the tissue can be checked for sperms. Has higher rate of sperm retrieval compared to TESA	Higher risk of risk hematocele, intra-testicular hemorrhage, or damaging the epididymis
Cutting needle biopsy (PERCUTANEOUS)	Testicular biopsy can also be obtained using a tissue-cutting biopsy needle. For example, Tru-cut™ needle	The needle once placed against the testis automatically enters the stroma and cuts a small piece of testicular tissue	Useful in men with testicular fibrosis in whom NAB may fail to retrieve sufficient tissue	More traumatic
Micro-TESE (OPEN)	A long incision is made in the tunica to expose the testicular parenchyma	The seminiferous tubules are gently separated and only selective tubules are examined under an operating microscope for sperms	Large area of testicular tissue can be visually evaluated and biopsied	More traumatic. Higher chances of devascularization and fibrosis of the testis
Single seminiferous tubule – biopsy (OPEN)	Testis is exposed and tunica is punctured and dilated with a 26-G needle to obtain a loop of seminiferous tubule that pops out from the puncture site	If seminiferous tubules are not obtained with just the puncture, the opening is widened a little so that both prongs of the micro-forceps can be pushed to obtain deeper testicular tissue for evaluation. (Extended SST technique)	Allows extensive sampling of the testis without opening the tunica. No need to suture the tunica since each opening is very small	In very small testes, which are mainly fibrous, no tubule may pop out

(PESA: percutaneous epididymal sperm aspiration; TESA: testicular sperm aspiration; NAB: needle aspiration; SST: single seminiferous tubule biopsy; Micro-TESE: microsurgical testicular sperm extraction; LA: local anesthesia)

SECTION 17

Advances in ART

- Assisted Hatching Indications—Technique
- Endometrial Receptivity Array/Analysis
- PGT and PGD
- Time-lapse Imaging of Preimplantation Embryos

Assisted Hatching Indications—Technique

Sujatha Ramakrishna

Zona pellucida (ZP) is a glycoprotein layer surrounding the plasma membrane of the embryo preventing its premature implantation in the fallopian tube. Once the blastocyst enters the uterine cavity, the proteolytic action of uterine secretions, helps in the lysis of the ZP, promoting adhesion and their by implantation of the embryo. Impairment in the desolution of the ZP reduces pregnancy rates. Assisted hatching is a laboratory micromanipulation technique that involves the disruption of the ZP to improve the implantation potential of the embryo.

A. *Assisted hatching—indications and methods:* Advanced maternal age, increased baseline follicle-stimulating hormone (FSH), previous failed attempts, cycles with poor quality embryos, uniformly thicker zona > 15 µm, and frozen thawed embryos are the common indications for assisted hatching.

   Two basic techniques of assisted hatching are breaching and thinning of ZP, which can be performed by mechanical, chemical, and laser methods. Choice of these methods depends on the availability of equipment, technical expertise, and stage of embryos.

B. *Mechanical hatching (MH):* MH is perforated tangentially through the space between blastomeres and ZP by a dissecting pipette or an injection pipette, at 2 o'clock position and exiting through the 10 o'clock position. Embryo is released from the holding pipette and the ZP trapped above the dissection pipette is rubbed on to the holding pipette until an opening is made. Lack of precision over the extent of breach in ZP, time taken to perform hatching, and inability to perform this technique on expanded blastocysts are the disadvantages of mechanical hatching.

C. *Chemical hatching:* Dissolving zona by the expulsion of a steady stream of acid Tyrode solution (pH 2.5 ± 0.3) forms the basis of chemical hatching. Assisted hatching dish is prepared by aliquoting two parallel rows of 20 µL droplets of HEPES (4-(2-hydroxyethyl)-1-piperazineethanesulfonic acid) media and acid Tyrode solution and covered with oil. Zona drilling pipette (10–12 µm ID) is loaded with acid Tyrode solution and placed in close proximity to the ZP at the 3 o'clock position of the embryo while applying minimal positive pressure. Acid Tyrode is gently released from the pipette directly onto the ZP in slow rubbing motion. A hole or trough of 25–30 µm area is created, which would be approximately the size of the outer diameter of the holding pipette. Once the outer layer of the ZP is thinned, acid solution is released only in the center of the thinned area. At the point when the inner layer of ZP bulges and collapses, further acid release is stopped and pipette lifted from the droplet. Hatched embryo is washed gently in successive droplets of fresh culture media and placed in culture. Acid Tyrode hatching is found to be detrimental when the ZP is less than 13 µm.

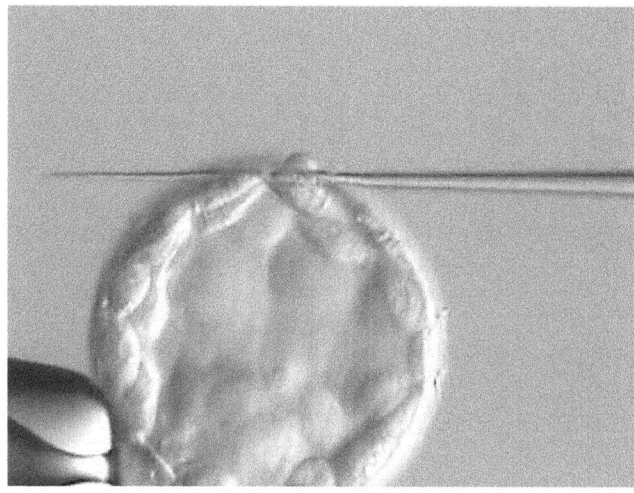

Mechanical hatching

D. If complete circumferential thinning of ZP of embryos post compaction is required, exposure to pronase enzyme is the preferred method. Embryos are transferred into the pronase (10 IU/mL) droplets and immediately observed under high magnification. Stretching and softening of ZP happens usually between 1.5 and 2 minutes of pronase exposure. Embryos are transferred to fresh culture media droplets and rinsed before the complete disappearance of ZP.

E. *Laser hatching:* Assisted hatching by laser involves dissolving ZP by thermal energy generated by a 1.48 μm laser beam focused through the conventional optics of an inverted microscope. Hole size is directly proportional to the laser intensity and pulse duration. On screen crosshair is positioned on the ZP, far away from the blastomeres and laser shots are fired according to the manufacturer's instruction.

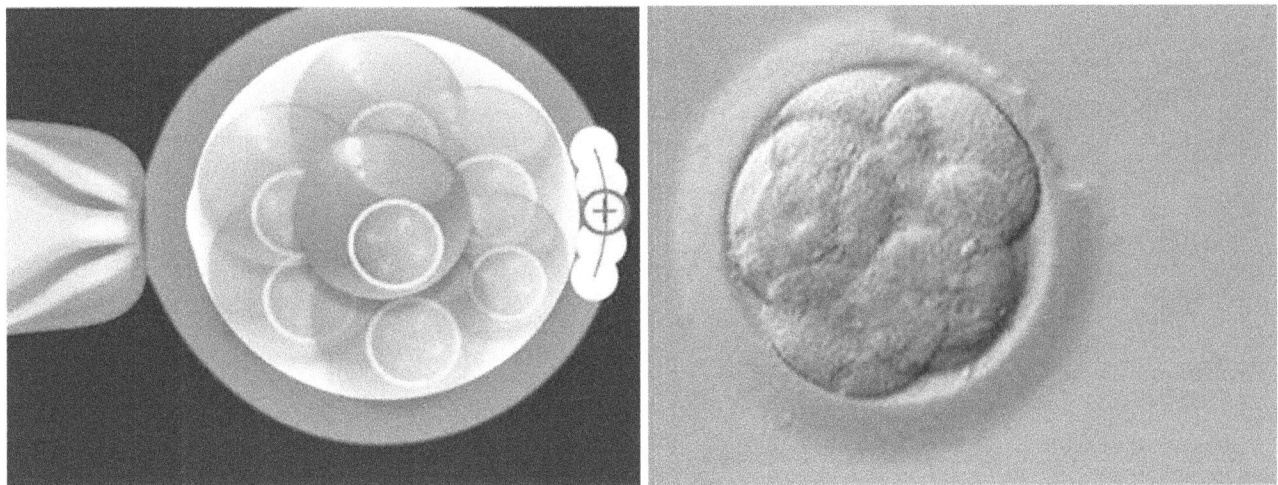

Laser assited hatching

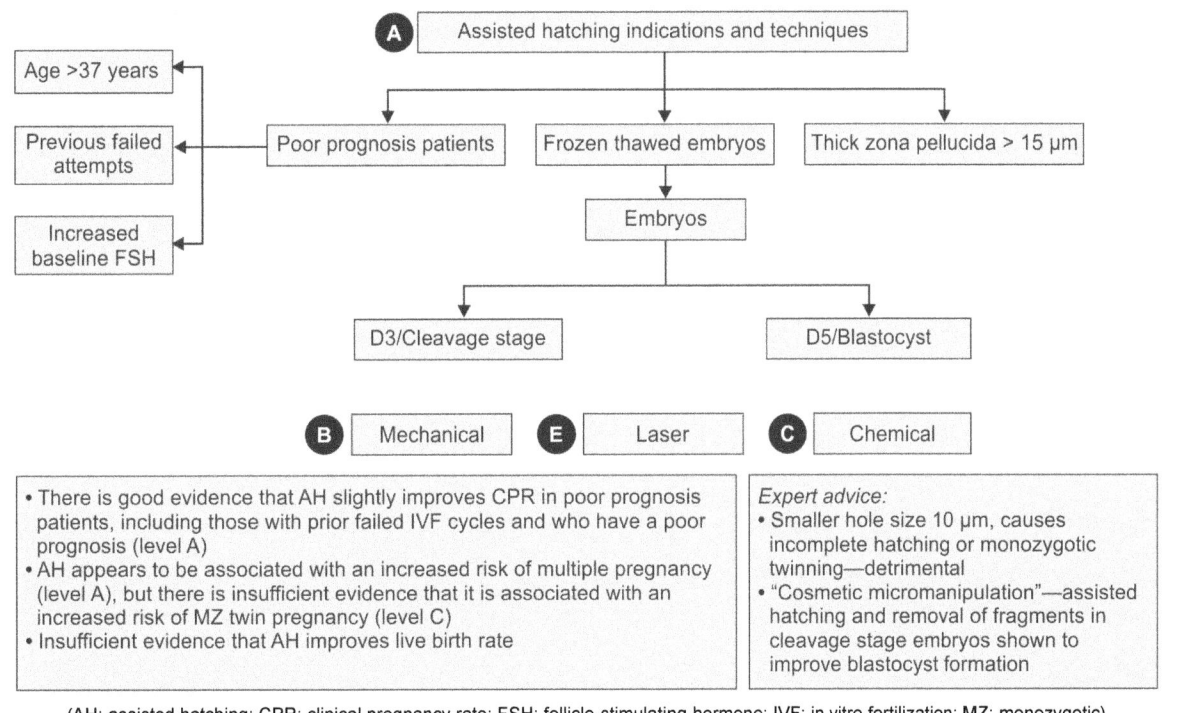

(AH: assisted hatching; CPR: clinical pregnancy rate; FSH: follicle-stimulating hormone; IVF: in vitro fertilization; MZ: monozygotic)

Section 17: Advances in ART

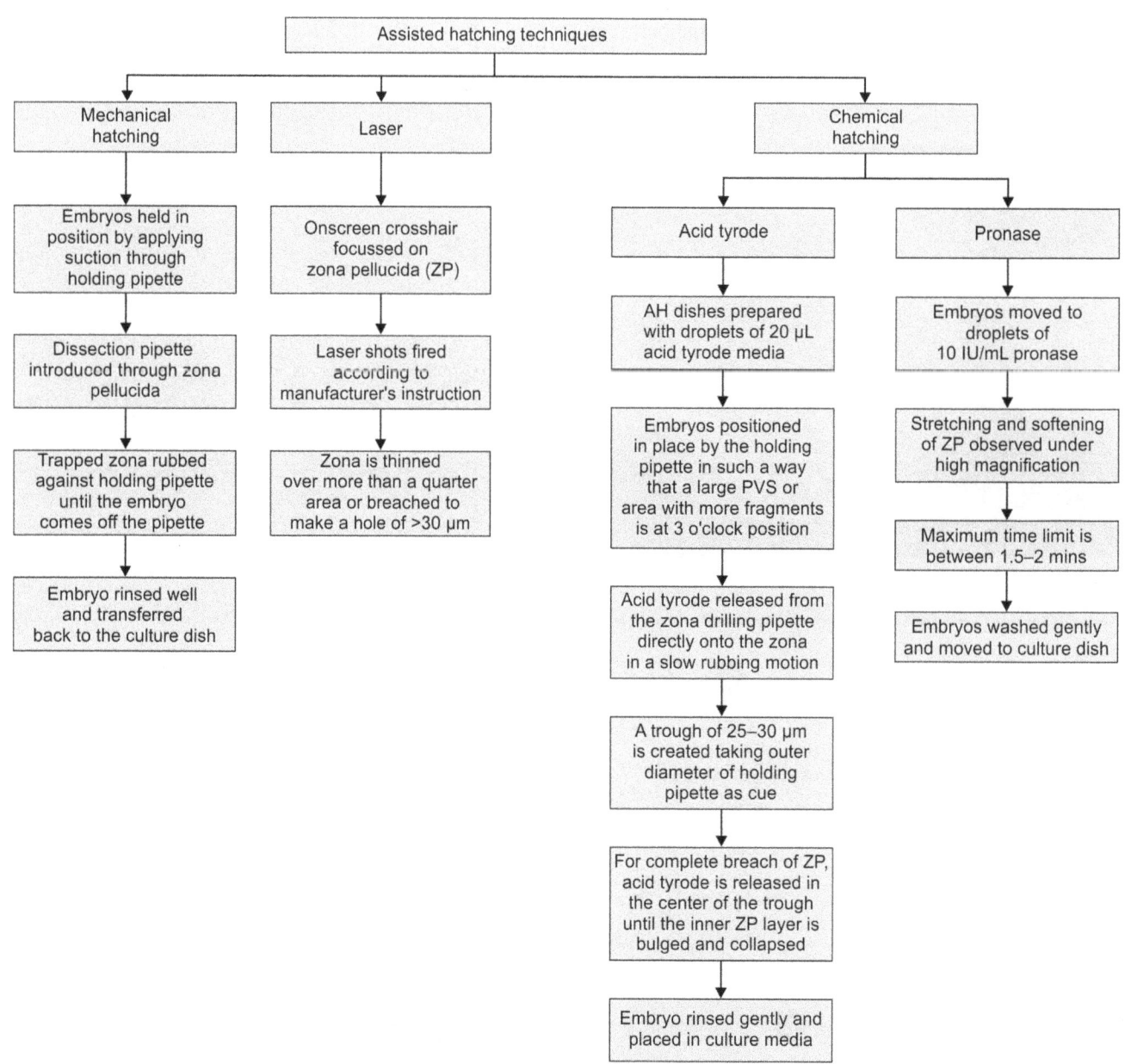

(AH: assisted hatching; PVS: penile vibratory stimulation)

CHAPTER 85

Endometrial Receptivity Array/Analysis

Swarnima Das, Rajeev Agarwal

A. Implantation is the final and the most important part of an assisted reproductive technique (ART) cycle. The endometrium under the hormonal influence of estrogen and progesterone coupled with many cytokines and growth factors enables the implantation of the embryo. If the endometrium is not primed sufficiently, despite the quality of the embryo, implantation fails to happen. Endometrial receptivity array (ERA) is a qualitative method that analyses the presence of 248 specific genes using new generation sequencing (NGS) which are deemed essential for the implantation process. This helps to determine the personalized window of implantation for each patient by evaluating the endometrial receptivity.

B. Although robust evidence is lacking, ERA may be indicated in cases of:
    – Recurrent implantation failure: More than two implantation failures with good quality own embryos or more than one failed implantation with good quality donor eggs
    – Patient with, atrophic (<6 mm) or hypertrophic (>12 mm) endometrium

C. Endometrial receptivity array involves taking a biopsy of the endometrium that is prepared for an embryo transfer. The endometrial preparation can be done using hormone replacement therapy or in a natural cycle.

D. In an hormone therapy (HT) cycle, endometrium is prepared using estradiol valerate from the day 2 of cycle. Progesterone supplementation is started once the endometrial thickness is more than 7 mm and the biopsy is taken from the fundus of uterus by pipelle technique after 5 full days of progesterone administration (P + 5) or 120 hours. In a natural cycle, biopsy is taken after 7 days of luteinizing hormone (LH) surge or 7 days after human chorionic gonadotropin (HCG) triggering (168 hours after HCG triggering).

E. *Methodology:* A separate kit is available for collection of ERA sample. Endometrial biopsy is taken using the pipette provided in the kit.

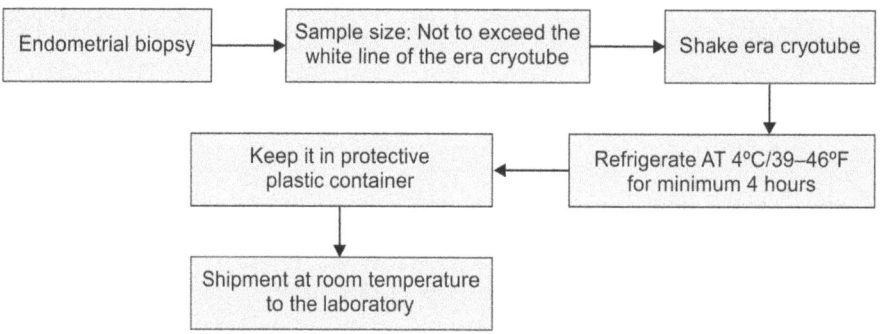

F. *Result Interpretation:* The turnaround time for the testing is around 7 days and the results are interpreted as receptive, prereceptive, and postreceptive.
    – *Receptive:* The gene expression profile is concordant with a receptive endometrium. Blastocyst transfer recommended using the same protocol.
        - *Early receptive:* The gene expression profile is concordant with an endometrium at the beginning of the receptive stage. Administer progesterone for 12 hours more before performing the blastocyst transfer.
        - *Late receptive:* The gene expression profile is concordant with an endometrium at the end of the receptive stage. Administer progesterone for 12 hours less before performing the blastocyst transfer.
    – *Prereceptive:* The gene expression profile is concordant with an endometrium at a prereceptive stage, could be due to displacement of window of implantation (>2 days—second endometrial biopsy). It is advised to transfer at a later time.

- *Postreceptive:* The gene expression profile is concordant with an endometrium at a postreceptive stage. Second endometrial biopsy is recommended. It is advised to transfer at an earlier time.
- *Proliferative:* The gene expression profile is concordant with an endometrium at a proliferative stage which means that progesterone effect has not been sufficient.

Factors that can cause improper reporting of the sample.
- High temperature (35°C) during shipment
- Sample size too small/large
- Too much blood.

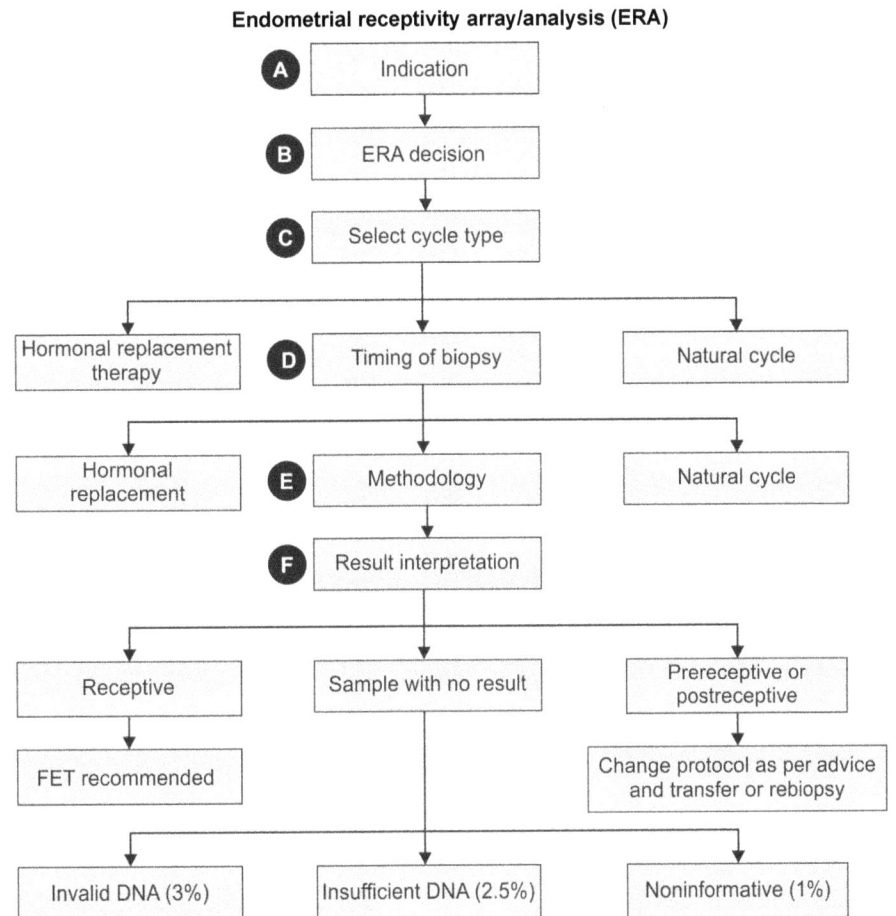

(DNA: deoxyribose nucleic acid; FET: frozen embryo transfer)

Section 17: Advances in ART

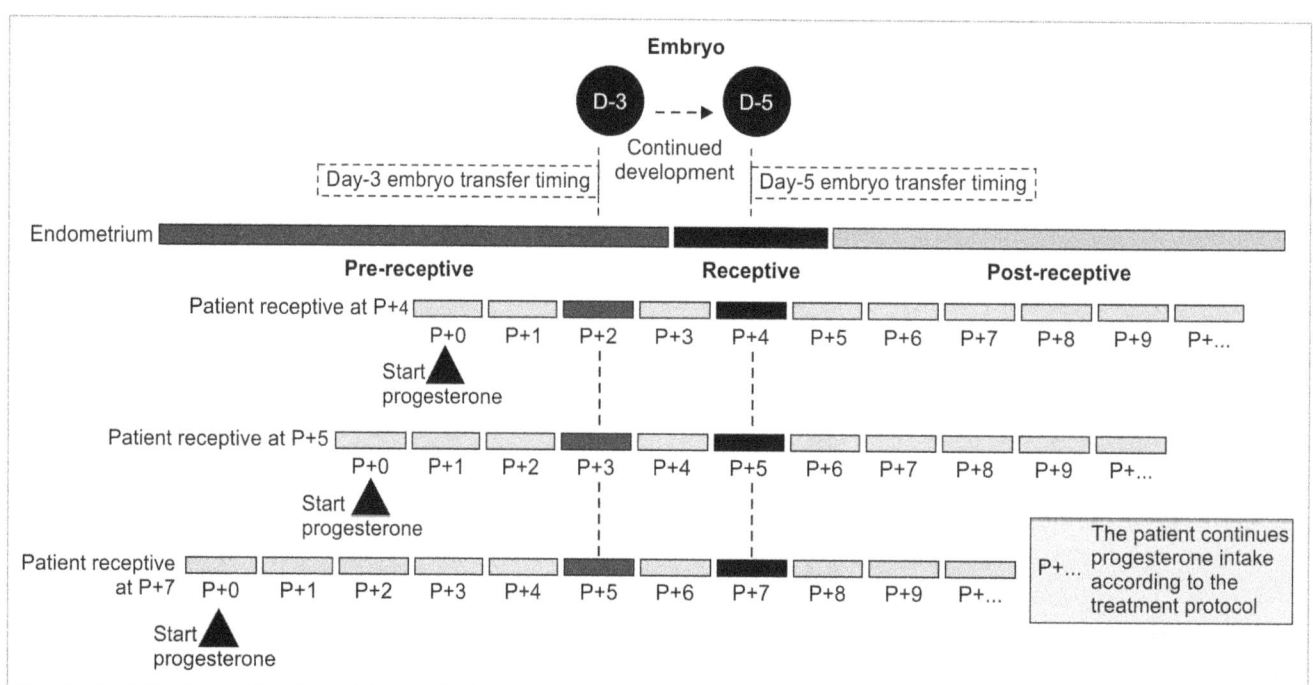

RECEPTIVE: LATE RECEPTIVE

Recommendation: The personalized embryo transfer (pET) of blastocyst/s should be performed with 107 ± 3 hours of progesterone administration (12 hours earlier than the time at which this endometrial biopsy was performed). A new endometrial biopsy is not required.**

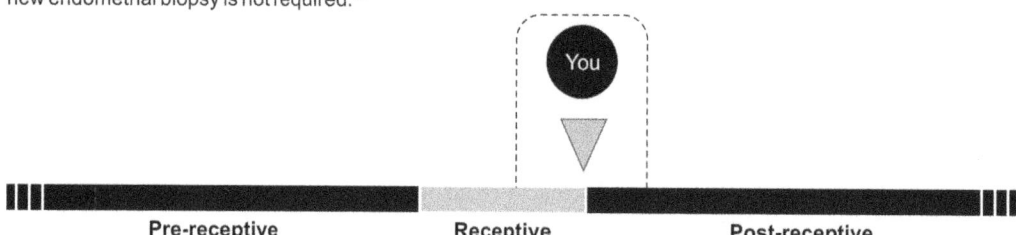

Inter pretation of your result:

The gene expression profile shows similarity to a late receptive stage. Blastocyst/s transfer is recommended with 107 ± 3 hours of progesterone administration (12 hours earlier than the time at which this endometrial biopsy was performed). Administration of progesterone can be delayed by 12 hours or the blastocyst transfer can be advanced by 12 hours relative to the timing used in the protocol for this endometrial biopsy.

For a day-3 embryo/s, the transfer should be performed two days earlier than indicated in the recommendation for blastocyst transfer above.

NON RECEPTIVE: POST-RECEPTIVE

Recommendation: To perform a new endometrial biopsy 1 day earlier than the time at which this endometrial biopsy was performed (110 ± 3 hours with progesterone administration)*

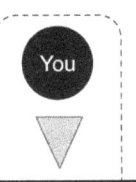

Pre-receptive   Receptive   Post-receptive

Inter pretation of your result:

The gene expression profile is concordant with an endometrium that has passed its receptive stage, meaning this patient may have a displaced window of implantation. A new endometrial biopsy is recommended to validate this displacement and to guide the personalized embryo transfer. The new biopsy should be performed 1 day earlier than the time at which this endometrial biopsy was performed.

* This recommendation is only applicable to the same type of cycle treatment as the one used for this endometrial biopsy and if the endogenous progesterone measured prior to the first progesterone intake is <1 ng/mL

NON RECEPTIVE: PRE-RECEPTIVE

Recommendation: To perform a new endometrial biopsy at P+6 (147 ±3 hours with progesterone administration)*

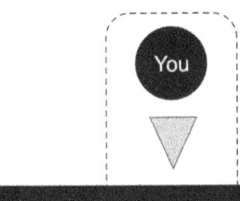

Pre-receptive   Receptive   Post-receptive

Inter pretation of your result:

The gene expression profile is concordant with an endometrium that has not yet reached its receptive stage, meaning this patient may have a displaced window of implantation. A new endometrial biopsy is recommended to validate this displacement and to guide the personalized embryo transfer. The new biopsy should be performed 1 day later than the time that this endometrial biopsy was taken (P+6).

CHAPTER 86

PGT and PGD

Keshav Malhotra, Neharika Malhotra Bora

A. Preimplantation genetic testing is a modality to test embryos for aneuploidy before they are transferred, it involves taking a biopsy from the embryo and running genetic tests like fluorescence in situ hybridization (FISH), array comparative genomic hybridization (CGH), or next-generation sequencing (NGS) on the biopsied product. The biopsy product can either be the polar body, blastomere from the cleavage embryo or trophectoderm cells from the blastocyst.

B. In patients for preimplantation genetic diagnosis (PGD), pre-PGD blood work is done for the couple and probe creation for the specific abnormality is created (2 weeks before start). This probe is used for the detection of similar genes in the embryonic biopsy. This step is absent for preimplantation genetic testing (PGT) process due to the presence of existing probes to detect various other commonly tested genetic abnormalities.

C. It is a good practice to do intracytoplasmic sperm injection (ICSI) for such embryos, when we do ICSI we are stripping off the maternal cumulus cells from the oocyte and also only one sperm is injected into the oocyte, with in vitro fertilization (IVF) there is a possibility of having either remnants of sperms or cumulus to contaminate the biopsied product thus can result in false positive results.

D. The list of common disorders to test with PGT is as follows:
   - Autosomal recessive:
     - Beta-thalassemia
     - Sickle-cell anemia
     - Cystic fibrosis
     - Tay-Sachs disease
     - Spinal muscular atrophy
     - Congenital adrenal hyperplasia
   - Autosomal dominant:
     - Myotonic dystrophy
     - Huntington's disease
     - Marfan syndrome
     - Familial adenomatous polyposis coli
     - Charcot-Marie-Tooth disease
   - X-linked:
     - Duchenne muscular dystrophy
     - Becker muscular dystrophy
     - Hemophilia
     - Fragile X syndrome
     - Lesch-Nyhan syndrome

E. Day 5 biopsy is associated with a higher implantation rate than day 3, a lower aneuploidy rate than day 3, and has a reduced chance of mosaicism and better chance of detection as more cells are available for diagnosis (Harton et al. 2011).

F. A high standard laboratory is essential to implement a PGT program, this means that the clinic should already have a validated culture system showing a high blastulation rate, should have trained embryologists, an efficient vitrification program, a good micro manipulation system equipped with a laser, and proper handling techniques so as to avoid contamination, false positives, and error rates.

G. Preimplantation genetic testing is still not recommended for universal practice but newer data is showing potential benefits in the form of an increased live birth rate with the transfer of single euploid embryos.

PGT and PGD

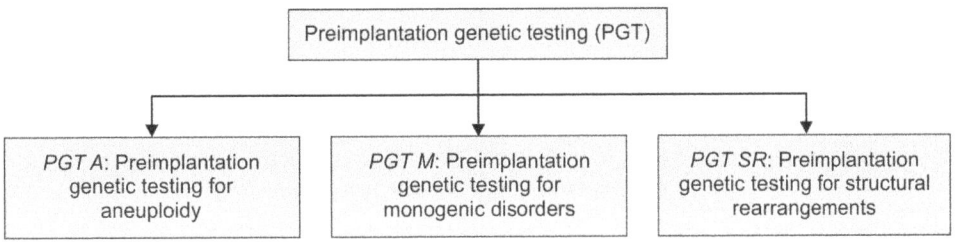

Preimplantation genetic testing for aneuploidy

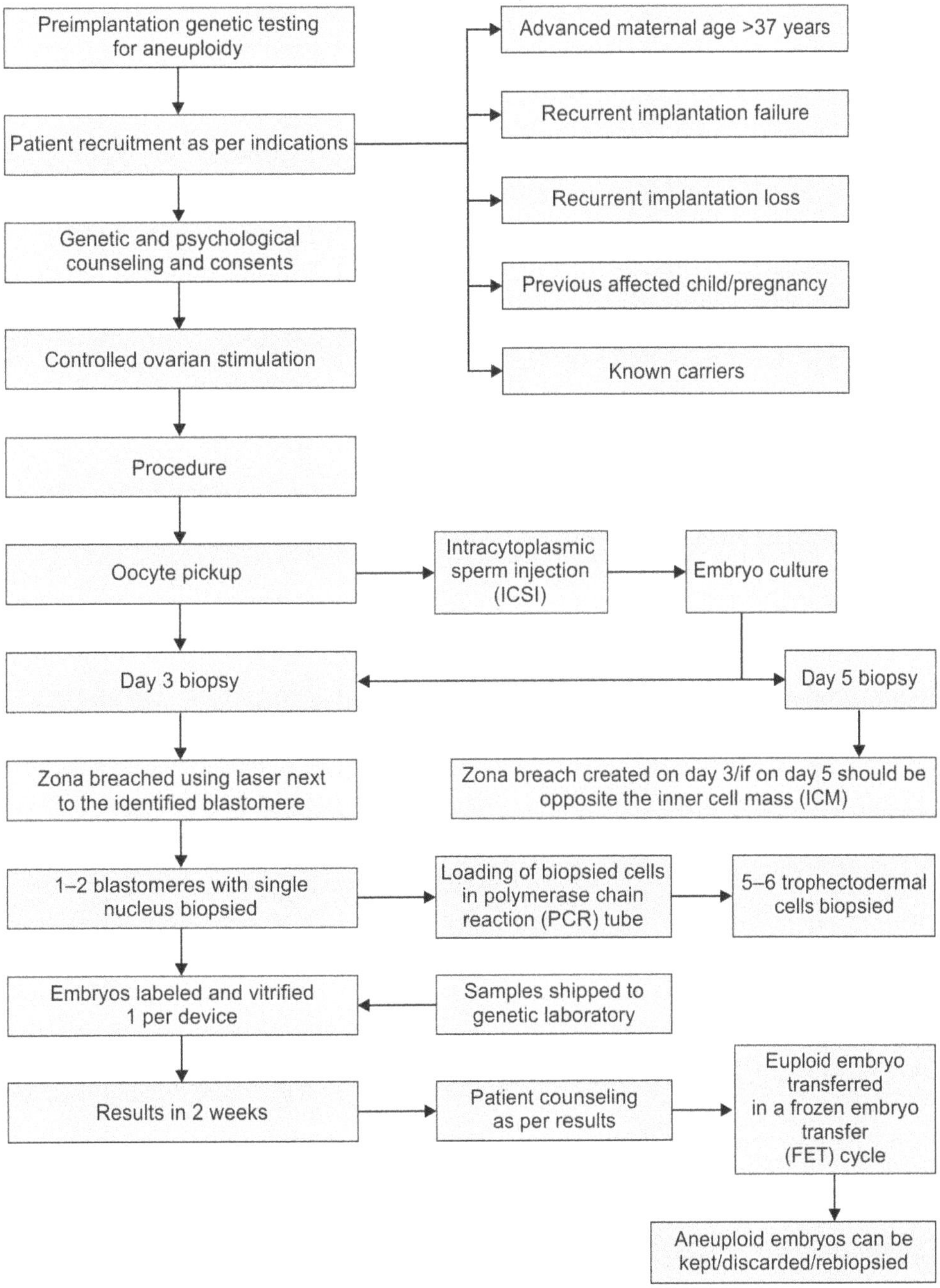

Preimplantation genetic diagnosis (PGD)

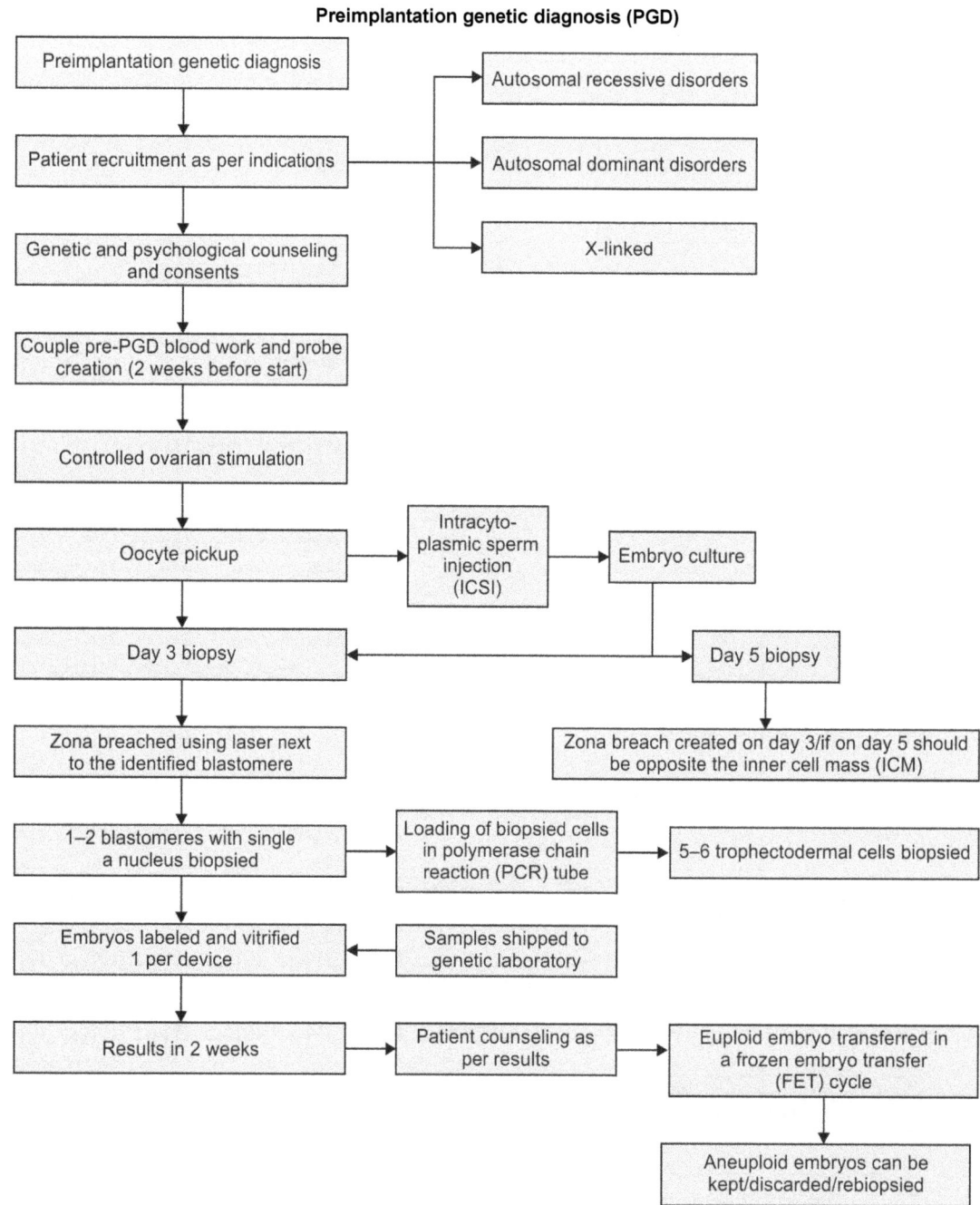

CHAPTER 87
Time-lapse Imaging of Preimplantation Embryos

Shubhashree Uppangala, Pratap Kumar, Satish Kumar Adiga

A. Enhancing the efficiency of assisted reproductive technique (ART) procedure by improving the pregnancy rate as well as decreasing multiple gestations are the primary objectives of the current ART treatment. If these goals have to be achieved, there is a need for improved selection method which can predict the implantation potential of the selected embryo accurately before its transfer. However, the current morphology-based evaluation method has been proven to be not robust always in predicting the embryo implantation as it is assessed at particular time point and also does not predict the genetic integrity of the embryos. Hence, new adjunct technologies have been introduced to assess embryo quality; one such technique is "time-lapse imaging" (TLI) of embryos.

B. The main principle of TLI based on the time-lapse photography. Several time-lapse systems to monitor embryo development are available in market, e.g. EmbryoScope (Vitrolife), PrimoVision (Vitrolife), EEVA (Aoxygen), and Miri (ESCO). The common features of all these systems are a digital camera attached to inverted microscope which comes with integrated incubator or can be kept inside the conventional incubator. The camera is programed to take pictures of the embryos at particular interval (usually 5–20 minutes). These images are processed and displayed on a computer. The pictures taken will be made into short films/video. These videos containing various events of embryo development that can be analyzed using the software to evaluate both morphology and developmental kinetics of the embryos, thus termed as morphokinetics.

C. In literature, various studies have developed distinct algorithms of embryo development to predict the embryo development/implantation potential. The time taken for first cytokinesis, time interval between first and second mitoses, and time interval between second and third mitoses have been correlated with blastocyst development. The timing of the cleavage to 5 cells (t5) has been correlated with implantation potential. Other parameter such as time to pronuclear fading (tPNf) has been associated with embryo developmental potential. The annotations such as time to start of blastoculation (tSB), time to blastocyst (tB) have been associated with chromosome status of the embryos and t5–t2 and cc3 (t5–t3) also been linked to chromosomal content of preimplantation human embryos.

D. The key advantages of TLI include the facility of a superior culture environment, which is based on the fact that embryo assessment is done without disturbing the culture inside the incubator itself, also the objective evaluation of embryos and the information collected are very accurate. Although, TLI-based embryo selection has many advantages, the results may be influenced by several factors such as the type of culture medium used, pH, oxygen, stimulation protocols, laboratory procedures, and type of infertility may affect the morphokinetic profile of embryos. As there are various confounding factors which can alter the developmental kinetics, recent study has recommended not to directly adapt already established algorithms in the in vitro fertilization (IVF) laboratory instead urges the need for in-house TLI selection algorithms. However, the field of ART is still waiting for the valuable quality proof to adapt TLI in its routine practice.

E. In summary, the current literature has defined time-lapse as an intervention that effectively involves undisturbed embryo culture and has robustness in objectively selecting embryos for transfer. However, there is a need for more randomized control trials before we consider TLI-based embryo selection in our routine practice. Also, it is important to develop in-house embryo selection algorithms adjusting all the confounding factors that can affect embryo developmental kinetics.

```
                There is a need for improved embryo selection procedure to enhance
                       pregnancy outcome in assisted reproductive technique (ART)

        (A)     As an adjunct technology, time-lapse imaging (TLI) of
                       embryos has been introduced

        (B)     All TLI systems are based on time-lapse photography and have
                       common features and assess morphokinetics of the embryos

        (C)     Generally, in TLI, standard embryo developmental timeline is taken
                as reference and compared with the observed timeline. The embryo
                       which follows reference timeline is selected
```

Embryo developmental stage	2 PN/2 PB	2 cell	4 cell	8 cell	Morula	Blastocyst
Reference timeline	16–18 hours	25–27 hours	43–45 hours	67–69 hours	90–94 hours	114–118 hours

```
        (D)     Various algorithms have been developed correlating embryo
                       development potential and implantation

                Although TLI is a better selection method, it is influenced by several
                factors including stimulation protocols, type of culture media, culture
        (E)                        conditions, and type of infertility

                • There is need for in-house developed algorithms
                • Need for more randomized control trials
```

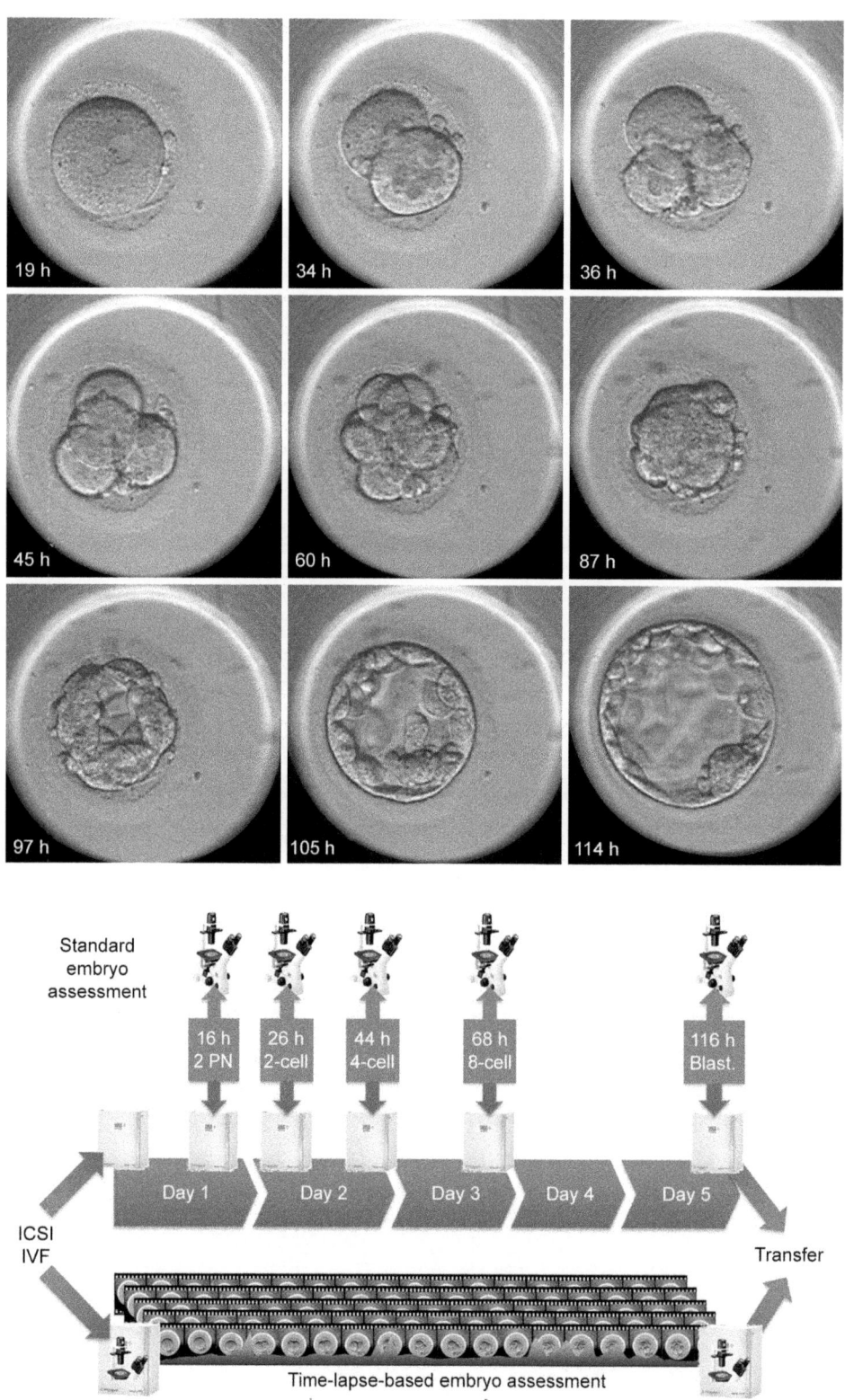

(ICSI: intracytoplasmic sperm injection)

SECTION 18

Difficult Scenarios

- Recurrent Implantation Failure
- Recurrent Implantation Failure: Evaluation
- Management of Recurrent Implantation Failure
- Recurrent Pregnancy Loss: Management
- Thin Endometrium
- Empty Follicular Syndrome

CHAPTER 88

Recurrent Implantation Failure

Divyashree PS, Surbhi Gupta

Recurrent implantation failure (RIF) remains an enigma in infertility practice. Despite many publications on this topic there is no universally accepted definition till date. Simon and Laufer defined RIF as the failure to obtain a clinical pregnancy after three consecutive in vitro fertilization (IVF) attempts, in which one or two embryos of high grade quality are transferred in each cycle. Somigliana et al. however has cautioned about over diagnosis of RIF, if diagnosis of RIF is drawn after only two to three IVF cycles. Indeed, the rate of false positive diagnosis remains above 50% in all sensitivity analyses, if diagnosis of RIF is considered after three IVF cycles. It is after six cycles that the diagnosis of RIF becomes more reliable. The actual prevalence of RIF is unidentified and randomly set at 10% (but then varied in sensitivity analyses from 5% to 25%). The etiology of RIF can be considered under three categories:

A. *Gamete and embryo factors:*
   - Impaired quality of either of the gametes (sperm or oocyte) is implicated in RIF. Advanced maternal age, poor response or hyper-response leads to impaired quality of oocytes and hence reduced implantation rates. Sperm quality is also important for fertilization and association between deoxyribonucleic acid (DNA) fragmentation and recurrent miscarriage has been proven, but its association with RIF is not clear. Embryogenesis can be impaired by chromosomal abnormalities of the male or female partner, the gametes or the developing embryo itself. Maternal cytoplasmic factors or mutations in cell cycle control genes can cause disruption of the normal sequence of chromosome replication and segregation in early human embryos, which can be a common cause for RIF. Defective hatching due to zona hardening as a cause for RIF has been suggested by a few studies.

B. *Factors affecting endometrial receptivity*:
   - Uterine factors such as myomas, polyps, adenomyosis, and synechiae lead to reduced implantation rates by affecting the vascular perfusion, impaired endometrial receptivity, and causing increased cellular apoptosis. Immunological factors like impaired Th1-Th2 balance, uterine natural killer cells and presence of autoantibodies have also been proposed as a cause of RIF. Altered endometrial microbiota; that is; nonlactobacillus-dominated microbiota has been correlated with adverse reproductive outcome like implantation failure and miscarriage.

C. *Multifactorial effects*:
   - Diseases like endometriosis, polycystic ovary syndrome (PCOS), and hydrosalpinx lead to altered folliculogenesis, impaired oocyte quality, altered expression of αvβ3 integrin, and *HOXA10* genes; thereby causing reduced implantation rates. Hydrosalpinx fluid, in addition has embryotoxic effect, which may lead to RIF.

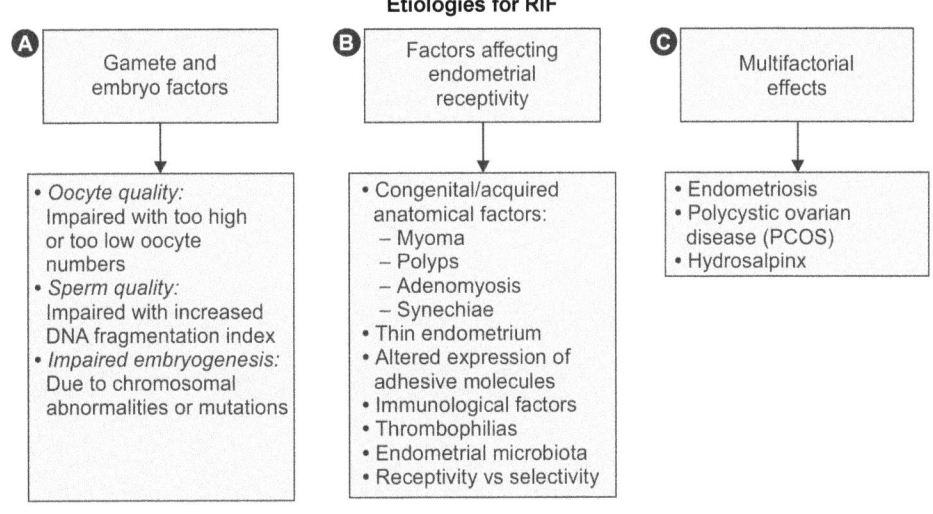

(DNA: deoxyribonucleic acid; RIF: recurrent implantation failure)

CHAPTER 88A

Recurrent Implantation Failure: Evaluation

Divyashree PS, Surbhi Gupta

EVALUATION FOR RECURRENT IMPLANTATION FAILURE

Recurrent implantation failure (RIF) is not a diagnosis but a mere clinical presentation, which requires appropriate phenotyping and etiological investigations. We have various tools to detect the cause of RIF, whether it is at the level of embryo, endometrium, or it is multifactorial, as depicted here in the Flowchart 1.

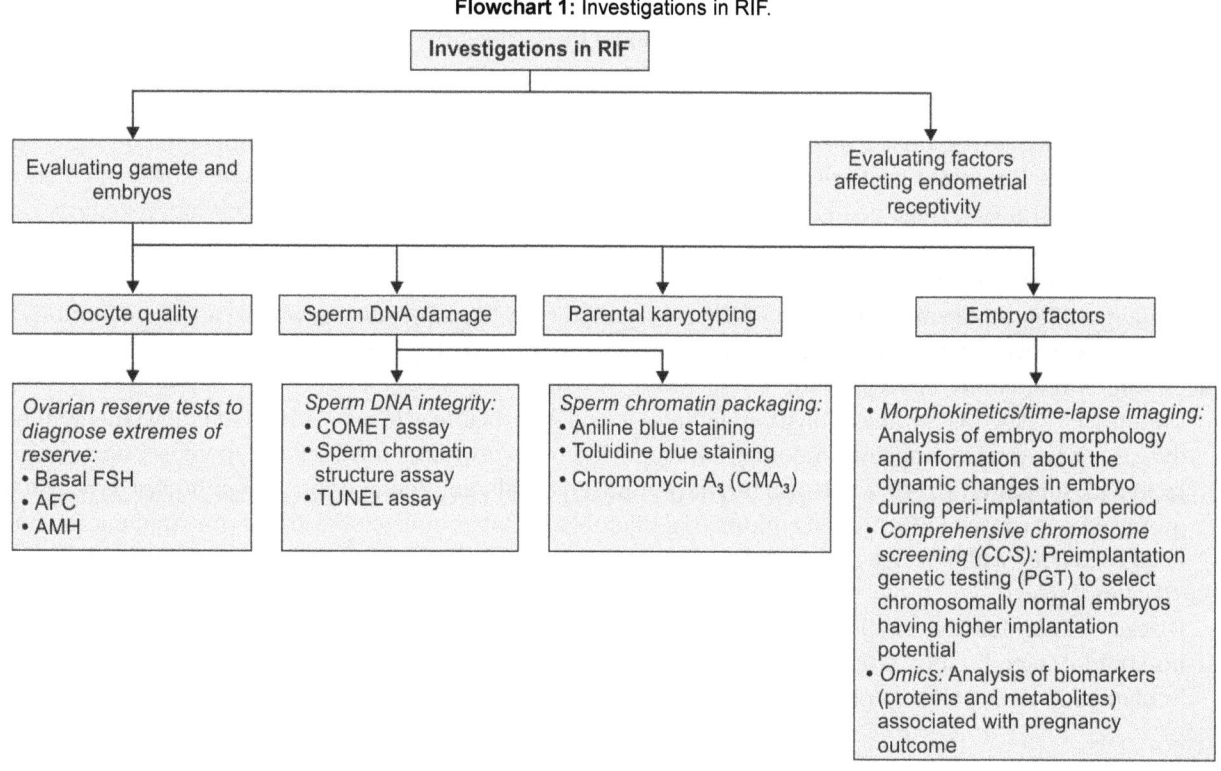

Flowchart 1: Investigations in RIF.

(AFC: antral follicle count; AMH: anti-Müllerian hormone; DNA: deoxyribonucleic acid; FSH: follicle-stimulating hormone; RIF: recurrent implantation failure)

Recurrent Implantation Failure: Evaluation

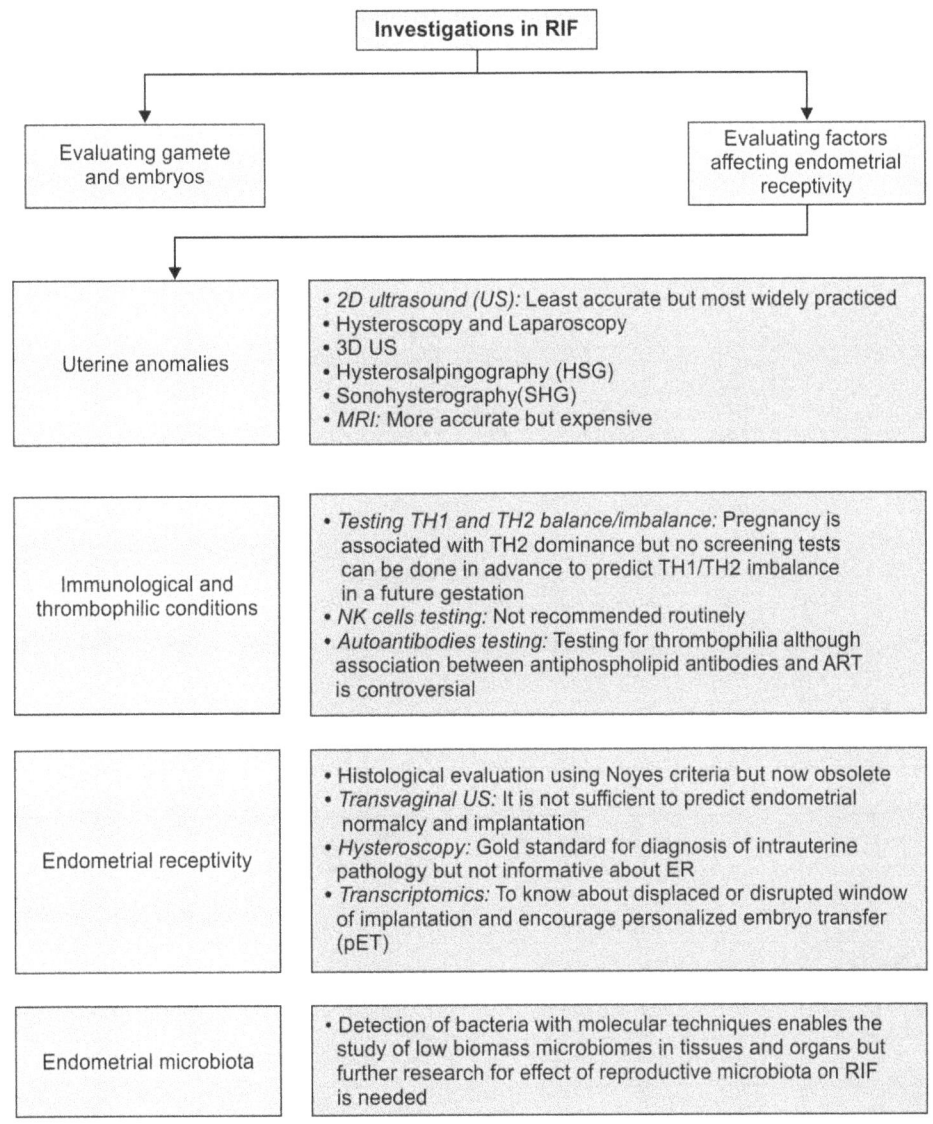

(2D: two-dimensional; 3D: three-dimensional; NK: natural killer; RIF: recurrent implantation failure; ART: assisted reproductive technique; ER: embryo transfer)

CHAPTER 88B

Management of Recurrent Implantation Failure

Divyashree PS, Surbhi Gupta

The role of multidisciplinary team in the management of recurrent implantation failure (RIF) cannot be overemphasized. The multidisciplinary team should comprise of Reproductive Medicine specialist, Embryologist, Counselor, Clinical Geneticist, Immunologist, and Endocrinologist. Couple with RIF should be evaluated by this team. There should be a local protocol agreed upon by this team as to how to investigate these couple with RIF which is based on robust evidence.

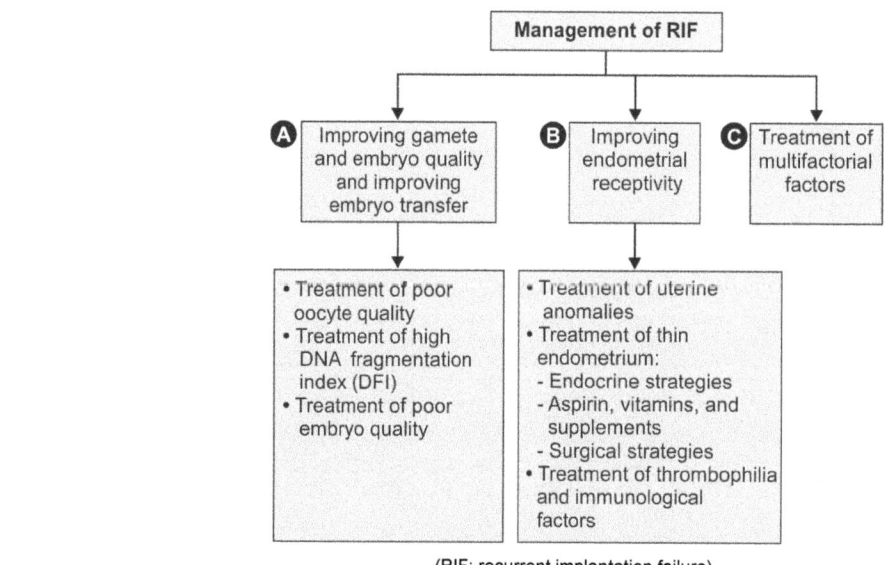

(RIF: recurrent implantation failure)

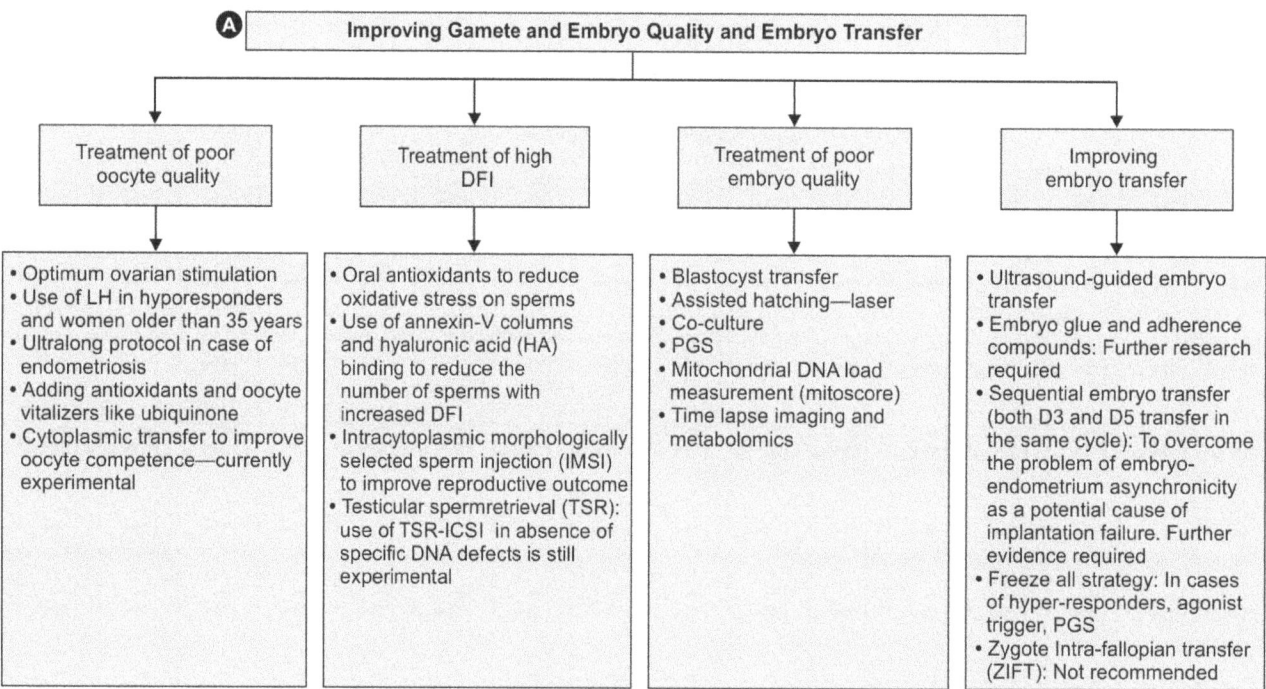

(DFI: DNA fragmentation index; LH: luteinizing hormone; PGS: preimplantation genetic screening)

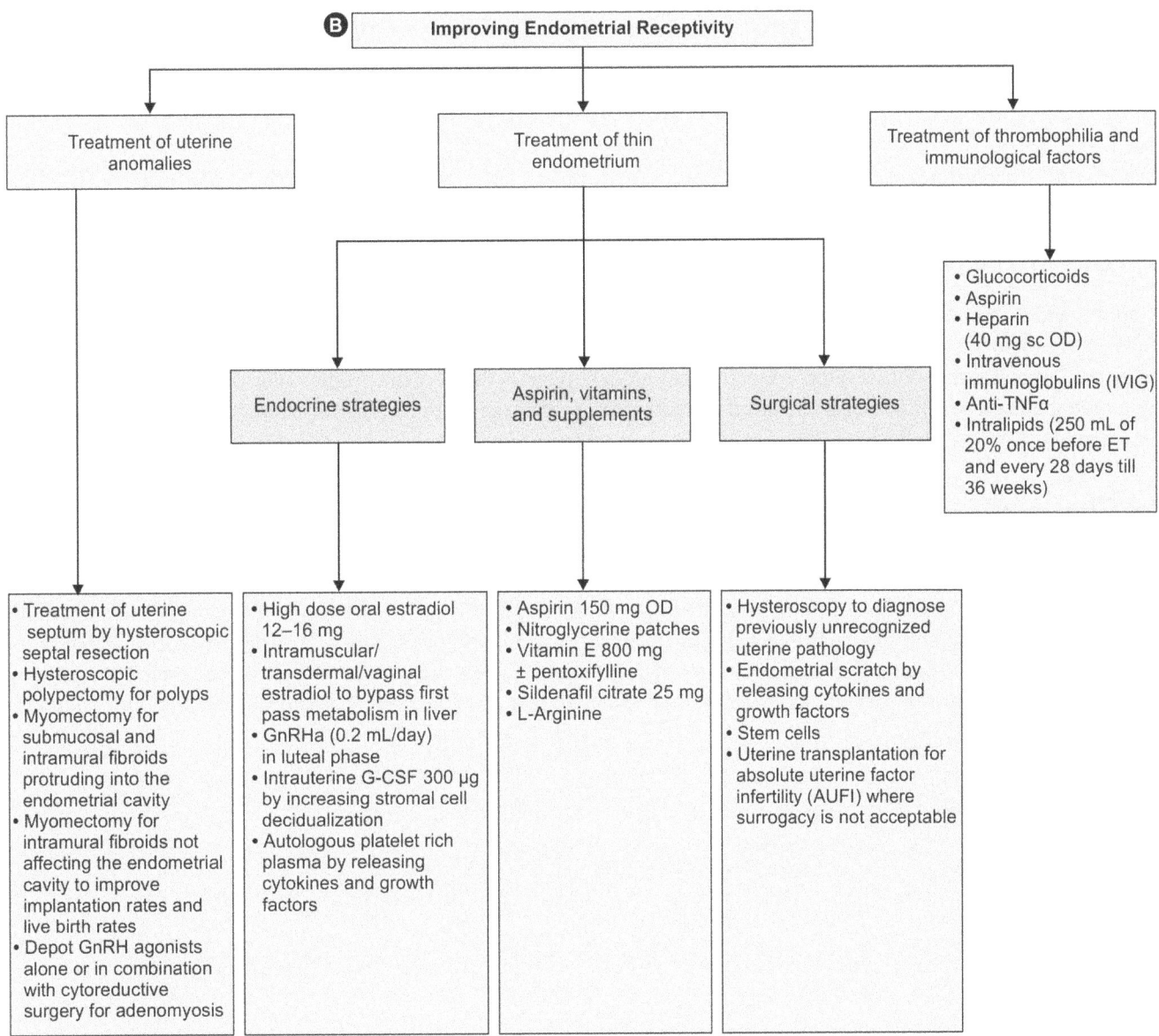

(ET: embryo transfer; G-CSF: granulocyte-colony stimulation factor; GnRHa: gonadotropin releasing hormone antagonist; OD: once a day; sc: subcutaneous; TNF: tumor necrosis factor)

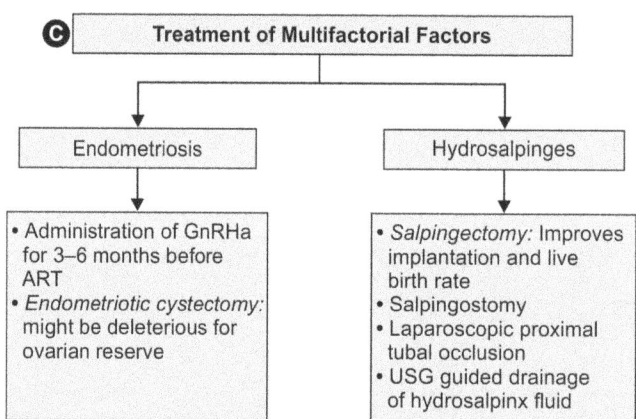

(ART: assisted reproductive technique; GnRHa; gonadotropin releasing hormone antagonist; USG: ultrasonography)

GAMETE DONATION AND SURROGACY

Couples with RIF need help on the aptness of ensuing with further in vitro fertilization (IVF) attempts. If implantation fails to occur in spite of repeated treatment attempts or if the prognosis of further IVF treatment is measured to be poor, alternative treatment options should to be reconnoitered. If the likely basis of the problem lies with the embryo, gamete donation should be recommended. On the other hand, if the problem lies in the uterus, for example multiple small fibroids or Asherman syndrome which has failed to react to surgical treatment, surrogacy must be discussed.

CONCLUSION

There are a lot of controversial issues in the field of reproductive medicine, starting from the definition of infertility, which moves on to the diagnosis of unexplained infertility, which entitles the couple to an unproven treatment, IVF. In those couple who do not conceive after three or more attempts of IVF, comes a fabricated diagnosis of RIF. Couples with infertility belong to a very vulnerable group. They will do almost anything to achieve a pregnancy. They deserve our dedicated care and evidence-based treatment. In case such an evidence base is lacking, the patients should be counseled accordingly and, if the occasion arises, they might be invited to participate in a carefully designed clinical trial. They should not be exploited.

CHAPTER 89

Recurrent Pregnancy Loss: Management

Kamini Patel, Vani Patel

A. Recurrent pregnancy loss (RPL) is common with 15% of all clinically recognized pregnancies resulting in miscarriage. Although conventionally RPL is defined as three consecutive pregnancy losses prior to 20 weeks from the last menstrual period as pregnancy loss is a significant negative life event as per European Society of Human Reproduction and Embryology (ESHRE) 2017 guidelines it is advised to considered the loss of two or more pregnancies as RPL. The risk of subsequent miscarriages is similar among women that have had two versus three miscarriages, and the probability of finding a treatable etiology is similar among the two groups, most experts agree that there is a role for evaluation after two losses.

B. Older women (> 40 years), maternal obesity, smoking, and excessive alcohol consumption are some risk factors associated with RPL.

C. Accepted etiologies for RPL include parental chromosomal abnormalities, untreated hypothyroidism, uncontrolled diabetes mellitus, certain uterine anatomic abnormalities, and the antiphospholipid antibody syndrome (APS). Other probable or possible etiologies include additional endocrine disorders, heritable and/or acquired thrombophilias, immunologic abnormalities, and environmental causes. After evaluation for these causes, more than 33% of all cases will remain unexplained.

D. *Genetic cause*: Routine genetic analysis of products of conception is not recommended. It may be done only for explanatory purposes. When performed, array-based comparative genomic hybridization (array-CGH) should be the preferred method of assessment. Parental karyotyping has its limitations and should be advised only after a detailed family history with risk assessment and not on a routine basis. Couples with genetic aberrations should receive appropriate genetic counseling and information regarding methods like preimplantation genetic diagnosis (PGD) for managing the specific genetic abnormality.

E. *Thrombophilias*: Thrombophilias are either hereditary [protein C, protein S, and antithrombin deficiency, abnormal factor V gene (factor V Leiden), and prothrombin gene variant 20210A] or acquired [anticardiolipin (aCL) antibodies and lupus anticoagulant (LA)]. Women with RPL should be investigated routinely for antiphospholipid antibodies (APLAs) [LA and aCL antibodies β2-glycoprotein I antibodies (ACA IgG and IgM) and not for inherited thrombophilias or homocysteine]. There is insufficient evidence to recommend routine testing of antinuclear antibodies (ANA) natural killer (NK) cell either in peripheral blood or in endometrial tissue. There is no role of use of low-molecular-weight heparin (LMWH) in women with hereditary thrombophilia unless indicated by a venous thromboembolism (VTE) risk. Starting low-dose aspirin (75–100 mg/day) before conception, and use of prophylactic dose heparin [unfractionated heparin (UFH) or LMWH] starting from date of a positive pregnancy test, in cases of RPL with a positive APLA laboratory criterion improves the live birth rate.

F. Thyroid screening is recommended through thyroid-stimulating hormone (TSH) and thyroid peroxidase (TPO) antibodies. An abnormal test should trigger testing of thyroxine (T4). There is limited evidence supporting the use of levothyroxine in cases of positive thyroid antibodies with normal TSH levels. Both overt and subclinical hypothyroidism should be corrected in pregnancy (7–9 weeks). Routine testing of fasting insulin, fasting glucose, and androgen testing in polycystic ovary syndrome (PCOS), prolactin, ovarian reserve or luteal phase insufficiency in RPL is not recommended unless associated with other symptoms. When elevated, prolactin should be controlled using bromocriptine to improve pregnancy rates. There is insufficient evidence to recommend the use of metformin, progesterone or human chorionic gonadotropin (hCG) in women with RPL to improve pregnancy rates. Prophylactic supplementation of vitamin D may be considered preconceptionally to improve reproductive outcome.

G. All women with RPL should be evaluated for uterine cavity preferably using a transvaginal sonography (TVS) with three-dimensional (3D) and when its not available, saline infusion sonography is a reasonable alternate. Routine use of magnetic resonance imaging (MRI) is not recommended. Metroplasty for bicornuate and uterine reconstruction for unicornuate uterus is not recommended. Hysteroscopic septal resection and myomectomy of submucous myoma are considered beneficial in a RPL setting. Women with suspected cervical incompetence should be offered serial ultrasonography (USG) after one loss less than 20 weeks and be advised prophylactic cerclage in case of more than one loss owing to cervical incompetence.

H. Assessing sperm deoxyribonucleic acid (DNA) fragmentation in male partner for couples with RPL may be considered for reasoning purposes.

I. Therapy should be directed toward any treatable etiology, and may include in vitro fertilization with PGD, use of donor gametes, surgical correction of anatomic abnormalities, correction of endocrine disorders, and anticoagulation or folic acid supplementation.

J. In cases of unexplained RPL, use of lymphocyte immunization therapy, intravenous immunoglobulin (IVIg), glucocorticoids, heparin or low dose aspirin or vaginal progesterone is not recommended routinely. There is some evidence that oral dydrogesterone may be of some benefit. There is insufficient evidence to recommend the use of intralipid therapy or granulocyte colony-stimulating factor (G-CSF) in women with unexplained RPL.

K. Antenatal counseling and psychological support should be offered to all couples experiencing RPL, as these measures have been shown to increase pregnancy success rates.

L. Prognosis will depend on the underlying cause for pregnancy loss and the number of prior losses. Patients and physicians can be encouraged by the overall good prognosis, as even after four consecutive losses a patient has a greater than 60–65% chance of carrying her next pregnancy to term.

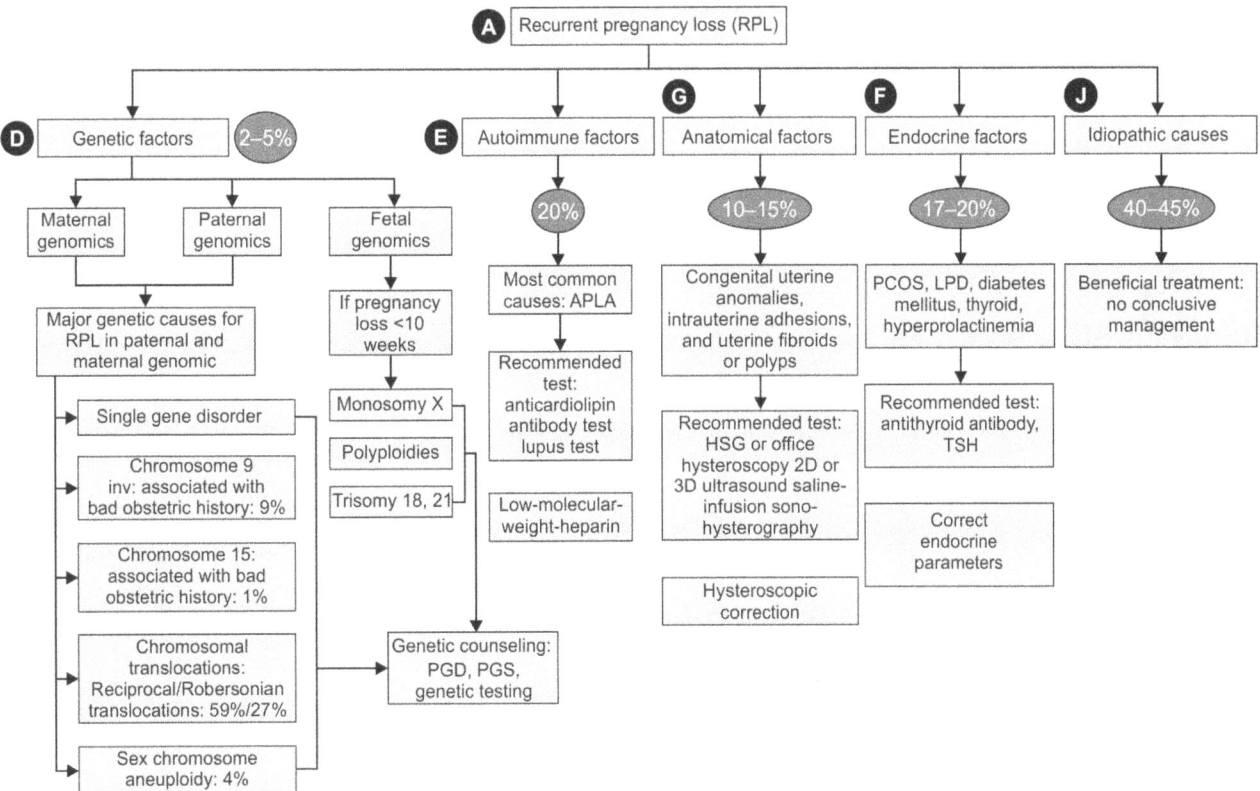

(APLA: antiphospholipid antibody; HSG: hysterosalpingogram; LPD: luteal phase defect; PCOS: polycystic ovary syndrome; PGD: preimplantation genetic diagnosis; PGS: preimplantation genetic screening; TSH: thyroid-stimulating hormone; 2D: two-dimensional; 3D: three-dimensional).

CHAPTER 90

Thin Endometrium

Pratik Tambe, Apoorva Pallam Reddy

A. The optimal endometrial thickness for conception remains debatable among clinicians despite all the research. Endometrial thickness (EMT) less than 7 mm on ultrasound is largely considered suboptimal for embryo transfer (ET) and is correlated to a decreased probability of pregnancy. Studies have shown that maximum conception rate is achieved if the thickness is in between 8 mm and 10 mm.

B. Scarring of the endometrial tissue due to infection, radiotherapy, previous surgical intervention, and reduced subendometrial vascularity may result in thin endometrium. However, most common causes for thin endometrium are idiopathic. The first line of management of thin endometrium includes treating the underlying cause. The rate of improvement in EMT however, is not consistent. Although multiple modalities have been tried to improve EMT in idiopathic cases there is no strong evidence supporting any single therapy.

C. If a diagnosis of intrauterine adhesions is made, hysteroscopic adhesiolysis is recommended before any other modality. Endometritis, specifically Koch's induced can result in subendometrial damage. Treating with anti tubercular therapy (ATT) at the right time reduces the risk of permanent damage.

D. Endometrium proliferates under the effect of estrogen. Increasing the dose and bioavailability of estrogen improve the endometrial thickness. Start with high doses (6–8 mg or up to 16 mg) continuously from cycle day 1. Maintaining high doses for long periods, for up to 9 weeks (Chen et al., 2006; Remohí et al., 1995), has no adverse effects, such as endometrial hyperplasia or bleeding. Endometrium is capable of maintaining its receptivity even in prolonged follicular phases. Transdermal/transvaginal routes should be considered when dealing with high-risk patients.

E. There is insufficient evidence to approve any single agent to definitively improve the vascularity and subsequently improve the endometrial thickness. However, multiple well-formulated observational studies have suggested the benefit of these agents in improving endometrial thickness. Sildenafil citrate is a selective inhibitor of cyclic guanosine monophosphate (cGMP)-specific phosphodiesterase type 5 (PDE5). It prevents breakdown of cGMP and potentiates effect of nitric oxide on vascular smooth muscle thus enhancing uterine blood flow. In a trial comparing sildenafil citrate 50 mg/day daily versus increasing doses of estradiol valerate, endometrial thickness ($p < 0.0001$), triple line patterns ($p > 0.0001$), and echogenic patterns were significantly higher ($p < 0.0001$) with sildenafil citrate. Use of low-molecular-weight heparin also improves subendometrial vascularity.

F. *Granulocyte colony-stimulating factor (G-CSF):* Patients with resistant thin endometrium unresponsive to estradiol, G-CSF administered on day of human chorionic gonadotropin (hCG) administration and repeated if ET still less than 7 mm 48 hours later via intrauterine catheter. ET increased from 6.4 ± 1.4 mm to 9.3 ± 2.1 mm ($p < 0.001$), average change was 2.9 ± 2.0 mm; CPR was 19.1% (n = 21) 26.

   In meta-analysis of 10 randomized controlled trials (RCTs), 1,016 cycles (521 in G-CSF group) showed improved clinical pregnancy rates with intrauterine infusion as well as with subcutaneous injection of G-CSF.

G. *Autologous platelet-rich plasma (PRP):* Fresh whole blood enriched with platelets many angiogenic and growth factors like vascular endothelial growth factor (VEGF), EGF, PDGF, TGF, IGF-I and II, IL-8, CTGF, and cytokines which stimulate proliferation and growth. On day 9/10 of cycle, 17.5 mL peripheral venous blood is collected in acid-citrate-dextrose (ACD) test tube with 2.5 mL ACD-A anticoagulant solution; centrifuged at 1,200 rpm for 12 minutes to separate RBCs. The supernatant plasma is again centrifuged at 3,300 rpm for 7 minutes. 0.5 mL of PRP is infused into the uterine cavity with an intrauterine insemination (IUI) catheter or injected into the subendometrial cavity under hysteroscopic guidance. Increase in the ET is noted as early as 48 hours after first infusion. A second infusion may be performed after 48 hours.

   PRP infusion may be repeated after 48 hours if there is no improvement in the EMT. Studies have shown significant improvement in not only EMT, but also in implantation rates, clinical pregnancy rates and lower cancellation rates.

H. Intrauterine administration of bone marrow stem cells and progenitor cells is showing promising results for endometrial regeneration especially in cases of subendometrial damage. The regenerative capacity of the functionalis layers of the endometrium every cycle is due to the presence of endometrial stem/progenitor cells in the basalis layer. It is shown that regeneration of the endometrium is influenced not only by local endometrial progenitor cells but also by the hematopoietic and nonhematopoietic bone marrow-derived stem cells (BMDSCs). In light of these findings, role of stem cell in regeneration of thin endometrium is being evaluated enthusiastically. Infusing autologous CD 133 + BMDSCs into the uterine cavity or into the spiral arterioles is shown to significantly increase the endometrial thickness.

I. In cases of persistent thin endometrium, use of natural cycle FET or modified natural cycle is reported to improve pregnancy results with or without change in the endometrial thickness.

J. *Tamoxifen:* Tamoxifen is a selective estrogen receptor modulator that stimulates the gpr30 estrogen receptor (GPER) that induces aromatase expression in endometrial cells, thus increases increases local estrogen biosynthesis in endometrial cells.

	Impact of endometrial thickness	
	Fresh embryo transfer	Frozen-thaw cycle
ET	LBR	LBR
4–4.9 mm	-	15%
5–5.9 mm	18.1%	21.2%
6–6.9 mm	24.6%	23.7%
7–7.9 mm	25.5%	27.4%
≥8 mm	33.7%	28.4%

Likelihood of achieving ET ≥8 mm with age	
<35 years	89.7%
35–39 years	87.8%
≥40 years	83.9%

(LBR: live birth rate; ET: embryo transfer)

Thin Endometrium

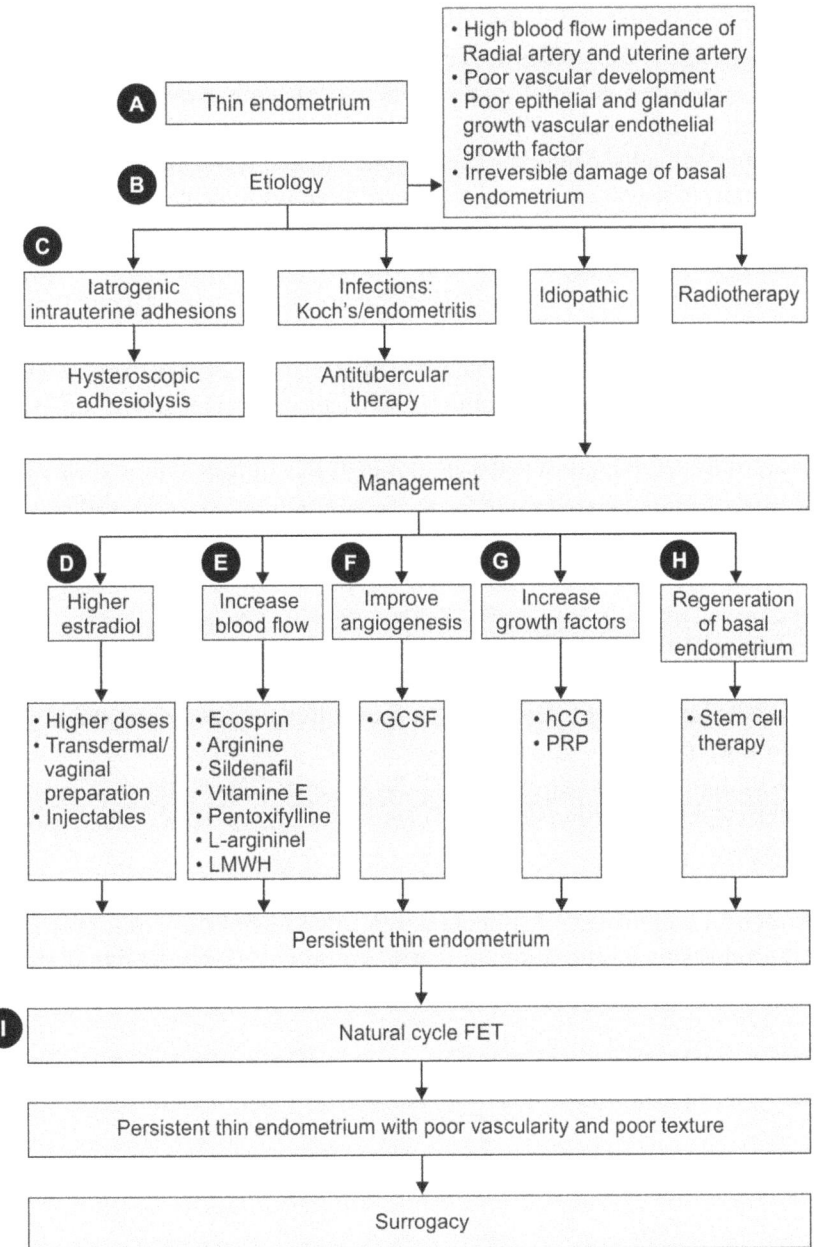

(FET: frozen embryo transfer; GCSF: granulocyte colony-stimulating factor; hCG: human chorionic gonadotropin; LMWH: low-molecular-weight heparin; PRP: platelet-rich plasma; VEGF: vascular endothelial growth factor)

Empty Follicular Syndrome

Kedar Ganla, Priyanka Vora, Rana Choudhary

A. Empty follicle syndrome (EFS) is defined as the complete inability to aspirate follicles after 36 hours from ovulation trigger seen after successful monitoring of controlled ovarian hyperstimulation for an assisted reproductive technique (ART) cycle. In any ART cycle, the number of oocytes obtained is usually lower then the number of follicles aspirated because even some mature follicles might not have an oocyte despite a normal follicular development (folliculogenesis) and estradiol levels (steroidogenesis). However, the incidence of inability to aspirate even one oocyte is less than 1%.

B. There are two types of empty follicular syndrome—(1) Genuine empty follicular syndrome or (2) False empty follicular syndrome. A genuine EPS is diagnosed after ruling out the cause for a false EFS (F-EFS). High maternal age, high basal follicle-stimulating hormone (FSH) level, and fall in serum estradiol level prior to trigger are certain risk factors for F-EFS. The most common cause of F-EFS is improper administration of trigger either with respect to timing or drug. Too early or too late pickup from trigger can result in failed aspiration. Lack of cold chain maintenance of the trigger or poor biological availability of certain batches or rapid clearance of the drug by the liver also can hamper the endogenous luteinizing hormone (LH) surge resulting in failed aspiration of follicles. Too low pressure of the aspiration system (ideal 100PSI) or incomplete aspiration of the follicle are also causes of F-EFS.

C. Obtaining immature oocytes [metaphase I (MI)] should not be confused with that of inability to retrieve oocytes. Aspirating higher number of immature oocytes can be seen in condition like polycystic ovary syndrome (PCOS), due to inadequate LH surge, derangement in oocyte cumulus complex, and intrinsic oocyte factor (aspirated oocytes did not reach M2 phase due to absent meiotic recombination in pachytene stage/inability to produce key cell regulating factors).

D. If EFS is suspected in an ongoing aspiration, a urinary human chorionic gonadotropin (hCG) level can be assessed using a urine pregnancy test (UPT) kit. If a strong positive is seen, continue to aspirate the other ovary. If the kit is negative, it indicates a failed trigger. Hence abandon the procedure, repeat trigger, and plan for oocyte pickup (OPU) 36 hours from the new trigger.

E. However, when a gonadotropin-releasing hormone (GnRH) agonist trigger is used, urinary LH kits are not favored for detection of serum LH levels because the endogenous LH surge occurs 10–12 hours before ovulation and the detection ability depends on the sensitivity of the kit.

F. The precautions to be taken in the subsequent cycle include giving a trigger from a different batch, preferring intramuscular route of injection instead of subcutaneous, using higher dose of trigger (10,000 IU or urinary hCG or 0.5 mg of rhCG), and checking for the serum progesterone and LH levels the day after trigger helps in ruling out any iatrogenic pathology. If the LH and P4 levels are low, it suggests failure of trigger and a repeat trigger should be considered.

G. Case reports have shown that, in case of G-EFS, giving a dual trigger with both hCG and GnRH agonist (5,000 IU or u-hCG + 2 mL of GnRH agonist) has been shown to not only retrieve mature oocytes but also result in healthy pregnancy.

H. Oocyte donation is the final resort for the women who fail to have oocyte retrieval in more than two attempts despite all rescue efforts.

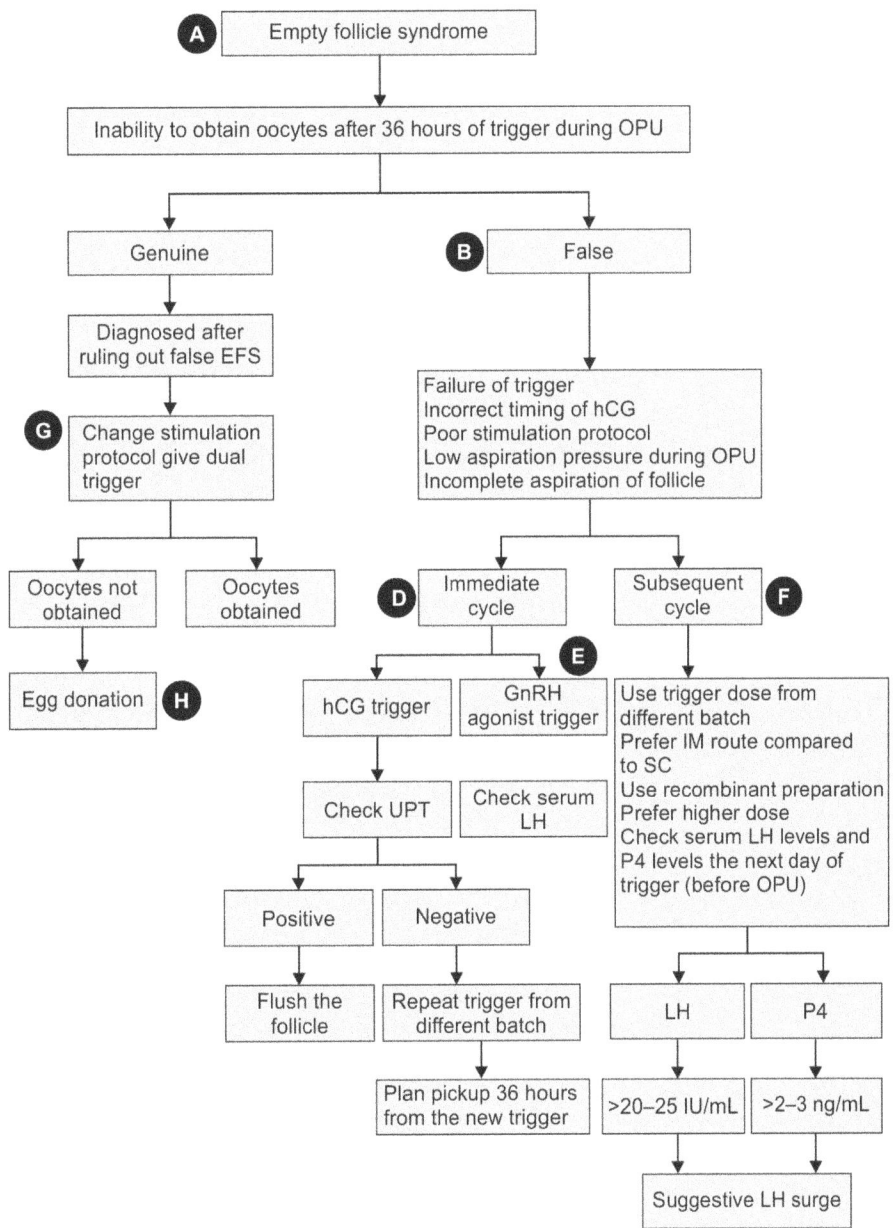

(EFS: empty follicle syndrome; GnRH: gonadotropin-releasing hormone; hCG: human chorionic gonadotropin; IM: intramuscular; LH: luteinizing hormone; OPU: oocyte pickup; SC: subcutaneous; UPT: urine pregnancy test)

SECTION 19

Pregnancy in ART

- Ectopic Pregnancy- Diagnosis
- Ectopic Pregnancy: Surgical Management
- Ectopic Pregnancy: Medical Management
- Fetal Reduction

Ectopic Pregnancy- Diagnosis

Astha Ubeja, Neharika Malhotra Bora

INTRODUCTION

Ectopic pregnancy is the implantation of a fertilized ovum outside the uterine cavity. The successful treatment of tubal pregnancy with salpingectomy was first reported by Robert Lawson Tait in 1884.

INCIDENCE AND SITES OF ECTOPIC IMPLANTATION

The overall incidence of ectopic pregnancies is around 1 in 100 pregnancies. Risk factors are only present in 25–50% of patients with an ectopic pregnancy. The risk factors include a history of the following:
- Previous pelvic inflammatory disease
- Tubal surgery
- Previous ectopic pregnancy
- Infertility
- Assisted reproductive technique
- Intrauterine contraceptive device
- Smoking
- Age above 40.

PRESENTATION

Typical presentation is a triad of amenorrhea, abdominal pain, and irregular vaginal bleeding. Pain is usually located at either lower quadrant of the abdomen or lower back. Rupture of an ectopic pregnancy causes a sharp pain in the iliac fossa, followed by abdominal distension, generalized abdominal tenderness, and guarding. The hemoperitoneum under the diaphragm cause referred pain to the shoulder. Massive intraperitoneal bleeding causes fainting or circulatory collapse. Vaginal bleeding in an ectopic pregnancy is usually dark and scanty in amount.

Type	Findings
Tubal	Tubal ring sign, ring of fire, pelvic hemorrhage
Interstitial	Eccentrically located gestational sac, interstitial line sign
Ovarian	Beta hCG >1,000, normal tubes, gestational sac/adnexal mass in ovary or a typical cyst
Cervical	Trophoblastic flow surrounding gestational sac within cervix, normal endometrium, ballooning of cervix, hourglass uterus
Scar pregnancy	Gestational sac within lower anterior segment of uterus, thinning of myometrium anterior to sac
Abdominal	Absence of intrauterine gestational sac, gestational sac located within intraperitoneal cavity, pelvic hemorrhage

(hCG: human chorionic gonadotropin)

Beta-human Chorionic Gonadotropin

In normal pregnancy, serum concentration of beta-human chorionic gonadotropin (hCG) will increase exponentially doubling every 2–3.5 days from the 4th to 8th week of gestation to reach a peak around 8th to 12th week. Therefore, estimate of serum hCG at 48 hours interval is helpful. If the increase of serum beta hCG is less than 63% or the level starts reaching a plateau or is decreasing, an ectopic pregnancy will be the most likely diagnosis.

Ultrasound

The ultrasonographic features of ectopic pregnancy are:

Uterine:
- An empty uterus
- Variable degree of thickening of endometrium
- A thin endometrium may exclude the possibility of an early intrauterine pregnancy as it is not compatible with an on-going early implantation
- An intrauterine pseudo sac—mere collection of variable amount of fluid with uterine cavity, is found in approximately 5% of all ectopic pregnancies

Adnexal:
- A hyperechogenic tubal ring ("doughnut" or "bagel" sign) is the most common finding on scan, probably due to early scanning
- A mixed adnexal mass–either tubal miscarriage or tubal rupture
- An ectopic sac with a yolk sac or an embryo with or without a heart beat in adnexa
- Fluid in the pouch of Douglas.

Increased blood flow in the adnexal mass seen on Doppler ultrasound scan is suggestive of ectopic pregnancy. The corpus luteum may be present on the ipsilateral side in 85% of cases.

Correlation of Beta hCG Level and Ultrasound Examination

In normal intrauterine pregnancy, a gestational sac can be visualized in uterine cavity via transvaginal ultrasound as early as 5-week period of amenorrhea or serum beta hCG level of 1,500 mIU/mL and via transabdominal ultrasound at 6-week period of amenorrhea or serum beta hCG level of 3,000 mIU/mL. The double ring or double deciduas sign of gestational sac is the hallmark of intrauterine pregnancy, whereas single layer (pseudo sac) would be seen inside the uterus in ectopic pregnancy.

MANAGEMENT OF ECTOPIC PREGNANCY

The treatment modalities available are:
- Expectant management
- Medical therapy with methotrexate
- Surgical intervention.

Ectopic Pregnancy- Diagnosis

Ectopic pregnancy flowchart

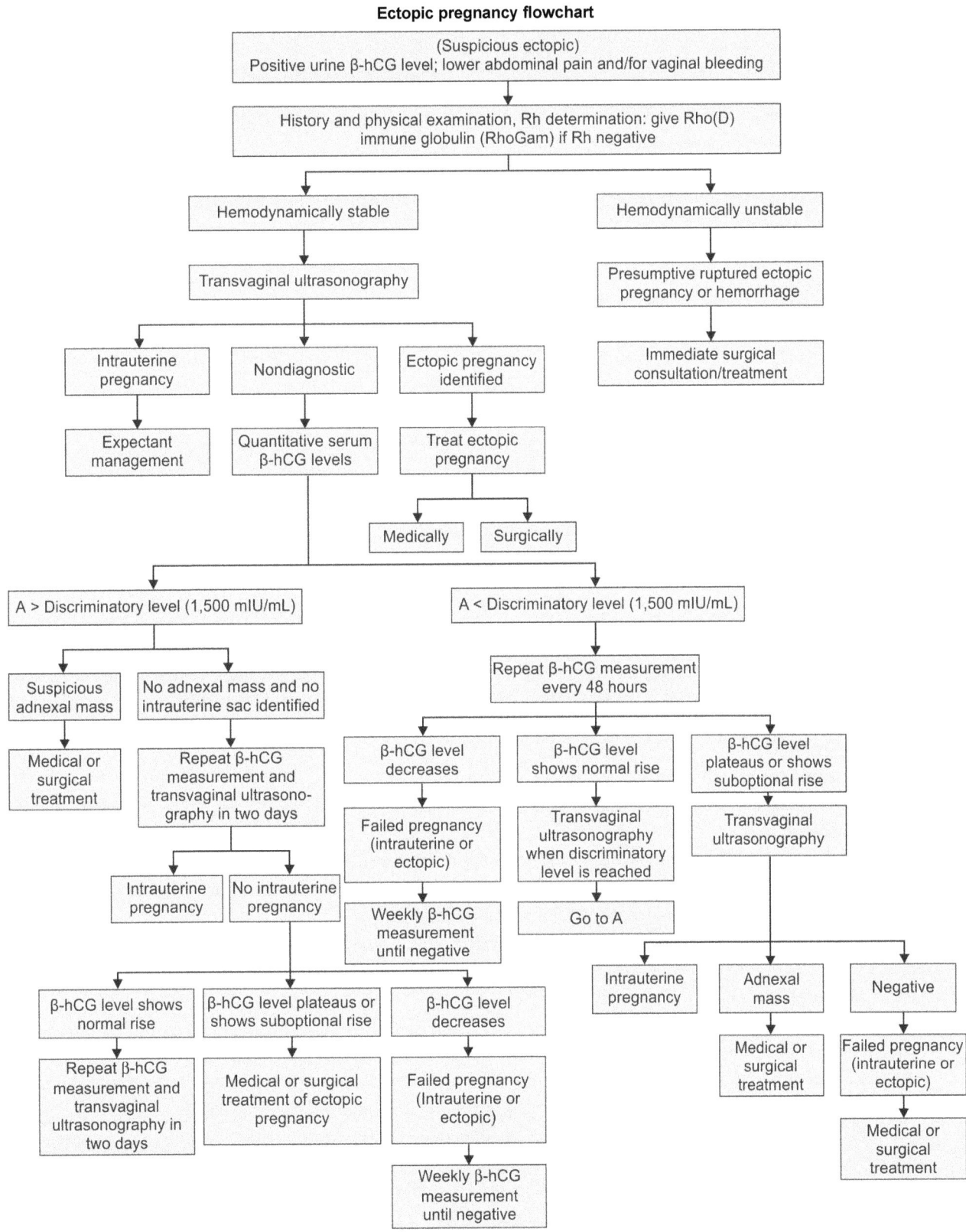

(hCG: human chorionic gonadotropin)

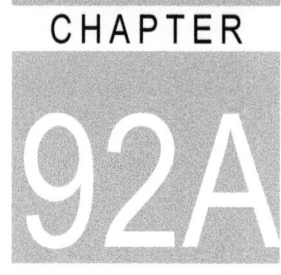

Ectopic Pregnancy: Surgical Management

Narendra Malhotra, Apoorva Pallam Reddy

A. Consider conservative management when the following criteria are met:
   - Adnexal mass less than 2 cm
   - Serum beta human chorionic gonadotropin (hCG) less than 1,000 and declining progressively
   - Asymptomatic patients
   - Absence of hemoperitoneum
   - No sign of rupture
   - No fetal parts.

   The beta hCG should fall progressively and the adnexal mass should decrease in size. Follow-up until beta hCG less than 10 IU/L.

B. For patients with beta hCG between 1,500 IU/L and less than 5,000 IU/L, one can offer both medical as well as surgical management if they also have the following:
   - No significant pain
   - Unruptured ectopic with an adnexal mass smaller than 35 mm with no visible heartbeat
   - No intrauterine pregnancy.

C. Surgery should be first-line management option for patients with:
   - An ectopic pregnancy and significant pain
   - Adnexal mass of 35 mm or more
   - Fetal heart seen on ultrasound
   - Serum beta hCG level of more than 5,000 IU/L.

D. Whenever surgery is decided, laparoscopy is the better way forward as compared to laparotomy taking into account the condition of the patient, the expertise of the surgeon, and the complexity of the procedure.

E. Laparoscopy advantage:
   - Shorter hospital stay
   - Adhesion formation and blood loss is lesser
   - Better pain profile
   - Quicker recovery
   - Recurrent ectopic pregnancy rate is lower (5%) compared to laparotomy (16.6%)
   - Chances of subsequent intrauterine pregnancy are higher (70%) than with laparotomy.

   Laparoscopy disadvantage: Higher risk of bowel or vascular damage.

F. Salpingectomy: Unless there are other risk factors, salpingectomy should be offered as first choice whenever surgery is decided. Fimbrial evacuation (milking) of the pregnancy from the fallopian tubes should be avoided as it might lead to persistence of the ectopic pregnancy.

G. Salpingostomy:
   - Consider salpingostomy for women with risk factors for infertility such as contralateral tubal damage.
   - Post the procedure, the histology should be followed-up. If there is no evidence of chorionic tissue the patient should be followed-up with weekly serum beta hCG until the levels are less than 10 IU/L.
   - Up to one in five women undergoing salpingostomy may need further methotrexate treatment or salpingectomy later.
   - Follow-up with weekly beta hCG levels. If the levels are rising or plateauing, consider further treatment with methotrexate or surgery if levels are more than 5,000 IU/L.
   - The recurrent ectopic pregnancy rate is about 20.5% and intrauterine pregnancy rate is about 5%.

Ectopic Pregnancy: Surgical Management

Management of nontubal ectopic pregnancies like heterotopic pregnancy, interstitial pregnancy, cervical pregnancy, ovarian pregnancy, pregnancy in a caesarean scar, and abdominal pregnancy are not straightforward and the treatment needs to be individualized based on the size of the pregnancy and its viability.

Ectopic Pregnancy. Clinic Guidelines Reg No 10121 NHS

Management of ectopic pregnancy

- Conservative management (A)
  - Primary medical management
    - Twice weekly beta hCG Scan weekly (B)
  - Primary surgical management (C)
    - Unruptured
      - Laparoscopy (E)
        - If contralateral tube damaged
          - Salpingectomy (F)
            - Urine test after 3 weeks. Report if positive
          - Salpingostomy (G)
            - May need methotrexate or salpingectomy later
              - Weekly serum beta hCG till negative
    - Ruptured
      - Laparoscopy/Laparotomy (D)
  - Medical or surgical management

(hCG: human chorionic gonadotropin)

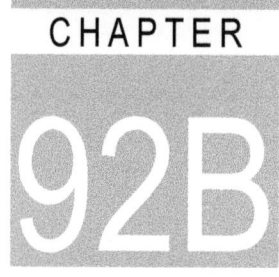

Ectopic Pregnancy: Medical Management

Apoorva Pallam Reddy, Aruna Siddharth

MEDICAL MANAGEMENT

Methotrexate is the most commonly used drug for medical management of ectopic pregnancy. It is a folic acid antagonist (antimetabolite) which prevents growth of rapidly dividing cells by interfering with DNA synthesis. A single injection is well tolerated and is effective in 90% of cases. Chances of recurrent ectopic pregnancy are about 10–20%, 80% of which turn out to be tubal in nature. For medical management, the patient must be willing for a prolonged follow-up and should not have medical problems like concurrent corticosteroid therapy, acute infection, severe anemia, renal or liver impairment, active peptic ulcer, blood disorders or active pulmonary disease.

Side effects of treatment: Nausea and vomiting, Stomatitis, Diarrhea, Abdominal discomfort, Photosensitivity, Reversible liver impairment, Hematosalpinx.

What the clinician should know:
- All the prerequisites mentioned in the algorithm should be matched. A normal full blood count (FBC), liver function test (LFT), renal function test (RFT) and electrolytes should be confirmed before administering methotrexate. If the values are abnormal medical management cannot be carried forward.
- Methotrexate is given as intramuscular in buttocks or lateral thigh. Patient rests for 1 hour. Check for any local reaction, BP, temperature, and pulse before discharge. If local reaction is present, give antihistamine or steroid cream.
- Up to 75% patients may complain of pain between days 3 and 7.
- The fall in the human chorionic gonadotropin (hCG) levels between day 4 and day 7 is important. If the fall is >15%, the patient is followed-up with weekly beta human chorionic gonadotropin (BhCG) without the need for repeat methotrexate dose. There might be an initial rise of hCG between days 1 and 4 (in up to 86% of patients).
- It takes about 35 days to resolve completely.
- 14% patients will need more than one dose of methotrexate. Each time methotrexate is administered, LFT, RFT, FBC, serum electrolytes should be repeated.
- Risk of tubal rupture is about 7%.
- If more than one dose of methotrexate is administered, folinic acid rescue in the dose of 0.1 mg/kg of leucovorin factor can be given 24 hours after methotrexate.
- If there is a raise in BhCG value at any point or if the patient becomes hemodynamically unstable, medical management should be abandoned and the patient is taken directly for surgical management.
- Avoid vaginal examination.
- Ovarian cysts may be found during treatment but resolve spontaneously.
- Do not give anti-D to patients who are being medically managed.

What the patient should know:
- Medical management is well established and 90% patients do not need surgery
- Prolonged follow-up is required
- Further dose of methotrexate may be needed
- Pain abdomen may happen between days 3 and 7
- Pregnancy should be avoided for 3 months from the *last* dose for possible teratogenic effect
- Ample fluid intake
- Avoid alcohol or folic acid containing vitamins. Avoid sexual intercourse till resolution of the ectopic pregnancy
- Avoid sunlight exposure, aspirin, and nonsteroidal anti-inflammatory drugs (NSAIDs).

Ectopic Pregnancy: Medical Management

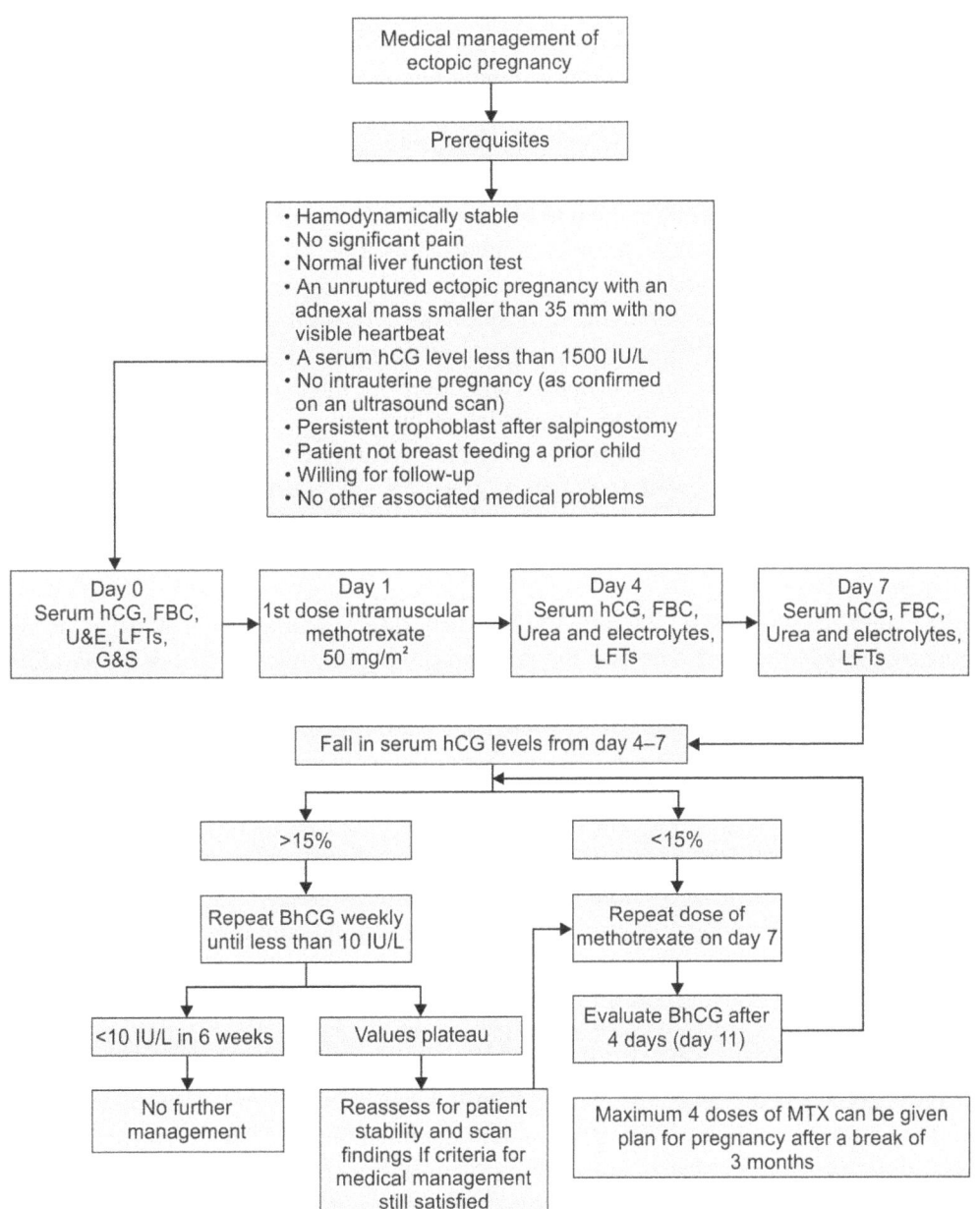

(FBC: full blood count; hCG: human chorionic gonadotropin; LFTs: liver function tests; MTX: methotrexate; U&E: urea and electrolyte; G&S: group and serum)

CHAPTER 93

Fetal Reduction

Meenu Batra

A. Fetal reduction (FR) is defined as reduction of selected fetus/fetuses in a multichorionic gestation as a therapeutic intervention to enhance the survival of other fetuses.
B. The term *multifetal pregnancy reduction (MFPR)* is used when couples decide to reduce an apparently normal fetus(es) (≥3) in order to increase the chance of survival of other fetuses of the same pregnancy.
C. When the procedure is performed to reduce or eliminate a fetus already identified with a birth defect or chromosomal abnormality, the term *selective reduction* is used.
D. The indications to perform the procedure include high-order multichorionic pregnancies (≥3), dichorionic (DC) triplets with a monochorionic (MC) pair, and an anomalous fetus. The relative indications include conditions such as previous history of cervical incompetence, maternal medical disorders complicating pregnancy, etc.
E. The initial step involves comprehensive and nondirective counseling done before the procedure. It is important to explain the specific risks, based on factors including the number of fetuses, age, any medical conditions/prior obstetrical history. The specific risks of the procedure like miscarriage, bleeding, infection, PPROM, etc. need to be explained in detail. The patient should be given freedom to make their own choices.
F. Multifetal pregnancy reduction is an outpatient procedure. It is commonly performed between 11 and 13 + 6 weeks. This allows for natural reduction to occur and provides a chance to identify fetal abnormalities. Also, there is less amount of postprocedural devitalized tissue and the risk of miscarriage is less. An ultrasound is performed to evaluate the uterus, chorionicity, and fetuses. If all the fetuses appear normal, the most technically accessible fetus(es) is/are targeted for reduction.
G. Transabdominal approach is the most preferred route. In dichorionic pregnancies, a 22-gauge needle is introduced through the mother's abdomen and then into the targeted pregnancy. Intracardiac or intrafunicular injection of 2–3 mL of 15% potassium chloride (KCL) is performed to stop fetal heart motion (Fig. 1). This procedure is repeated for each fetus to be reduced and is usually performed through a separate needle insertion. When the diagnosis is made in the second trimester, women might opt for late selective termination. In monochorionic pregnancies, cord occlusion or intrafetal coagulation (laser or radiofrequency ablation) is the preferred method. A repeat ultrasound should be done the next day after the procedure for confirmation of viability in the remaining fetuses.
H. In dichorionic triplets, the options include reduction of the monochorionic pair using KCl or ablation of the pelvic vessels of one of the twins of the monochorionic pair with the help of intrafetal laser.
I. Reduction of dichorionic triplet pregnancies to dichorionic twins by ultrasound-guided laser ablation of the pelvic vessels of one of the monochorionic twins has been proposed. Local anesthesia is administered at the site of insertion. Under continuous ultrasound visualization, an 18-G needle is inserted into the fetal abdomen adjacent to the pelvic vessels. A 400-μm laser fiber is inserted into the needle and advanced to a few millimeters beyond the tip of the needle and laser coagulation is performed using an Nd:YAG laser with 40 W. This results in hyperechogenicity of tissues in the lower abdomen and cessation of blood flow in the iliac arteries and umbilical vein. Fetal heart activity usually continues for several minutes. A repeat ultrasound examination is carried out the next day to confirm death of one monochorionic twin and survival of a dichorionic pair. The patient is discharged the next day and a follow-up ultrasound examination is performed the next day. Antibiotic cover is advised for 5 days.
J. The procedure-related risks of fetal reduction include the risk of complete abortion which is 4.5% for triplets and can increase up to 15% for sextuplets, abortion of the wrong (normal) fetus, damage without death to a fetus, preterm labor less than 34 weeks, intrauterine growth restriction (IUGR) in surviving fetus (12.4%), and maternal infection/hemorrhage.
K. Outcome of the procedure depends on various factors which include the original number of fetuses, route of the needle, number of fetuses terminated, and which fetus is terminated. Most losses were observed several weeks after the procedure. As noted by Papageorghiou and colleagues, most of the excess loss with fetal reduction is likely to be the consequence of the resorbing dead fetoplacental tissue rather than faulty MFPR technique. It is recommended to avoid reduction of the lower lying fetus, intending not to leave necrotic tissue as a nidus to infection in close proximity to the cervical canal.

CONCLUSION

Multifetal pregnancy reduction is a vital procedure which when done at the right time helps us to increase the duration of pregnancy, decrease incidence of prematurity and prolonged neonatal intensive care unit (NICU) stay, and improve maternal outcome.

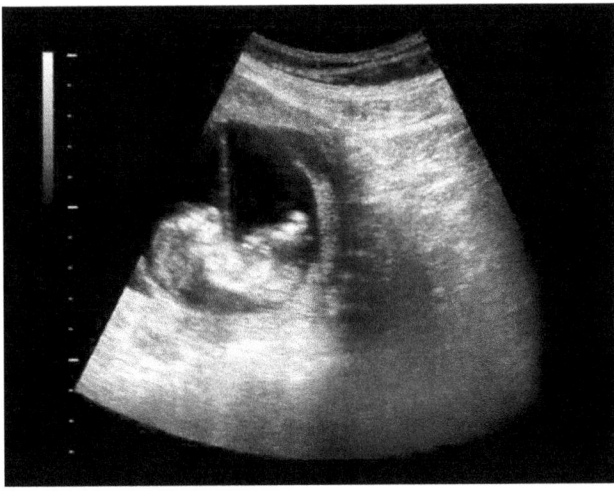

Fig. 1: Dichorionic diamniotic twins with one fetus having anencephaly. The needle can be seen inserted into the thorax to inject potassium chloride (KCL).

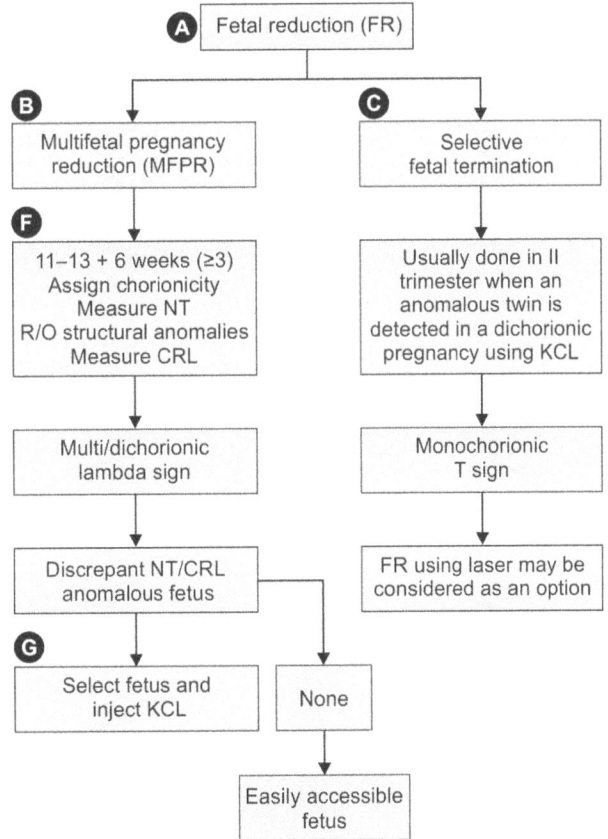

(CRL: crown rump length; NT: nuchal translucency; R/O: rule out; KCL: potassium chloride)

SECTION 20

Other Factors in ART

- Unconsummated Marriage
- Male Sexual Dysfunction
- Failure to Respond to Gonadotropins
- Unruptured Follicular Syndrome
- Diet and Lifestyle in Infertility
- Endometrial Scratching
- Medical Management of Oligoasthenoteratozoospermia

CHAPTER 94

Unconsummated Marriage

Vijayasarathi Ramanathan

A. Inability to have penetrative sex (unconsummated marriage—UCM) is one of the most common sexual difficulties with which couples present to a fertility center or referred to a specialist in sexual medicine by gynecologists.
B. In couples presenting with UCM, often the male partner presents with erectile difficulties. Eliciting sexual history from partner is a vital element in the process of diagnosis of erectile dysfunction (ED) inability to have penetrative sex and (mis)diagnosis of ED in the male partner makes it a very stressful journey for the couple which in turn could lead to resentment.
C. Some couples explicitly state that they could not have penetrative sex while others have doubt whether they had penetrative sex or not. In both these situations, taking a targeted sexual history is critical in the assessment of unconsummated marriage due to inability of having penetrative sex. It is advisable to take history from the individual partners (one at a time) and then together. At this stage of history taking or at a later stage of assessment, a number of sexuality (e.g. sexual identity) and relationship (extramarital affairs, marital disharmony) issues could unfold and a clinician should be able to make a referral to an appropriate professional. Should the history suggest that the male partner had erectile difficulties with other sexual partners and/or during masturbation, then there is a possibility of ED which needs to be managed accordingly.
D. Vaginismus is defined as an *involuntary* spasm of the pelvic muscles (perineal muscles and the levator ani) surrounding the outer third of the vagina causing pain and penetration virtually impossible. It is characterized by *fear and anxiety* concerning penetration combined with *anticipatory pain* upon penetration. Women with vaginismus generally experience shame, disgust, and dislike toward their genitals and some women do have phobias and/or history of sexual abuse or unwanted sexual experience in the past. Their sexual partners are usually characterized as kind, gentle, considerate, and passive who lack of assertiveness.
E. Assessment—general views about sex (best friends' opinion about pain and bleeding are very strong); sexual history (any traumatic experience); psychological assessment (childhood brought-up, aversion); vaginal examination—preferred but *not* mandatory. Pelvic floor tonicity assessment—physiotherapist. Vaginismus questionnaire (if needed).
F. For optimal outcomes, the management strategy should involve a multidisciplinary team (minimum involving a physiotherapist and a psychologist/counselor) and an integrated, person-centered approach (meaning all health professionals have an equal weighting and contribute to the overall management).
G. The role of a (female) physiotherapist with adequate training in pelvic floor and basic understanding of vaginismus is of paramount importance in the management of vaginismus. It is this retraining of pelvic floor using a hands-on approach that contributes much to the desired outcome. A physiotherapist could teach how to relax pelvic floor and the whole body (tight contraction can cause pain).
H. Education and self-management: Educate the couple about the problem and actively involve them in every step throughout the journey.
I. It is integral to challenge some of the irrational beliefs, negative thinking patterns and address the emotional status of women with vaginismus. Reinforce that *avoidance* is not helpful in long term. Encourage the male partner to be more assertive and motivate his wife but not to demonstrate aggressiveness. Injecting 100–150 units of muscle relaxants like bolulinum toxin into the tense pelvic floor muscles can be considered for vaginismus. The effect usually lasts for about 6 months during which vaginal dilators can be use to increase the confidence.
J. Vulvodynia (vulval pain arising fro a trigger point) should be differentiated from vaginismus.
K. For women with severe vaginismus or men with ED seeking pregnancy vaginal insemination of the semen around ovulation or intrauterine insemination under anesthesia should be offered.
L. Establish from the beginning that there is no magic fix to most sexual problems and that regular follow-up is the most critical aspect of any management approach. In order for your patients to follow-up, it is essential that you have built good rapport and won their trust and confidence in you.

Unconsummated Marriage

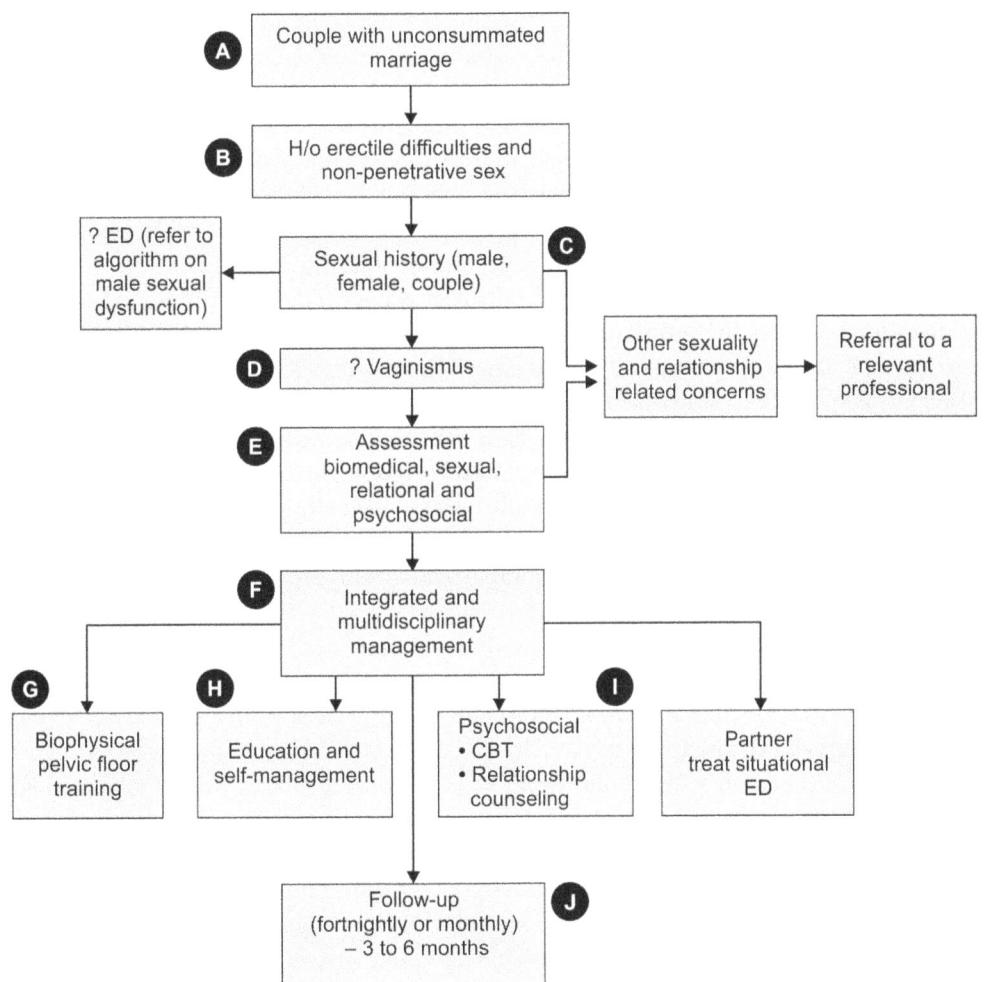

(CBT: cognitive behavioral therapy; ED: erectile dysfunction; H/o: history of)

CHAPTER 95

Male Sexual Dysfunction

Vijayasarathi Ramanathan

A. There are many barriers for a person not to raise the topic of sexual function with a health professional such as emotional factors (shame, anxiety, guilt or embarrassment), perception (that sexual function is not an important medical problem), lack of trust, fear of rejection, and/or concerns around confidentiality. It is important that you reassure about confidentiality and the purpose of asking questions about sexual function is to "help" and *not* judge them.

B. Healthy sexual functioning is the ability to experience sexual pleasure and satisfaction and is an integral part of overall sexual health which includes fertility. It is important to recognize that there is no such thing called "normal" sexual function (referred to as "sex" in lay terms). Concerns and problems with sexual functioning could be a cause and/or a consequence of subfertility and is highly vital to address the issue of sexual functioning as part of your fertility consultation. Practice tip: *Do not* be in a rush to diagnose a pathology without taking a thorough history.

C. In my clinical experience, many men have been misdiagnosed (and mismanaged) with a sexual dysfunction mainly because sexual history was never obtained from the index person's sexual partner.

D. A number of medical conditions (cancer, endocrine disorders, psychiatric conditions, cardiovascular disorders, neurological disorders, urinary incontinence, chronic pain, recent surgery) and medications [antipsychotics, antiepileptic drugs, opioids, antihypertensive drugs (especially beta blockers), antidepressants and antiandrogens] could have sexual dysfunction as a side-effect. Examination of penis, scrotum, and testicles is highly important but not required on a routine basis for all men. Assess for signs of hypogonadism (if required). In terms of blood tests, the bare minimums are glycosylated hemoglobin (HbA1c), fasting blood glucose (FBG), lipid profile, serum prolactin, and thyroid profile. Serum testosterone (8–11 am sample only), serum albumin, and sex hormone-binding globulin (SHBG). Bioavailable and free testosterone levels need to be manually calculated by going to the link http://www.issam.ch/freetesto.htm. Special tests (Penile Doppler and Nocturnal Penile Tumescence) are useful but not required on a routine basis.

E. There are a number of psychological and interpersonal dimensions of sexual function. Taking a targeted sexual and relationship history is an art but you do not have to be an expert in sexology. For rapid and convenient questioning, you could use selected sexual function measures (International Index of Erectile Function-5; Premature Ejaculation Diagnostic Tool) that are well validated.

F. While taking sexual history, bear in mind about the 4 Ps—predisposing factors (why this person got the problem), precipitating factors (why this person is having the problem now), perpetuating factors (what is sustaining the problem despite treatment and effort), and finally protective factors (what is helpful and working in this person).

G. Oral medications for erectile dysfunction (phosphodiesterase type 5 inhibitors—sildenafil, tadalafil or vardenafil) and premature ejaculation [selective serotonin reuptake inhibitor (SSRI)—dapoxetine] are available. A common pitfall in the use of these drugs is that clinicians do not provide adequate instructions on how to use it. It is advisable to seek opinion from or refer to medical specialists in sexual medicine for consideration of other medical management options (penile injections), testosterone replacement, and surgical procedures (*rarely*).

H. Many men with or without sexual dysfunction do have unrealistic expectations around sexual performance partly because they never had any sex education and due to strong influence of pornography. In the management of sexual concerns/dysfunctions, it is highly critical to provide some basic advice on sexual anatomy and sexual function. It is recommended to make appropriate referral to any mental health professional (psychiatrist clinical psychologist, counseling psychologist) who specializes in psychosexual therapy. Some of the options are sexcercise (mindfulness sexual practice/sensate focus), cognitive behavior therapy, relationship counseling, and emotional management.

I. Establish from the beginning that there is no magic fix to most sexual problems and that regular follow-up is the most critical aspect of any management approach. In order for your patients to follow-up, it is essential that you have built good rapport and won their trust and confidence in you.

Male Sexual Dysfunction

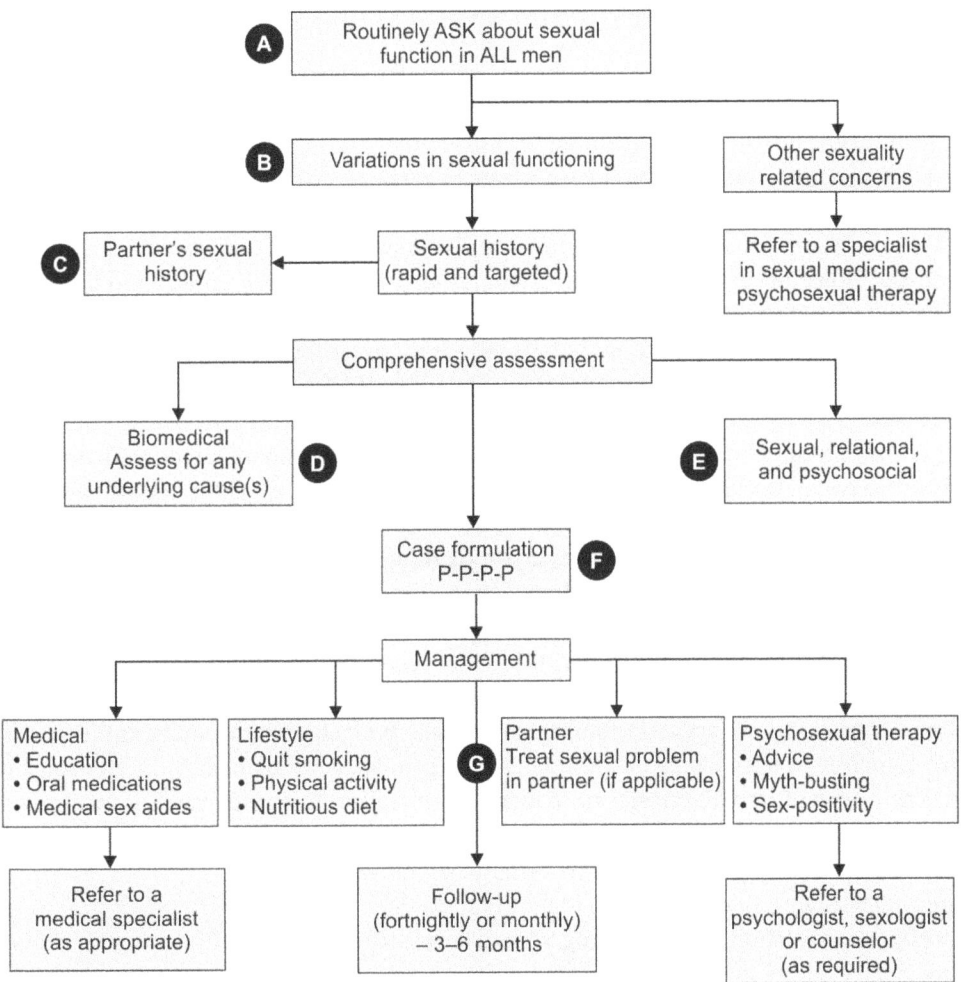

CHAPTER 96

Failure to Respond to Gonadotropins

Kedar Ganla, Priyanka Vora, Rana Choudhary

A. Gonadotropins are frequently used in assisted reproductive technique (ART) cycles for controlled ovarian stimulation (COS). The response to a COS can be predicted using various ovarian reserve markers like age, anti-Müllerian hormone (AMH), and antral follicular count (AFC). However, on occasions, despite anticipating a specific response the patient might fail to achieve the same. This can be the result of a poor choice of ovarian stimulation protocol or very rarely due to receptor deficiency. The various causes of poor response to ovarian stimulation despite normal ovarian reserve are discussed below.

B. *High FSH threshold:* Variation in the endogenous hormonal profile affects the hypothalamic-pituitary-ovarian (HPO) axis and thus alters the ovarian response to external androgens. There is failure of aromatization of androgens into estrogens. Each antral follicle has a follicle-stimulating hormone (FSH) threshold, the minimum dose of FSH required for it to reach a preovulatory status. When the exogenous FSH does not exceed the FSH threshold, then the antral follicles fail to achieve dominance. In such cases, increasing the dose of FSH to a maximum of 600 IU might induce response. In case of smaller antral follicles (2–5 mm) on day 2 starting a step-down protocol might be beneficial as compared to having larger antral follicles (5–9 mm) when a step-up protocol is considered beneficial (Fig. 1).

C. *High LH:FSH ratio:* As per the two-cell–two-gonadotropin theory, luteinizing hormone (LH) stimulation of the theca cells causes androgen synthesis and FSH stimulation of the granulosa cells causes conversion of these androgens into estrogen. An estrogen dominant milieu is essential for a healthy follicle. In case of LH hypersecretion, intrinsic FSH deficiency or increased LH sensitivity [LH receptors are seen at 4 mm in polycystic ovary syndrome (PCOS) patients and 11 mm in normoresponders], the follicle becomes androgen predominant resulting in atresia. Suppressing the endogenous LH with one or two cycles of oral contraceptive pill (OCP) or using 2–3 doses of gonadotropin-releasing hormone (GnRH) antagonist from D2 to 3 can improve the ovarian response.

D. *Low endogenous FSH and LH levels:* When the endogenous FSH and LH levels are severely suppressed like in a long agonist protocol, longer and higher doses of FSH may be required to evoke a normal response.

E. *FSH receptor polymorphism:* FSH and LH secreted by the pituitary, act by binding to their receptors, which are localized in the gonads, i.e. the FSH receptor (FSHR) and LH/hCG receptor (LHCGR). Polymorphism in the genes coding for FSH receptor alters the response of ovaries to stimulation. Most of these polymorphisms are localized to single nucleotide of the sequence. The inactivating mutations result in poor ovarian response, higher basal FSH, prolonged menstruation, premature ovarian failure or sometimes even primary amenorrhea. The activating mutations result in hyper-response of the receptors to FSH resulting in increased chances of ovarian hyperstimulation syndrome (OHSS) even at lower doses (Fig. 2).

Types of single nucleotide polymorphism (SNP) FSH receptor mutation:

- *Asn 680 Ser polymorphism*:
  - It is a heterozygous mutation where asparagine replaces serine and it is consistent with reduced sensitivity to endogenous FSH. Carriers of this trait have higher FSH levels throughout the menstrual cycle and this leads to increase in AFC and total menstrual cycle length.
- *Ser 680 Ser polymorphism*:
  - It is a homozygous mutation where decreased estradiol levels are found while stimulation.
- *Asn 680 Asn (Wild-type mutation)*:
  - 680th SNP which leads to poor ovarian response
  - 307th SNP which leads to OHSS—which is not widely studied.

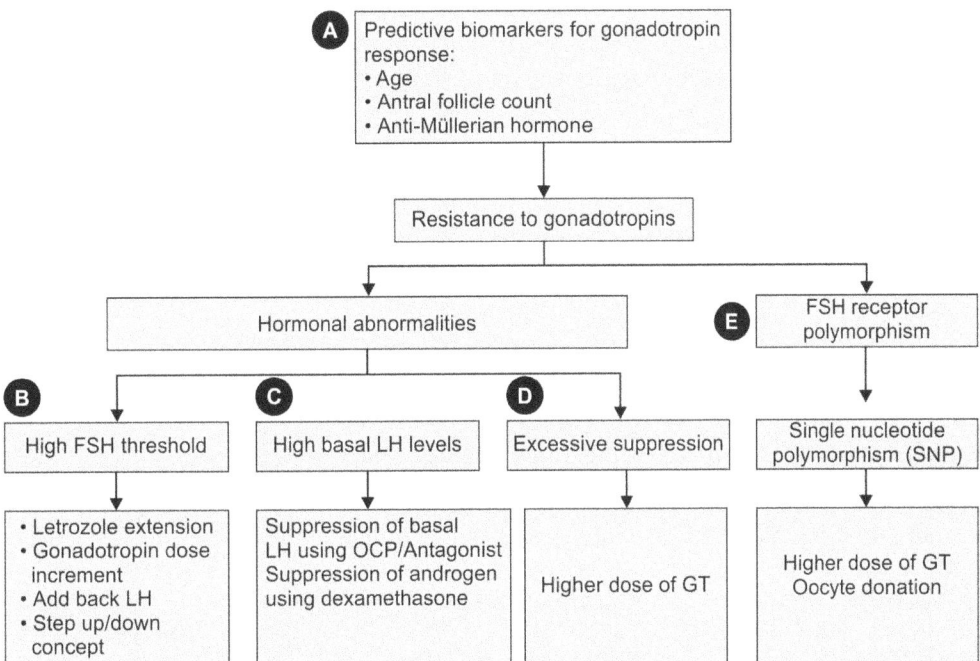

(FSH: follicle-stimulating hormone; LH: luteinizing hormone; OCP: oral contraceptive pill; GT: gonadotropins)

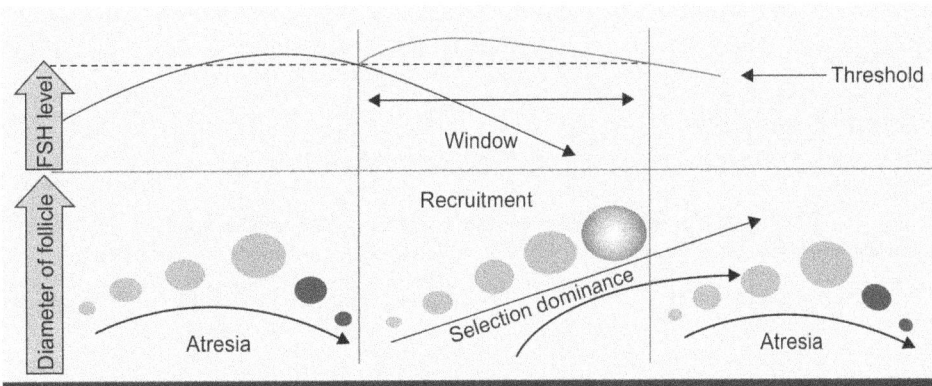

The longer and higher the FSH is above threshold more follicles are recruited

Fig. 1: Follicle-stimulating hormone (FSH) threshold and recruitment window.

FSH Response panel for women

In brief

Significance	Result
FSH dosage requirement for IVF stimulation protocol	Increased FSH dosage may give optimal response
Clomiphene citrate response prediction	Poor responder to Clomiphene citrate

Results

Gene/Marker	Function	Result
FSHR FSHR 2039A>G, Ser680Asn	Cellular receptor of FSH, follicle stimulating hormone	GG: subfertile function of FSH receptor Two variants, homozygous
ESR1 ESR1 453-397C>T	Cellular receptor type I of the hormone estrogen	CC: fully functional estrogen receptor No variants, homozygous

In detail

Significance	Gene/Marker (Evidence)	Result
FSH dosage requirement for IVF stimulation protocol	FSHR (5*) ESR1 (4*)	Increased FSH dosage may give optimal response

Response to gonadotropin stimulation
Optimal response is NOT likely to standard FSH dosage in ovarian stimulation because of subfunctional hormone receptor. Subfunctional hormone receptor gene is likely to be the cause of clinical infertility.

FSH dosage in ovarian stimulation
Standard FSH dosage is not likely to be sufficient for optimal response to ovarian stimulation. A higher dosage of rh-FSH from Day 1 of controlled ovarian stimulation has been shown to achieve good response and outcome in terms of days of stimulation, antral follicle count, and the quality and quantity of eggs retrieved.

Risk of Ovarian hyperstimulation syndrome (OHSS)
There is not enough evidence to make a statement regarding OHSS based on these genetic variations. Standard precautions are needed.

Significance	Gene/Marker (Evidence)	Result
Clomiphene citrate response prediction	FSHR (3*)	Poor responder to Clomiphene citrate

Clomiphene response prediction
Normal response to ovulation induction by clomiphene citrate is NOT likely based on this gene. Studies have shown that women with two FSH receptor gene variations may be resistant to clomiphene citrate, and may benefit from gonadotropin stimulation instead.

Fig. 2: FSH receptor polymorphism panel for women sample report.
(FSH: follicle-stimulating hormone; CC: clomiphene citrate; FSHR: FSH receptor; ESR1: erythrocyte sedimentation rate 1; GG: G genotype)

CHAPTER 97

Unruptured Follicular Syndrome

Kedar Ganla, Rana Choudhary, Priyanka Vora

A. Luteinized unruptured follicle (LUF) syndrome is defined as a failure of ovulation in which, despite the absence of follicular rupture and release of the oocyte, an unruptured follicle undergoes luteinization under the action of luteinizing hormone (LH). In such cases, normal production of progesterone and duration of the luteal phase of the cycle could be seen. This form of anovulation is considered a subtle cause of female infertility.

B. Luteinized unruptured follicle is seen in 10% of menstrual cycles of normal fertile women. A higher incidence has been reported in infertile women.

C. The only evidence available, that the LUF syndrome is a cause of infertility, is the finding that the syndrome occurs statistically more frequently in women with unexplained infertility than in a control group of women. The occurrence of LUF has been linked to many conditions such as unexplained infertility, endometriosis, pelvic adhesions, and the use of nonsteroidal anti-inflammatory drugs (NSAIDs). There is a relationship between the LUF syndrome and luteal phase insufficiency. Another study hypothesizes that the LUF syndrome might be caused by stress thus constituting a "psychological infertility" and this could explain the spontaneous cure rate.

D. The precise mechanism by which the ovulatory follicle fails to rupture is unclear. It has been postulated that LUF is a consequence of a chronic follicular inflammatory-like reaction involving inhibition of synthesis of prostaglandins. Others postulated that the aberrant prolactin release and luteal phase defect might be contributory factors in the pathophysiology of this syndrome. More recently, studies suggested that a primary granulosa cell defect might be the responsible mechanism for this syndrome.

E. Different methods have been used to predict and detect the time of ovulation. Of these, only the mid-cycle LH surge was found to be the most reliable predictor. LUF is the failure of the ovulatory follicle to rupture on ultrasound examination performed daily from day 10 to 20 of the cycle despite normal indices of ovulation. Ultrasound has been demonstrated to be the method of choice for diagnosing LUF.

F. Studies have shown that diagnosis of LUF syndrome can be made by laparoscopic inspection of the ovaries and by the assay of 17 beta-estradiol and progesterone, in peritoneal fluid between day 14 and 20 of the cycle, but this may not be practically possible.

Following are practical diagnostic methods for LUF:
- Failure of follicular rupture with serum progesterone more than 1.5 ng/mL
- Larger follicles of more than or equal to 22 mm diameter—higher incidences of LUF
- Lower systemic LH concentration at early stages of follicle development.

G. Two distinct types of LUF syndrome are identified: Mature follicle LUF, in which release of an ovum was not demonstrated after a follicle attained maturity (serum estradiol reached 200 pg/mL while serum progesterone remained less than 2.5 ng/mL), versus premature luteinization LUF, where the serum progesterone increased above 2.5 ng/mL before follicular maturation was attained.

H. The use of either human chorionic gonadotropin (hCG) alone or hCG in combination with human menopausal gonadotropin (hMG) in a single injection at the time of follicular maturation (as trigger) successfully corrected mature follicle LUF in around 46%. A combination of ovulation-inducing drugs like clomiphene citrate or letrozole plus trigger with hCG can also correct the ovulation in up to 12–15% patients using clomiphene citrate and 22–25% using letrozole. Some studies have shown that clomiphene citrate may in fact lead to LUF in some patients and hence is not a good choice of drug for LUF. Hence, letrozole is better than clomiphene citrate in reducing incidence of LUF (22% vs 12%). When hMG is given for ovulation induction in combination with hCG trigger, this syndrome (LUF) is corrected in up to 96% of patients.

Thus, hMG-hCG therapy is the most efficacious for mature follicle LUF, but because release can occur spontaneously on occasion by an appropriately timed single gonadotropin injection, one could offer the less costly options first.

I. For premature luteinization, speeding up follicular maturation with gonadotropin therapy is effective. Upon failure of this technique, the more costly endogenous gonadotropin suppression followed by hMG can be employed. Recent studies have demonstrated that granulocyte colony-stimulating factor (GCSF) 100 µg during ovulation induction and 300 µg at the time of trigger along with hCG successfully corrects LUF in majority of the patients (95–96%).

Unruptured Follicle Syndrome—Diagnosis

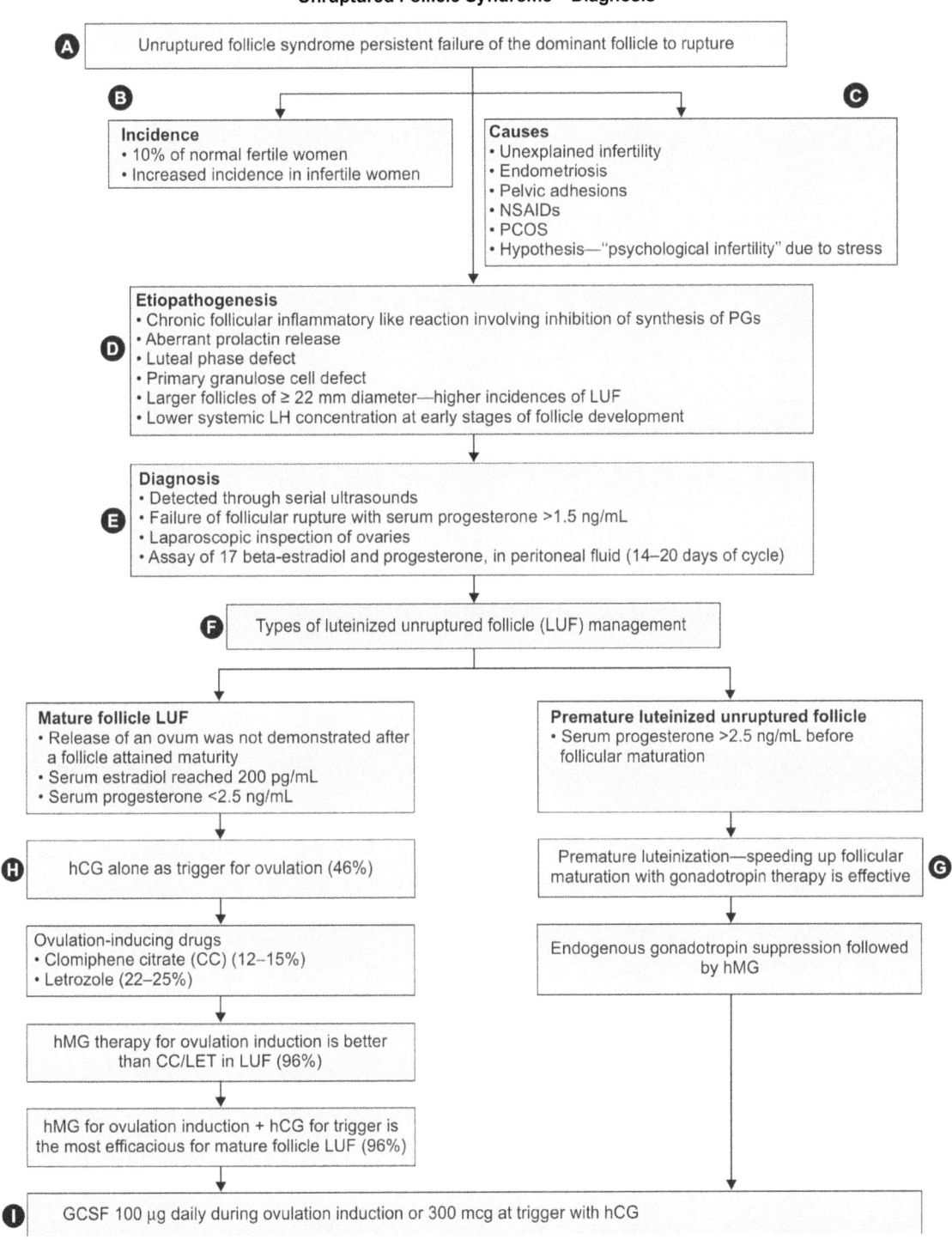

(LH: luteinizing hormone; LUF: luteinized unruptured follicle; PCOS: polycystic ovary syndrome; PGs: prostaglandins; NSAIDs: nonsteroidal anti-inflammatory drugs; GCSF: granulocyte colony-stimulating factor; hCG: human chorionic gonadotropin; hMG: human menopausal gonadotropin; LET: letrozole)

CHAPTER 98

Diet and Lifestyle in Infertility

Prashanth K Adiga, Anjali M

Lifestyle factors are important modifiable factors which greatly influence overall health and well-being; this is applicable to infertility as well. Poor diet, lack of physical activity, smoking, and alcohol intake are some of the important risk factors which increase preponderance to chronic diseases. In this chapter, we have discussed the influence of these lifestyle factors on infertility.

OBESITY

As per the World Health Organization (WHO), obesity is defined as body mass index (BMI) of greater than 30. Obesity causes insulin resistance, which in turn results in hyperinsulinemia, elevated androgens, low sex hormone–binding globulin, accentuated peripheral conversion of androgens to estrogens, high free insulin-like growth factor 1, and elevated leptins. The compounding effect of these changes results in hypothalamic dysfunction, abnormal gonadotropin secretion, impaired folliculogenesis, and lower luteal phase progesterone. Reduced response to gonadotropins has been observed in obese patients. BMI over 30 demands higher gonadotropin-releasing hormone (GnRH) requirements, prolonged GnRH stimulation, lower peak estradiol (E2) levels, and fewer large and medium size follicles. There is decline in number of oocytes retrieved and the number of high quality embryos that can be produced as the BMI rises over 40. With increasing severity of obesity, implantation, clinical pregnancy, and live birth rates all decline gradually. However, the absolute decline in pregnancy rates is small. Overall likelihood of a live birth per cycle start declined from 31.4% in women with a normal BMI, to 28% in women with BMI 30–34.9, to 24.3% in women with a BMI 40–44.5, and down to 21.2% in women with a BMI > 50.

SMOKING

Cigarette smoking has deleterious effects on fertility rates. Cigarette smoking contributes to about 13% of female infertility. There is a detrimental impact of smoking on fecundity among women attempting to conceive without medical assistance. Early menopause has been observed in women who smoke than those who do not. Excessive smoking may cause ovarian follicular reduction; impact escalates with smoking pack years. Young smokers have significantly higher basal follicular-stimulating hormone (FSH) than in nonsmokers. Current smoking is also associated with lower anti-Müllerian hormone (AMH) levels in late reproductive age and perimenopausal women. It was observed that smokers take longer to impregnate compared to nonsmokers because there will be higher gonadotropin requirement for ovarian stimulation, lower peak E2 levels, and higher testosterone levels. It also causes lower oocyte retrieval, thicker zona pellucida, lower implantation rates, and number of canceled cycles. It is well documented that smokers require approximately twice the number of in vitro fertilization (IVF) attempts to conceive as compared to nonsmokers.

CAFFEINE AND ALCOHOL

Evidences of effects of caffeine on fertility are inconsistent. There is no documented negative impact on time to pregnancy in normal women who consume caffeine. Klonoff et al. observed lower conceptional rates in IVF patients who consumed caffeine of 50 mg/day. At present, little evidence supports a detrimental effect of caffeine consumption on reproductive outcomes among women undergoing assisted reproductive technique (ART) treatments.

Maternal alcohol consumption during pregnancy can have negative impacts on multiple fetal organ systems, the best studied being the adverse effects on the developing brain. It is uncertain whether intake of alcohol reduces the ability to achieve a pregnancy. Moderate alcohol intake in the year before ART treatment do not seem to have an appreciable impact on the success of ART; however, current alcohol intake immediately before the start of (and during) treatment may be harmful. Center for Disease Control and Prevention reiterated that "there is no known safe amount of alcohol use during pregnancy or while trying to get pregnant".

EXERCISE

Exercising regularly will have positive effect on improving ovarian morphology, both ovarian volume and number of follicles, in women with polycystic ovary syndrome (PCOS). A study by Gaskins et al. concluded that overall physical activity in the year before starting fertility treatment was unlikely to have a deleterious effect on outcomes of IVF. Moreover, certain forms of physical activity may be beneficial and certain subgroups of women such as those of normal BMI may benefit from vigorous physical activity before IVF treatment initiation. Table 1 shows the exercise recommendations for PCOS women derived from major international guidelines.

- 150 minutes of exercise weekly, including 90 minutes of moderate-to-high intensity aerobic activity at 60–90% of maximal heart rate
- Exercise recommended for all women, especially if overweight/obese.

AE-PCOS Society (Androgen Excess-PCOS) recommends:

- 30 minutes of moderate-intensity physical activity daily with slow increase according to exercise tolerance. Personal goals to target weight loss, e.g. if walking, daily aim should be 15,000 steps or 45-minutes duration
- Exercise recommended for all women, especially if dyslipidemia.

DIET

The literature on the relationship between diet and human fertility has greatly expanded over the last decade, resulting in the identification of a few clear patterns. The influence of diet on female infertility has been summarized in Table 1.

TABLE 1: Diet and fertility.

Variables	What is the bottom line	What are the gaps in the evidence?
Antioxidant supplements	Most likely do not make a difference	Too few studies have tested the exact same intervention, so it is difficult to draw strong conclusions
Folic acid and Vitamin B	Folic acid may increase fertility and live birth rates in ART. Doses higher than recommended for NTD prevention may offer the greatest benefit as might the additional intake of Vitamin B	No randomized trials have tested the doses related with greatest benefit in observational studies
Vitamin D	Vitamin D does not have a major impact on fertility within the observed range of supplementation/adequate serum levels	Most published work has focused on women with vitamin D intakes or serum concentrations within or very close to normal range; an adverse effect of severe deficiency on fertility cannot be ruled out
Dairy	Dairy foods probably do not have an important influence on fertility	Very few studies have addressed this question
Meats	Intake of red meats and fish with high levels of environmental contamination may be of concern	Very few studies have addressed this question
Soy, isoflavone	Soy intake does not help or hurt couples trying to conceive on their own; however, isoflavone intake may increase live birth rates in ART	Only one study to date among pregnancy planners. Vast range of doses in ART studies yet all show similar effects
Dietary fats	Higher 3 PUFA and lower trans fatty acid intake may enhance female fertility	Trials of omega-3 fatty acid supplementation are needed
Diet patterns	Healthy diets have been consistently related to better fertility and higher live birth rates in ART across multiple studies. Unhealthy diets have consistently had the opposite relationship	Definition of healthy and unhealthy diets changes slightly from study to study. No randomized trials to date
Alcohol and caffeine	Most large, well-designed studies have not detected associations between higher alcohol or caffeine intake and lower fertility	Because randomized trials of alcohol/caffeine will likely be judged as unethical, there is a need for more large, high-quality prospective cohort studies to clarify this issue

(ART: assisted reproductive technique; PUFA: polyunsaturated fatty acid; NTD: neural tube defect)
(*Source:* Modified from Gaskins et al.)

Diet and Lifestyle in Infertility

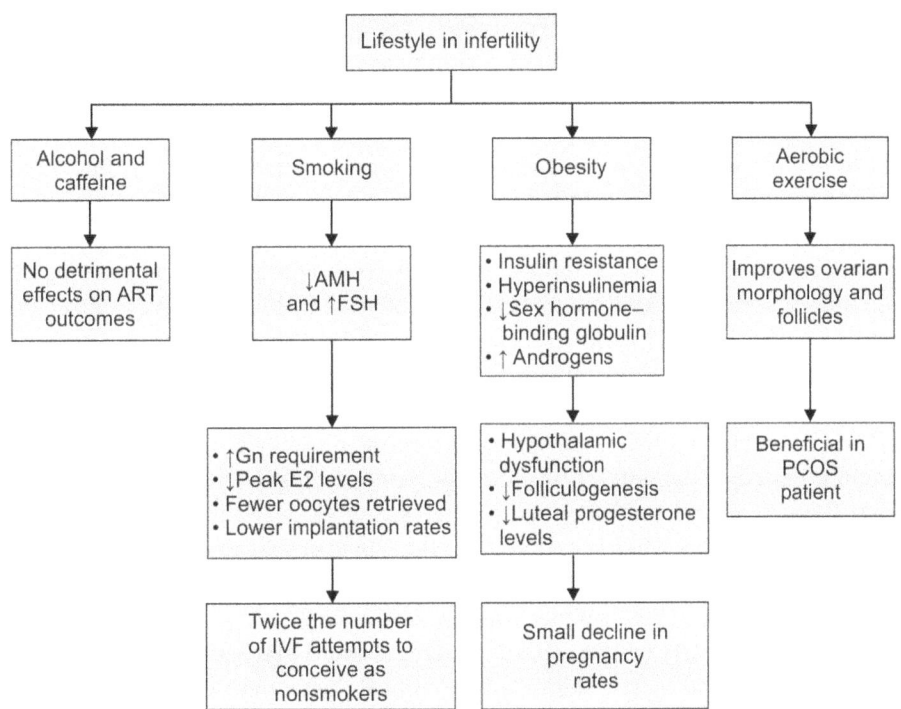

(AMH: anti-Müllerian hormone; ART: assisted reproductive technique; E2: estradiol; FSH: follicle-stimulating hormone; IVF: in vitro fertilization; PCOS: polycystic ovary syndrome; Gn: gonadotropin)

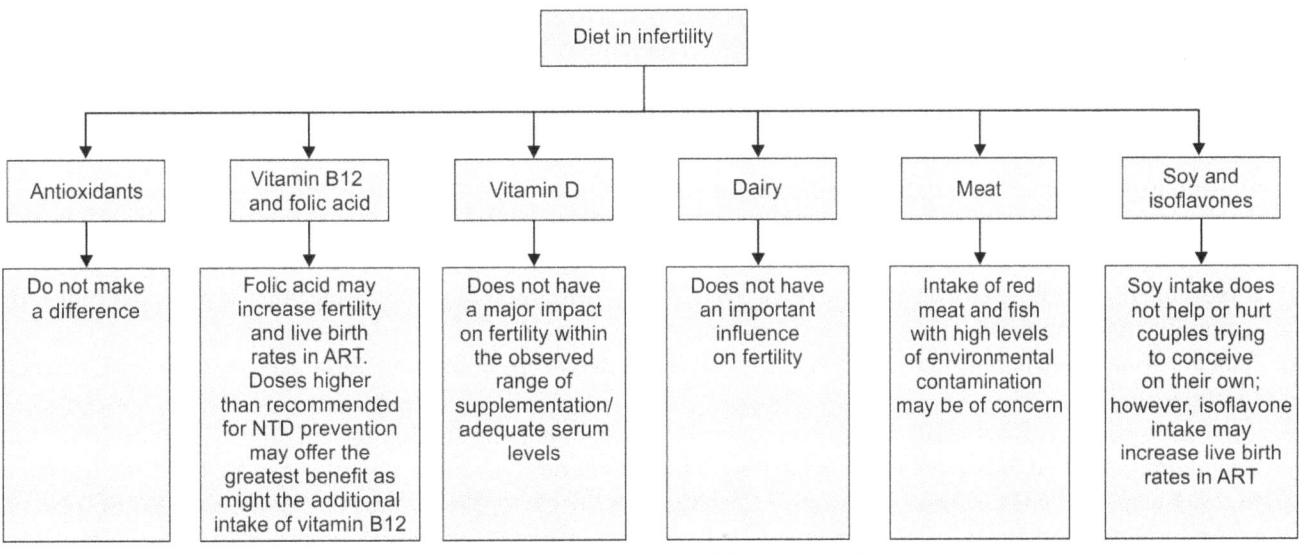

(ART: assisted reproductive technique; NTD: neural tube defect)

CHAPTER 99

Endometrial Scratching

Kanti Bansal, Meenu Handa

A. Creating a mild mechanical endometrial injury by scratching was suggested to improve the pregnancy rates in women. It is hypothesized to work by:
   - Facilitating decidualization
   - Injury leading to healing with activation of an immune response with cytokines, interleukins, growth factors, macrophages, and natural killer (NK) cells being released
   - It slows endometrial maturation to improve synchrony.
B. Despite being practiced since ages and accepted widely, there is conflicting evidence regarding the efficacy of endometrial scratching over reproductive outcomes. It may be used in a natural, intrauterine insemination (IUI) or assisted reproductive technique (ART) cycle. In a survey done with 143 clinicians from Australia, New Zealand, and United Kingdom, 83% recommended scratching for in vitro fertilization (IVF) but only 4% agreed that it would benefit patients trying to conceive naturally or undergoing IUI.
C. In 2016 another Cochrane review with nine randomized controlled trials (RCTs) with 1,512 patients concluded that endometrial scratching benefited patients trying naturally or undergoing IUI, but this was again based on low or very low evidence. In 2017 Vitagliano et al. published an updated systematic review and meta-analysis which included four new studies. His results showed that when scratching was done in the cycle preceding IUI, there was no difference in the pregnancy rates, but when it was done in the same cycle, the pregnancy rates were significantly higher (OR 2.57, $P < 0.00001$). However, the quality of the evidence was low here as well.
D. A 2015 Cochrane analysis of 14 RCTs with 2,128 IVF patients showed that scratching in the preceding luteal phase or early follicular phase of a fresh IVF cycle improved the clinical pregnancy rates (RR 1.34, 95% confidence interval 1.21–1.61; $P = 0.002$). However, the study was based on moderate evidence quality. In 2019, Sarah Jensen et al. presented details of their randomized trial of endometrial scratching done for both fresh as well as frozen embryo transfer. It was done between day 3 of the cycle preceding the embryo transfer to day 3 of the embryo transfer cycle. A total of 1,354 women underwent randomization. The endometrial scratching did not produce higher live birth rates. Thus, the role of endometrial scratching is being criticized with the more recent papers stating that it does not improve reproductive outcomes. There are two large trials whose results are awaited and they may help in solving the mystery. The final nail in the coffin is an editorial published in New England Journal of Medicine which is titled as "Scratching the Endometrium in IVF—Time to Stop".
E. The timing of endometrial scratch, when decided, is equally controversial. Studies have tried to evaluate the efficacy of an early follicular phase in a concurrent cycle or in the luteal phase of previous cycle. The SCRaTCH study is a Dutch multicenter—both academic and nonacademic—RCT of woman undergoing IVF with scratching in the luteal phase preceding the transfer cycle. When done in the luteal phase, disruption of an early pregnancy is principally the only substantial risk associated.
F. Mild injury has been performed using a Pipelle or during hysteroscopy or in some studies even using a small Karman cannula.
G. The controversies will hopefully end once the results of some ongoing studies are out. The SCRaTCH-OFO trial, originating in Netherlands looks at how scratching can help natural conception. A multicenter RCT will be conducted in Dutch academic and nonacademic hospitals starting from November 2017. A total of 792 women with unexplained infertility and a good prognosis for spontaneous conception less than 12 months (Hunault > 30%) will be included, of whom half will undergo endometrial scratching in the luteal phase of the natural cycle.
H. Keeping in mind the available evidence, routine use of endometrial scratching is not advised.

Endometrial Scratching

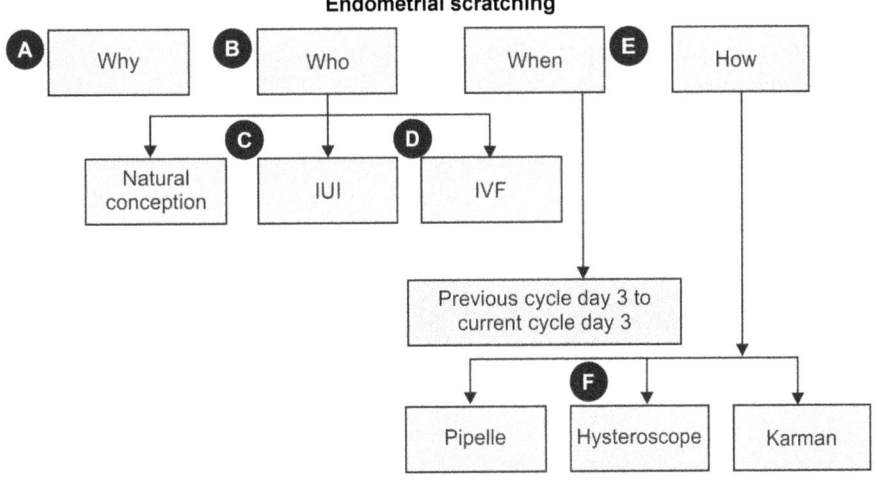

(IUI: intrauterine insemination; IVF: in vitro fertilization)

CHAPTER 100

Medical Management of Oligoasthenoteratozoospermia

Kedar Ganla, Rana Choudharay, Priyanka Vora

A. *Oligoasthenoteratozoospermia* (OATS) is a condition that includes oligozoospermia (low number of sperm), asthenozoospermia (poor sperm movement), and teratozoospermia (abnormal sperm shape). It is the most common cause of male subfertility.

B. Lower limit of normal reference values for different sperm parameters (WHO 2010 GUIDELINES)

Parameter	Lower reference limits (WHO 2010)
Semen volume	1.5 mL
Sperm concentration	15 million sperm/mL
Progressive motility	32%
Total motility	40%
Vitality	58% live
Morphology (strict criteria)	4% normal form

C. OAT can be secondary to a pre-existing condition like varicocele, infections, occupational exposure, smoking, impaired collection or idiopathic in nature.

D. Adapting a healthier lifestyle is always the first line of advice of men with poor sperm parameters. Regular exercise, abstaining from smoking and alcohol, reducing exposure to heat, chemical or radiation from electronic devices, ejaculation of minimum twice a week, cutting down caffeine intake, strict control of blood sugar levels, practice of calming activities like yoda or meditation to reduce stress etc are a part of adapting healthier lifestyle.

E. Managing asthenospermia: A variety of antioxidants, sperm vitalizers and nutritional supplements are used for reducing the reactive oxygen species (ROS) levels and thus improving the motility. There is no role of routine antioxidant therapy for all men, however, vitalizers do increase sperm motility in oligospermic men. In the presence of pus cells, a semen culture is indicated and appropriate antibiotic therapy for a minimum of 14 days is required. A repeat culture may be performed to confirm complete clearance of infection. Presence of infection in semen not only reduces sperm motility, but also reduces fertility potential and increases chances of pelvic infections in women.

F. Managing oligospermia:

G. Varicocele correction may help improve sperm parameters in selected cases.

H. The effectiveness of the therapy depends on multiple factors like severity of OAT, age, lifestyle, body mass index (BMI), compliance to therapy etc. If no improvement in sperm parameters is seen after 3 months of therapy or if pregnancy is not achieved within 6 months of improved sperm parameters, other therapeutic options should be considered.

I. Managing asthenospermia: There is no specific therapy to manage poor sperm morphology. Intracytoplasmic sperm injection (ICSI) is considered the best option for morphology <4%.

CONCLUSION

- Give patients a very clear road map of therapy
- Individualized treatment, with timeline and endpoints established beforehand
- Treatment should be of at least 3 months to incorporate full 74-day spermatogenesis cycle, followed by semen analysis
- Patient should be counseled about realistic expectations
- Do not waste time and money over medical therapy if the circumstances call for assisted reproductive therapy.

Medical Management of Oligoasthenoteratozoospermia

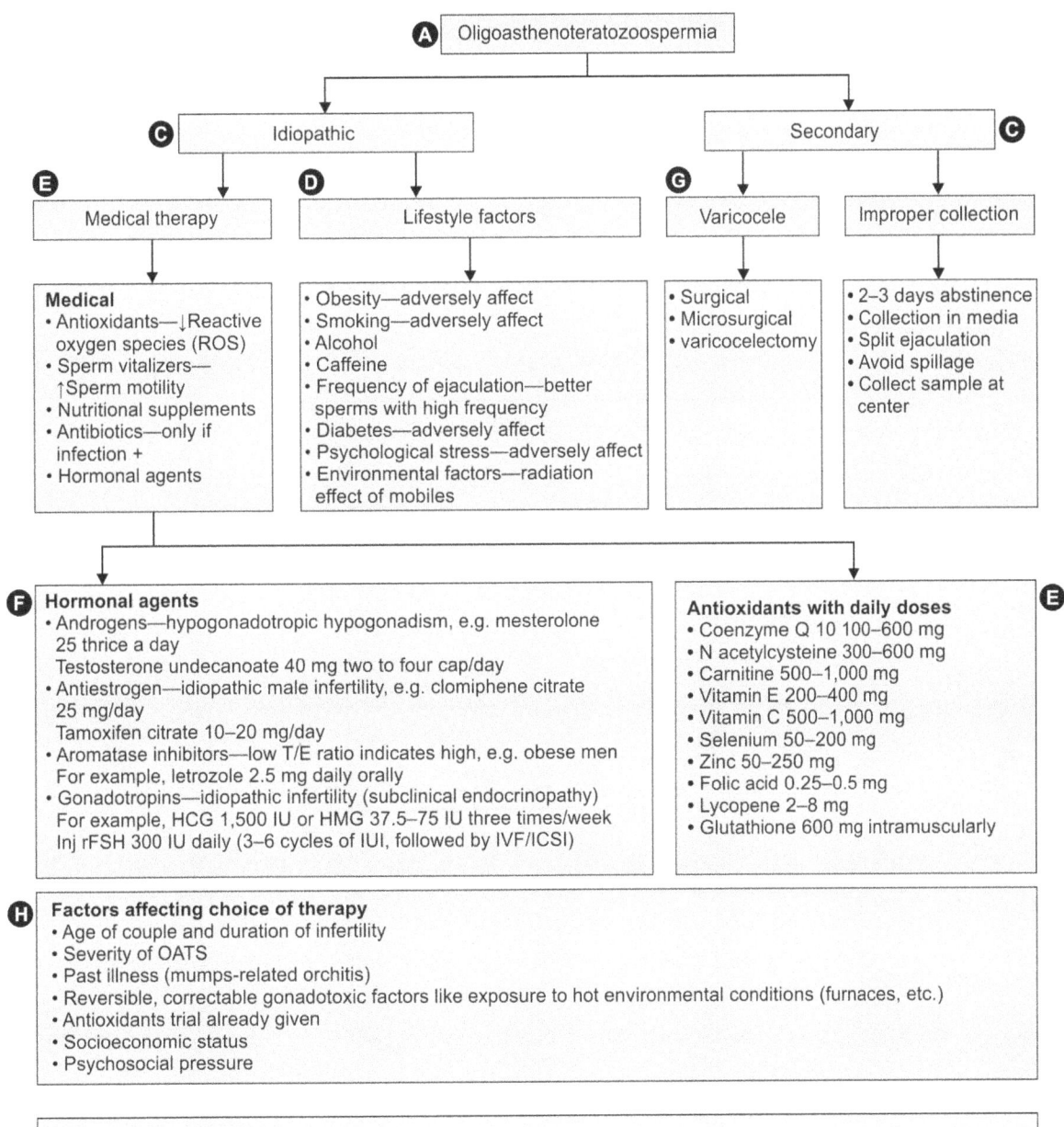

(HCG: human chorionic gonadotropin; HMG: human menopausal gonadotropin; ICSI: intracytoplasmic sperm injection; IUI: intrauterine insemination; IVF: in vitro fertilization; OATS: oligoasthenoteratozoospermia; rFSH: recombinant follicle-stimulating hormone; T/E: testosterone/epitestosterone; DNA: deoxyribonucleic acid)

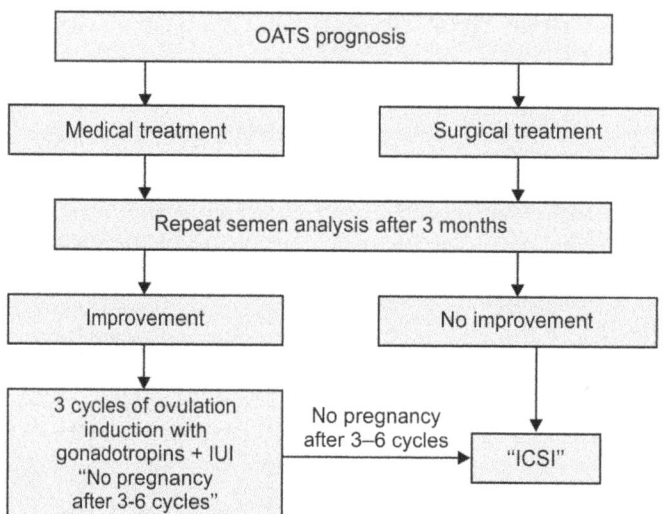

(ICSI: intracytoplasmic sperm injection; IUI: intrauterine insemination; OATS: oligoasthenoteratozoospermia)

Bibliography

Chapter 1

1. Adisa J, Egbujo EM, Yahaya BA, et al. Primary infertility associated with schitosoma mansoni: a case report from the Jos plateau, north central Nigeria. Afr Health Sci. 2012;12(4):563-5.
2. Akande V, Turner C, Horner P, et al. Impact of Chlamydia trachomatis in the reproductive setting: British fertility society guidelines for practice. Hum Fertil. 2010;13(3):1-18.
3. Ashok A, Aspinder S, Alaa H, et al. Cell phones and male infertility: a review of recent innovations in technology and consequences. Int Braz J Urol. 2011;37(4):432-54.
4. Hickman RA, Gordon C. Causes and management of infertility in systemic lupus erythematosus. Rheumatology. 2011;50(9):1551-8.
5. Honig SC, Lipshultz LI, Jarow J. Significant medical pathology uncovered by a comprehensive male infertility evaluation. Fertil Steril. 1994;62:1028-34.
6. Jaiswal D, Trivedi S, Agrawal NK, et al. Association of polymorphism in cell death pathway gene FASLG with human male infertility. Asian Pac J Reprod. 2015;4(2):112-5.
7. Jensen T, Heitmann BL, Blomberg JM, et al. High dietary intake of saturated fat is associated with reduced semen quality among 701 young Danish men from the general population. Am J Clin Nutr. 2013;97(1):411-8.
8. Li C, Meng CX, Zhao WH, et al. Risk factors for ectopic pregnancy in women with planned pregnancy: a case-control study. Eur J Obstet Gynecol Reprod Biol. 2014;181:176-82.
9. Nodine PM, Hastings-Tolsma M. Maternal obesity: improving pregnancy outcomes. MCN Am J Matern Child Nurs. 2012;37(2):110-5.
10. Practice Committee of American Society for Reproductive Medicine. Definitions of infertility and recurrent pregnancy loss: a committee opinion. Fertil Steril. 2013;99:63.
11. Richardson WR. Inguinal hernia of the internal genitalia in female infants and children. Am Surg. 1963;29:446.
12. Sabarre KA, Khan Z, Whitten AN, et al. A qualitative study of Ottawa university students' awareness, knowledge and perceptions of infertility, infertility risk factors and assisted reproductive technologies (ART). Reprod Health J. 2013;10(41):1-10.
13. Sarvari A, Naderi MM, Heidari M, et al. Effect of environmental risk factors on human fertility. J Reprod Infertil. 2010;11(4):211-25.
14. Vessey MP. Results of epidemiological studies of the return of fertility in ex-users of the pill. The Regulation of Fertility Evaluation and Perspectives. Paris: Institut National de la Santé et de la Recherche; 1979. p. 185.
15. West Z. Fertility and conception: The Complete Guide to Getting Pregnant. UK: Dorling Kindersley; 2003. p. 36.

Chapter 1B

1. Ahmed B. Factors influencing the success rate of IUI. J Women's Health Care. 2017;6(5):402.
2. El-Toukhy T. Role of hysteroscopy surgery in the management of female infertility. Surg Res Pract. 2014:Article ID 105412.
3. NICE Fertility Guidelines. No 11. 2004.

Chapter 4

1. Deligeoroglou E, Athanasopoulos N, Tsimaris P, et al. Evaluation and management of adolescent amenorrhea. Ann N Y Acad Sci. 2010;1205:23-32.
2. Klein DA, Poth MA. Amenorrhea: an approach to diagnosis and management. Am Fam Physician. 2013;87(11):781-8.
3. Ko JKY, King TFJ, Williams L, et al. Hormone replacement treatment choices in complete androgen insensitivity syndrome: an audit of an adult clinic. Endocr Connect. 2017;6(6):375-9.

Chapter 5

1. *Fertility:* Assessment and treatment for people with fertility problems. National Collaborating Center for Women's and Children's health commissioned by the National Institute for Health and Clinical Excellence February 2013.

Chapter 6

1. Jirge PR. Poor ovarian reserve. J Hum Reprod Sci. 2016;9(2):63-9.
2. Practice Committee of the American Society for Reproductive Medicine. Testing and interpreting measures of ovarian reserve: a committee opinion. Fertil Steril. 2015;103(3):e2-e9.
3. Tal R, Seifer DB. Ovarian reserve testing: a user's guide. Am J Obstet Gynecol. 2017;217(2):129-40.

Chapter 8

1. Campo S. Ovulatory cycles, pregnancy outcome and complications after surgical treatment of polycystic ovary syndrome. Obstet Gynecol Surv. 1998;53(5):297-308.
2. Carranza-Mamane B, Havelock J, Hemmings R, et al. The management of uterine fibroids in women with otherwise unexplained infertility. J Obstet Gynaecol Can. 2015;37(3):277-85.
3. Cohen J, Audebert A, de Brux J, et al. Sterility due to dysovulation: prognostic and therapeutic role of ovarian biopsy during calioscopy. J Gynecol Obstet Biol Reprod (Paris). 1972;1(7):657-71.
4. Gjönnaess H. Polycystic ovarian syndrome treated by ovarian electrocautery through the laparoscope. Fertil Steril. 1984;41(1):20-5.
5. Hassa H, Aydin Y. The role of laparoscopy in management of infertility. J Obstet Gynaecol. 2014;34(1):1-7.
6. Kamal N, Sanad Z, Elkelani O, et al. Changes in ovarian reserve and ovarian blood flow in patients with polycystic ovary syndrome following laparoscopic ovarian drilling. Gynecol Endocrinol. 2018;34(9):789-92.
7. O'Flynn N. Assessment and treatment for people with fertility problems: NICE guideline. Br J Gen Pract. 2014;64(618):50-1.
8. Practice Committee of the American Society for Reproductive Medicine. Role of tubal surgery in the era of assisted reproductive technology: a committee opinion. Fertil Steril. 2015;103(6):e37-43.
9. Practice Committee of the American Society for Reproductive Medicine. Uterine septum: a guideline. Fertil Steril. 2016;106(3):530-40.
10. Thessaloniki ESHRE/ASRM-Sponsored PCOS Consensus Workshop Group. Consensus on infertility treatment related to polycystic ovary syndrome. Hum Reprod. 2008;23:462-77.

Chapter 9

1. American Association of Gynecologic Laparoscopists (AAGL), Advancing Minimally Invasive Gynecology Worldwide. AAGL practice report: practice guidelines for the diagnosis and management of submucous leiomyomas. J Minim Invasive Gynecol. 2012;19(2):152-71.
2. En-Lan Xia, Tin-Chiu Li, Sze-Ngar Sylvia Choi, et al. Reproductive Outcome of Transcervical Uterine Incision in Unicornuate Uterus. Chin Med J (Engl). 2017;130(3):256-61.
3. National Institute for Health and Clinical Excellence, 2013.
4. National Institute for Health and Clinical Excellence: Guidance. Fertility: Assessment and Treatment for People with Fertility Problems. London: RCOG Press; 2004.
5. Preutthipan S, Linasmita V. A prospective comparative study between hysterosalpingography and hysteroscopy in the detection of intrauterine pathology in patients with infertility. J Obstet Gynaecol Res. 2003;29(1):33-7.
6. Shalev J, Meizner I, Bar-Hava I, et al. Predictive value of transvaginal sonography performed before routine diagnostic hysteroscopy for evaluation of infertility. Fertil Steril. 2000;73(2):412-7.

Chapter 10

1. Ahmadi F, Rashidy Z, Haghighi H, et al. Uterine cavity assessment in infertile women: Sensitivity and specificity of three-dimensional hysterosonography versus hysteroscopy. Iran J Reprod Med. 2013;11(12):977-82.
2. Moreno I, Cicinelli E, Garcia-Grau I, et al. The diagnosis of chronic endometritis in infertile asymptomatic women: a comparative study of histology, microbial cultures, hysteroscopy, and molecular microbiology. Am J Obstet Gynecol. 2018;218(6):602.

Chapter 11

1. Moreno I, Cicinelli E, Garcia-Grau I, et al. The diagnosis of chronic endometritis in infertile asymptomatic women: a comparative study of histology, microbial cultures, hysteroscopy, and molecular microbiology. Am J Obstet Gynecol. 2018;218(6):602.e1-602.e16.

Chapter 13

1. Kasapoglu T, Kasapoglu D, Deren O. Successful management of the recurrent uterine rupture after the uterine septum resection. Case Rep Womens Health. 2015;8:13-6.
2. Kashyap M. Hysteroscopic septum resection. In: Agarwal M, Mettler L, Alkatout I (Eds). A Manual of Minimally Invasive Gynecological Surgery. New Delhi: Jaypee Brothers Medical (P) Ltd.; 2015. pp. 260-9.
3. Practice Committee of the American Society for Reproductive Medicine. Uterine septum: a guideline. Am Soc Reprod Med. 2016;106(3):530-40.

Chapter 14

1. Al Chami A, Saridogan E. Endometrial polyps and subfertility. J Obstet Gynaecol India. 2017;67(1):9-14.
2. DeVita JM, Merriam K, Usadi RS, et al. Incidence and recurrence of uterine polyps in women undergoing embryo transfer. Fertil Steril. 2016;106(3):e16-e17.
3. Stadtmauer L, Waud K, Cohen DP, et al. Ultrasonography in assisted reproduction. In: Garner DK, Weissman A, Howlws CM, Shoham Z (Eds). Textbook of Assisted Reproductive Techniques. Boca Raton: CRC, Press; 2017.

Chapter 16

1. Mol BW, Collins JA, Burrows EA, et al. Comparison of hysterosalpingography and laparoscopy in predicting fertility outcome. Hum Reprod. 1999;14(5):1237-42.
2. Panchal S, Nagori C. Imaging techniques for assessment of tubal status. J Hum Reprod Sci. 2014;7(1):2-12.
3. Practice Committee of the American Society for Reproductive Medicine. Role of tubal surgery in the era of assisted reproductive technology: a committee opinion. Fertil Steril. 2015;103(6):e37-43.

Chapter 17

1. Practice Committee of the American Society for Reproductive Medicine. Role of Tubal surgery in the era of assisted reproductive technology: a committee opinion. Fertil Steril. 2015;103(6):e37-43.

Chapter 19

1. Monash University. International evidence-based guideline for the assessment and management of polycystic ovary syndrome 2018. [online] Available from https://www.monash.edu/medicine/sphpm/mchri/pcos/guideline [Last accessed February 2019].

Chapter 20

1. Cho MK. Thyroid dysfunction and subfertility. Clin Exp Reprod Med. 2015;42(4):131-5.
2. Garber JR, Cobin RH, Gharib H, et al. Clinical practice guidelines for hypothyroidism in adults: cosponsored by the American Association of Clinical Endocrinologists and the American Thyroid Association. Endocr Pract. 2012;18:988-1028.
3. Ross DS, Burch HB, Cooper DS, et al. 2016 American Thyroid Association Guidelines for diagnosis and management of hyperthyroidism and other causes of thyrotoxicosis. Thyroid. 2016;26(10):1343-21.

Chapter 21

1. Ferriman D, Gallwey JD. Clinical assessment of body hair growth in women. J Clin Endocrinol Metab. 1961;21:1440-7.
2. Friedman CI, Schmidt GE, Kim MH, et al. Serum testosterone concentrations in the evaluation of androgen-producing tumors. Am J Obstet Gynecol. 1985;153:44-9.
3. Kahraman K, Sukur YE, Atabekoglu CS, et al. Comparison of two oral contraceptive forms containing cyproterone acetate and drospirenone in the treatment of patients with polycystic ovary syndrome: a randomized clinical trial. Arch Gynecol Obstet. 2014;290:321-8.
4. Loriaux DL. An approach to the patient with hirsutism. J Clin Endocrinol Metab. 2012;97(9):2957-68.
5. Martin KA, Chang RJ, Ehrmann DA, et al. Evaluation and treatment of hirsutism in premenopausal women: an endocrine society clinical practice guideline. J Clin Endocrinol Metab. 2008;93:1105-20.
6. Mofid A, Seyyed Alinaghi SA, Zandieh S, et al. Hirsutism. Int J Clin Pract. 2008;62:433-43.
7. Rosenfield RL, Clinical practice. Hirsutism. N Engl J Med. 2005;353:(24)2578-88.

Chapter 22

1. Casanueva FF, Molitch ME, Schlechte JA, et al. Guidelines of the Pituitary Society for the diagnosis and management of prolactinomas. Clin Endocrinol (Oxf). 2006;65(2):265-73.
2. Gillam MP, Molitch ME, Lombardi G, et al. Advances in the treatment of prolactinomas. Endocr Rev. 2006;27(5):485-534.
3. Glezer A, Bronstein MD. Approach to the patient with persistent hyperprolactinemia and negative sellar imaging. J Clin Endocrinol Metab. 2012;97(7):2211-6.
4. Huang W, Molitch ME. Evaluation and management of galactorrhea. Am Fam Physician. 2012;85(11):1073-80.
5. Melmed S, Casanueva FF, Hoffman AR, et al. Diagnosis and treatment of hyperprolactinemia: an Endocrine Society clinical practice guideline. J Clin Endocrinol Metab. 2011;96(2):273-88.

Chapter 23

1. Bankowski BJ, Zacur HA. Dopamine agonist therapy for hyperprolactinemia. Clin Obstet Gynecol. 2003;46(2):349-62.
2. Kinon BJ, Ahl J, Liu-Seifert H, et al. Improvement in hyperprolactinemia and reproductive comorbidities in patients with schizophrenia switched from conventional antipsychotics or risperidone to olanzapine. Psychoneuroendocrinology. 2006;31(5):577-88.
3. Klibanski A. Clinical practice. Prolactinomas. [published correction appears in N Engl J Med. 2010;362(22): 2142]. N Engl J Med. 2010;362(13):1219-26.
4. Schlechte J, Dolan K, Sherman B, et al. The natural history of untreated hyperprolactinemia: a prospective analysis. J Clin Endocrinol Metab. 1989;68(2):412-8.
5. Thomson JA, Gray CE, Teasdale GM. Relapse of hyperprolactinemia after transsphenoidal surgery for microprolactinoma: lessons from long-term follow-up. Neurosurgery. 2002;50(1):36-9.
6. Webster J, Piscitelli G, Polli A, et al. A comparison of cabergoline and bromocriptine in the treatment of hyperprolactinemic amenorrhea. Cabergoline Comparative Study Group. N Engl J Med. 1994;331(14):904-9.
7. Zacur HA. Indications for surgery in the treatment of hyperprolactinemia. J Reprod Med. 1999;44(12 Suppl):1127-31.

Chapter 24

1. Allahbadia GN. Clomiphene citrate for ovarian stimulation. Manual of Ovulation Induction. New Delhi: Jaypee Brothers Medical Publishers (P) Ltd.; 2005.
2. Bhatnagar AS. The discovery and mechanism of action of letrozole. Breast cancer Res Treat. 2007;105(1):7-17.
3. Purata JR. What is the ideal starting dose for patients utilizing letrozole for ovulation induction? Fertil Steril. 2015;104(3):e107-8.

Chapter 25

1. Manuel FS, Visnova H, Yuzpe A, et al. Individualization of the starting dose of follitropin delta reduces the overall OHSS risk and/or the need for additional preventive interventions: cumulative data over three stimulation cycles. Reproductive BioMedicine Online. 2019;38(4):528-37.
2. Martin KA, Hall JE, Adams JM. Gonadotropin preparations: past, present, and future perspectives. Fertil Steril. 2008;90(5):S13-S20.

Chapter 26

1. Basirat Z. Impact of dexamethasone on pregnancy outcome in PCOs women candidate for IVF/ICSI, a single-blind randomized clinical trial study. Middle East Fertil Soc J. 2016;21(3):184-8.
2. International evidence-based guideline for the assessment and management of polycystic ovary syndrome. 2018.
3. Regidor PA. Management of women with PCOS using myo-inositol and folic acid. New clinical data and review of the literature. Horm Mol Biol Clin Investig. 2018;34(2):2017-67.
4. Shah D. Consensus Statement on the Use of Oral Contraceptive Pills in Polycystic Ovarian Syndrome Women in India. J Hum Reprod Sci. 2018.

Chapter 27

1. Agrawal R, Burt E, Gallagher AM, et al. Prospective randomized trial of multiple micronutrients in subfertile women undergoing ovulation induction: a pilot study. Reprod BioMed 2012;24(1):54-6.
2. Ubaldi F, Vaiarelli A, D'Anna R, et al. Management of poor responders in IVF: Is there anything new? BioMed Res Int 2014:Article ID 352098.

Chapter 28

1. Kuznetsov L, Dworzynski K, Davies M, et al. Diagnosis and management of endometriosis: summary of NICE guidance. BMJ. 2017;358:j3935.
2. Practice Committee of the American Society for Reproductive Medicine. Endometriosis and infertility. Fertil Steril. 2006;86(5 Suppl 1):S156-60.
3. Schenken RS, Asch RH, Williams RF, et al. Etiology of infertility in monkeys with endometriosis: luteinized unruptured follicles, luteal phase defects, pelvic adhesions, and spontaneous abortions. Fertil Steril. 1984;41(1):122-30.

Chapter 29

1. De Graaff AA, D'Hooghe TM, Dunselman GA, et al. The significant effect of endometriosis on physical, mental and social well-being: results from an international cross-sectional survey. Hum Reprod. 2013;28(10):2677-85.
2. Eskenazi B, Warner ML. Epidemiology of endometriosis. Obstet Gynecol Clin North Am. 1997;24:235-58.
3. Kennedy S, Bergqvist A, Chapron C, et al. ESHRE guideline for the diagnosis and treatment of endometriosis. Hum Reprod. 2005;20:2698-704.
4. May KE, Conduit-Hulbert SA, Villar J, et al. Peripheral biomarkers of endometriosis: a systematic review. Hum Reprod Update. 2010;16:651-74.
5. NICE Guideline NG73. (2017). The NICE guidance that was used to create this part of the interactive flowchart; Endometriosis: diagnosis and management. [online] Available from https://www.nice.org.uk/guidance/ng73/resources/endometriosis-diagnosis-and-management-pdf-1837632548293 [Last accessed May, 2019].
6. Pascual MA, Guerriero S, Hereter L, et al. Diagnosis of endometriosis of the rectovaginal septum using introital three-dimensional ultrasonography. Fertil Steril. 2010;94:2761-5.
7. Stratton P, Winkel C, Premkumar A, et al. Diagnostic accuracy of laparoscopy, magnetic resonance imaging, and histopathologic examination for the detection of endometriosis. Fertil Steril. 2003;79:1078-85.

Chapter 30

1. National Institute of Health and Care Excellence. (2017). Endometriosis: Diagnosis and management. NICE guideline NG73. [online] Available from https://www.nice.org.uk/guidance/ng73 [Last accessed February 2019].
2. Stratton P, Winkel C, Premkumar A, et al. Diagnostic accuracy of laparoscopy, magnetic resonance imaging and histopathologic examination for the detection of endometriosis. Fertil Steril. 2003;79:1078-85.

Chapter 31

1. Adamson GD, Pasta DJ. Endometriosis fertility index: the new, validated endometriosis staging system. Fertil Steril. 2010;94:1609-15.
2. Boujenah J, Cedrin-Durnerin I, Herbemont C, et al. Use of the endometriosis fertility index in daily practice: A prospective evaluation. Eur J Obstet Gynecol Reprod Biol. 2017;219:28-34.
3. Revised American society for reproductive medicine classification of endometriosis. Fertil Steril. 1996;67:817-21.

Chapter 32

1. Adamson GD, Pasta DJ. Endometriosis fertility index: the new, validated endometriosis staging system. Fertil Steril. 2010;94(5):1609-15.
2. Pabuccu R, Onalan G, Kaya G. GnRH agonist and antagonist protocols for stage I-II endometriosis and endometrioma in in vitro fertilization/intracytoplasmic sperm injection cycles. Fertil Steril. 2007;88(4):832-9.
3. Practice Committee of the American Society for Reproductive Medicine. Endometriosis and infertility: a committee opinion. Fertil Steril. 2012;98(3):591-8.

Chapter 33

1. Dunselman GA, Vermeulen N, Becker C, et al. ESHRE guideline: management of women with endometriosis. Hum Reprod. 2014;29(3):400-12.
2. Hoo WL, Hardcastle R, Louden K. Management of endometriosis-related pelvic pain. Obstet Gynaecol. 2017;19(2):131-8.
3. NICE. (2017). Endometriosis: diagnosis and management. Guidance and guidelines. [online] Available from https://www.nice.org.uk/guidance/ng73 [Accessed April, 2019].
4. Somigliana E, Vercellini P, Viganó P, et al. Should endometriomas be treated before IVF-ICSI cycles? Hum Reprod Update. 2006;12(1):57-64.

Chapter 34

1. Working group of ESGE, ESHRE, and WES, Saridogan E, Becker CM, et al. Recommendations for the surgical treatment of endometriosis—part 1: ovarian endometrioma. Gynecol Surg. 2017;14(1):27.

Chapter 35

1. Donnez J, Tatarchuk TF, Bouchard P, et al. Ulipristal acetate versus placebo for fibroid treatment before surgery. N Engl J Med. 2012;366(5):409-20.
2. Purohit P, Vigneswaran K. Fibroids and infertility. Curr Obstet Gynecol Rep. 2016;5:81-8.
3. RANZCOG Board and Council. Fibroids in Infertility 2018 consensus.
4. Yang JH, Chen MJ, Chen CD, et al. Optimal waiting period for subsequent fertility treatment after various hysteroscopic surgeries. Fertil Steril. 2013;99(7):2092-6.

Chapter 36

1. Dueholm M. Uterine adenomyosis and infertility, review of reproductive outcome after in vitro fertilization and surgery. Acta Obstet Gynecol Scand. 2017;96(6):715-26.
2. Niu Z, Chen Q, Sun Y, et al. Long-term pituitary downregulation before frozen embryo transfer could improve pregnancy outcomes in women with adenomyosis. Gynecol Endocrinol. 2013;29(12):1026-30.

Chapter 37

1. van Schalkwyk J, Yudin MH. Infectious Disease Committee. Vulvovaginitis: screening for and management of trichomoniasis, vulvovaginal candidiasis, and bacterial vaginosis. J Obstet Gynaecol Can. 2015;37(3):266-74.

Chapter 39

1. World Health Organization. (2016). Index TB Guidelines. Guidelines on extrapulmonary tuberculosis for India. [online] WHO website. Available from http://www.icmr.nic.in/guidelines/TB/Index-TB%20Guidelines%20-%20green%20colour%202594164.pdf [Accessed February 2019].

Chapter 40

1. Badawy A, Wageah A, Gharib ME, et al. Prediction and diagnosis of poor ovarian response: The dilemma. J Reprod Infertil. 2011;12(4):241-8.
2. Grynberg M, Labrosse J. Understanding Follicular Output Rate (FORT) and its Implications for POSEIDON Criteria. Front Endocrinol (Lausanne). 2019;16(10):246.
3. Jirge PR. Poor ovarian reserve. J Hum Reprod Sci. 2016;9(2):63-9.
4. Poseidon Group (Patient-Oriented Strategies Encompassing IndividualizeD Oocyte Number); Alviggi C, Andersen CY, et al. A new more detailed stratification of low responders to ovarian stimulation: from a poor ovarian response to a low prognosis concept. Fertil Steril. 2016;105(6):1452-3.

Chapter 41

1. Duffy JM, Ahmad G, Mohiyiddeen L, et al. Growth hormone in in vitro fertilization. Cochrane Database Syst Rev. 2010;(1):CD000099.
2. Humaidan P, Schertz J, Fischer R. Efficacy and safety of pergoveris in assisted reproductive technology—ESPART: Rationale and design of a randomised controlled trial in poor ovarian responders undergoing IVF/ICSI treatment. BMJ Open. 2015;5(7):e008297.
3. Jeve YB, Bhandari HM. Effective treatment protocol for poor ovarian response: A systematic review and meta-analysis. J Hum Reprod Sci. 2016;9(2):70-81.
4. Keane KN, Hinchliffe PM, Rowlands PK, et al. DHEA supplementation confers no additional benefit to that of growth hormone on pregnancy and live birth rates in IVF patients categorized as poor prognosis. Front Endocrinol (Lausanne). 2018;9:14.
5. Nagels HE, Rishworth JR, Siristatidis CS, et al. Androgens (dehydroepiandrosterone or testosterone) for women undergoing assisted reproduction. Cochrane Database Syst Rev. 2015;(11):CD009749.
6. Practice Committee of the ASRM. Comparison of pregnancy rates for poor responders during IVF with mild ovarian stimulation vs. conventional IVF: a guideline. Fertil Steril. 2018;109(6):993-9.
7. Xu Y, Nisenblat V, Lu C, et al. Pretreatment with coenzyme Q10 improves response and embryo quality in low prognosis young women with decreased ovarian reserve: a randomised controlled trial. Reprod Biol Endocrinol. 2018;16(1):29.

Chapter 42

1. Darbandi M, Darbandi S. Three-parent IVF methods in aged oocytes and oocytes with mitochondrial problems. Cresco J Reprod Sci. 2016;1(1):1-2.
2. Kristensen SG, Pors SE, Andersen CY. Improving oocyte quality by transfer of autologous mitochondria from fully grown oocytes. Hum Reprod. 2017;32(4):725-32.

3. Labarta E, de Los Santos MJ, Herraiz S, et al. Autologous mitochondrial transfer as a complementary technique to intracytoplasmic sperm injection to improve embryo quality in patients undergoing in vitro fertilization—a randomized pilot study. Fertil Steril. 2019;111(1):86-96.
4. Tanaka A, Nagayoshi M, Tanaka I, et al. Successful drug-free IVA (in vitro activation) approach with laparoscopy to increase viable embryos in poor responder (POR) patients. Fertil Steril. 2018;110(4):e325.

Chapter 43

1. Male Infertility Best Practice Policy Committee of the American Urological Association, Practice Committee of the American Society for Reproductive Medicine. Report on optimal evaluation of the infertile male. Fertil Steril. 2006;86(5 Suppl 1):S202-9.

Chapter 45

1. Gunasekaran K, Pandiyan N. Male Infertility: A Clinical Approach, 1st edition. New York: Springer; 2017.
2. Parekattil SJ, Agarwal A. Male Infertility: Contemporary Clinical Approaches, Andrology, ART, and Antioxidants, 1st edition. New York: Springer; 2012.
3. World Health Organization (WHO). (2010). WHO Laboratory Manual for the Examination and Processing of Human Semen. [online] Available from https://apps.who.int/iris/bitstream/handle/10665/44261/9789241547789_eng.pdf;jsessionid=460F9CDBCEB85C6BA38761EBF023C7CE?sequence=1. [Last accessed March, 2019].

Chapter 47

1. Caroppo E, Colpi EM, Gazzano G, et al. Testicular histology may predict the successful sperm retrieval in patients with nonobstructive azoospermia undergoing conventional TESE: a diagnostic accuracy study. J Assist Reprod Genet. 2017;34(1):149-54.
2. Carpi A, Sabanegh E, Mechanick J. Controversies in the management of nonobstructive azoospermia. Fertil Steril. 2009;91(4):963-70.
3. Esteves SC. Clinical management of infertile men with nonobstructive azoospermia. Asian J Androl. 2015;17(3):459-70.
4. Gudeloglu A, Parekattil SJ. Update in the evaluation of the azoospermic male. Clinics (Sao Paulo). 2013;68(Suppl 1):27-34.
5. Khourdaji I, Lee H, Smith RP. Frontiers in hormone therapy for male infertility. Transl Androl Urol. 2018;7(Suppl 3):S353-66.
6. Lotti F, Maggi M. Ultrasound of the male genital tract in relation to male reproductive health. Hum Reprod Update. 2015;21(1):56-83.
7. Lotti F, Maseroli E, Fralassi N, et al. Is thyroid hormones evaluation of clinical value in the work-up of males of infertile couples? Hum Reprod. 2016;31(3):518-29.
8. Schoor RA, Elhanbly S, Niederberger CS, et al. The role of testicular biopsy in the modern management of male infertility. J Urol. 2002;167(1):197-200.
9. Tanaka T, Itoh N, Sasao T, et al. Prediction of candidates for seminal tract reconstructive surgery among patients with clinically suspected idiopathic or inflammatory obstructive azoospermia. Reprod Med Biol. 2006;5(3):211-4.
10. Van Saen D, Vloeberghs V, Gies I, et al. When does germ cell loss and fibrosis occur in patients with Klinefelter syndrome? Hum Reprod. 2018;33(6):1009-22.
11. Velasquez M, Tanrikut C. Surgical management of male infertility: an update. Transl Androl Urol. 2014;3(1):64-76.

Chapter 48

1. Colpi G, Weidner W, Jungwirth A, et al. EAU working party on male infertility. EAU guidelines on ejaculatory dysfunction. Eur Urol. 2004;46:555-8.
2. Emery M, Senn A, Wisard M, et al. Ejaculation failure on the day of oocyte retrieval for IVF: case report. Hum Reprod. 2004;19(9):2088-90.
3. Gopalakrishnan R, Thangadurai P, Kuruvilla A, et al. Situational psychogenic anejaculational: a case study. Indian J Psychol Med. 2014;36(3):329-31.
4. Meacham R. Management of psychogenic anejaculation. J Androl. 2003;24(2):170-1.
5. Okohue JE, Ikimalo JI, Onuh SO. Ejaculation failure on the day of oocyte retrieval for IVF: A report of five cases. 2011;16(2):159-62.
6. Tur-Kaspa I, Segal S, Moffa F, et al. Viagra for temporary erectile dysfunction during treatment with assisted reproductive technologies. Hum Reprod. 1999;14(7):1783-4.

Chapter 49

1. Esteves S, Miyaoka R, Agarwal A. An update on the clinical assessment of the infertile male. Clinics (Sao Paulo). 2011;66(4):691-700.
2. Plaseska-Karanfilska D, Noveski P, Plaseski T, et al. (2012). Genetic Causes of Male Infertility. Balkan Journal of Medical Genetics :BJMG. 2012;15(Suppl):31-4.
3. WHOManual-2010 Update.

Chapter 50

1. Chohan KR, Griffin JT, Lafromboise M, et al. Comparison of chromatin assays for DNA fragmentation evaluation in human sperm. J Androl. 2006;27(1):53-9.
2. Fernandez JL, Muriel L, Rivero MT, et al. The sperm chromatin dispersion test: a simple method for the determination of sperm DNA fragmentation. J Androl. 2003;24(1):59-66.
3. Gold R, Schmied M, Rothe G, et al. Detection of DNA fragmentation in apoptosis: application of in situ nick translation to cell culture systems and tissue sections. J Histochem Cytochem. 1993;41(7):1023-30.
4. Gosálvez J, López-Fernández C, Fernández JL, et al. Unpacking the mysteries of sperm DNA fragmentation: Ten frequently asked questions. J Reprod Biotechol Fertil. 2015;4:1-16.
5. Herrero MB, Gagnon C. Nitric oxide: a novel mediator of sperm function. J Androl. 2001;22(3):349-56.
6. Shafik AA, El Sibai O, Shafik I. Sperm DNA Fragmentation. Arch Androl. 2006;52(3):197-208.
7. Spanò M, Bonde JP, Hjøllund HI, et al. Sperm chromatin damage impairs human fertility. The Danish First Pregnancy Planner Study Team. Fertil Steril. 2000;73(1):43-50.

Chapter 51

1. Current practice from BMJ. 2019.
2. Male Infertility Best Practice Policy Committee of the American Urological Association; Practice Committee of the American Society for Reproductive Medicine. Report on Varicocele and infertility. 2004;82(Suppl 1):S142-5.

Chapter 54

1. ASRM. Testing and interpreting measures of ovarian reserve: a committee opinion. Fertil Steril. 2015;103(3):e9-17.
2. Coelho Neto MA, Ludwin A, Borrell B, et al. Counting ovarian antral follicles by ultrasound: a practical guide. Ultrasound Obstet Gynecol. 2018;51(1):10-20.
3. Panchal S, Nagori CB. Ultrasound in infertility. Donald School J Ultrasound Obstet Gynecol. 2015;9(1):100-10.
4. Sheikh M, Plavsic SK. Role of ultrasound in the assessment of female infertility. Donald School J Ultrasound Obstet Gynecol. 2014;8(2):184-200.

Chapter 55

1. Pandey S, Khanna G, Bajpai A, et al. Emerging role of Color Doppler in Infertility Management: A Public Health perspective. Fertil Sci Res. 2014;1:87-91.
2. Sonal Panchal, Nagori CB. Follicular Monitoring. Donald School Journal of Ultrasound in Obstetrics and Gynecology. 2012;6(3):300-12.

Chapter 56

1. Khan MS, Shaikh A, Ratnani R. Ultrasonography and Doppler Study to Predict Uterine Receptivity in Infertile Patients Undergoing Embryo Transfer. JOGI. 2016;66(Suppl 1):377-82.

Chapter 57

1. European Recombinant LH Study Group. Human recombinant luteinizing hormone is as effective as, but safer than, urinary human chorionic gonadotropin in inducing final follicular maturation and ovulation in in vitro fertilization procedures: results of a multicenter double-blind study. J Clin Endocrinol Metab. 2001;86(6):2607-18.
2. Griesinger G, Diedrich K. GnRH agonist for triggering final oocyte maturation in GnRH antagonist ovarian hyperstimulation protocol: a systematic review and meta-analysis. Hum Reprod Update. 2006;12:159-68.
3. Griesinger G, Kolibianakis E. Triggering final maturation. In: Aboulghar M (Ed). Ovarian Stimulation. Cambridge: Cambridge University Press; 2011.
4. Humaidan P, Bredkjaer HE, Bungum L, et al. GnRH agonist (buserelin) or hCG for ovulation induction in GnRH antagonist IVF/ICSI cycles: a prospective randomized study. Hum Reprod. 2005;20(5):1213-20.
5. Kolb B, Frederick JL, Miller C, et al. Does a reduced HCG trigger dose compromise outcomes in a large prospective trial of vaginal progesterone for luteal phase support? 2015;103(2):e28.
6. The International Recombinant Human Chorionic Gonadotropin Study Group. Induction of ovulation in World Health Organization group II anovulatory women undergoing follicular stimulation with recombinant human follicle-stimulating hormone: a comparison of recombinant human chorionic gonadotropin (rhCG) and urinary hCG. Fertil Steril. 2001;75:1111-8.
7. Youssef M, Griesinger G. GnRH agonist versus HCG for oocyte triggering in antagonist ART cycles. A systematic review and meta-analysis. Hum Reprod. 2009;24:1241-1530.

Chapter 59

1. ASRM practice guideline: 2008 guidelines for gamete and embryo donation. Fertil Steril. 2008;90:S30-44.
2. Critser JK, Huse-Benda AR. Cryopreservation of human spermatozoa. The effect of cryoprotectants on motility. Fertil Steril. 1988;50:314-20.
3. Martines, O. Lascano, M. Charaso, et al. Intrauterine insemination using donor sperm: a report of 2 years of experience. Fertil Steril. 2008;90:S463.
4. Quinn PH. Principle of membrane stability and phase behaviour under extreme conditions. J Bioenerg Biomemb. 1989;21:3-19.

Chapter 60

1. Gün I, Özdamar O, Yılmaz A. Luteal phase support in intrauterine insemination cycles. Turk J Obstet Gynecol. 2016;13(2):90-4.
2. Rashidi BH, Tanha FD, Rahmanpour H. Luteal phase support in the intrauterine insemination (IUI) cycles: A randomized double blind, placebo controlled study. J Family Reprod Health. 2014;8(4):149-53.

Chapter 65

1. Al-Inany HG, Youssef MA, Aboulghar M, et al. Gonadotrophin-releasing hormone antagonists for assisted reproductive technology. Cochrane Database Syst Rev. 2011;5:CD001750.
2. Chen Q, Wang Y, Sun L, et al. Controlled ovulation of the dominant follicle using progestin in minimal stimulation in poor responders. Reprod Biol Endocrinol. 2017;15:71.
3. ESHRE Reproductive Endocrinology Guideline Group. (2019). Controlled Ovarian Stimulation for IVF/ICSI. [online] Available from https://www.eshre.eu/-/media/sitecore-files/Guidelines/COS/ESHRE-COS-guideline_for-stakeholder-review.pdf?la=en&hash=C9FC98E92C426B5AC7677C1618EB1C443B3995B4. [Last accessed from February, 2019].
4. Hamdi K, Farzadi L, Ghasemzadeh A, et al. Comparison of medroxyprogesterone acetate with cetrotide for prevention of premature luteinizing hormone surges in women undergoing in vitro fertilization. Int J Women Health Reprod Sci. 2018;6:187-91.

Chapter 66

1. Bider D, Ben-Rafael Z, Shalev J, et al. Pituitary and ovarian suppression rate after high dosage of gonadotropin-releasing hormone agonist. Fertil Steril. 1989;51:578-81.
2. Hughes EG, Fedorkow DM, Daya S, et al. The routine use of gonadotropin-releasing hormone agonists prior to in vitro fertilization and gamete intrafallopian transfer: a meta-analysis of randomized controlled trials. Fertil Steril. 1992;58:888-96.

Chapter 67

1. Schumacher BM, Mersereau JE, Stiener AZ. Cycle day, estrogen level, and lead follicle size: analysis of 27,790 in vitro fertilization cycles to determine optimal start criteria for gonadotropin-releasing hormone antagonist. Fertil Steril. 2018;109:633-7.
2. Toftager M, Bogstad J, Løssl K, et al. Cumulative live birth rates after one ART cycle including all subsequent frozen-thaw cycles in 1050 women: secondary outcome of an RCT comparing GnRH-antagonist and GnRH-agonist protocols. Hum Reprod. 2017;32:556-67.

Chapter 68

1. ESHRE Reproductive Endocrinology Guideline Group. (2019). Controlled Ovarian Stimulation for IVF/ICSI. [online] Available from https://www.eshre.eu/-/media/sitecore-files/Guidelines/COS/ESHRE-COS-guideline_for-stakeholder-review.pdf?la=en&hash=C9FC98E92C426B5AC7677C1618EB1C443B3995B4. [Last accessed from February, 2019].
2. Kwan I, Bhattacharya S, McNeil A, et al. Monitoring of stimulated cycles in assisted reproduction (IVF and ICSI). Cochrane Database Syst Rev. 2008;2:CD005289.
3. La Marca A, Sunkara SK. Individualization of controlled ovarian stimulation in IVF using ovarian reserve markers: from theory to practice. Hum Reprod Update. 2014;20:124-40.

Chapter 69

1. Alper MM, Fauser BC. Ovarian stimulation protocols for IVF: is more better than less? Reprod Biomed Online. 2017;34(4):345-53.
2. Jungheim ES, Meyer MF, Broughton DE. Best practices for controlled ovarian stimulation in IVF. Semin Reprod Med. 2015;33(2):77-82.
3. Nargund G, Datta AK, Fauser BCJM. Mild stimulation for in vitro fertilization. Fertil Steril. 2017;108(4):558-67.
4. Verpoest W, Fauser BC, Papanikolaou E, et al. Chromosomal aneuploidy in embryos conceived with unstimulated cycle IVF. Hum Reprod. 2008;23(10):2369-71.

Chapter 70

1. Alviggi C, Conforti A, Esteves SC, et al. Recombinant luteinizing hormone supplementation in assisted reproductive technology: a systematic review. Fertil Steril. 2018;109:644-64.

Chapter 71

1. Al-Inany HG, Abou-Setta AM, Aboulghar M. Gonadotropin releasing hormone antagonists for assisted conception. Cochrane Database Sys Rev. 2006;CD001750.
2. Griesinger G, Diedrich K. GnRH agonist for triggering final oocyte maturation in GnRH antagonist ovarian hyperstimulation protocol: a systematic review and meta analysis. Hum Reprod Update. 2006;12:159-68.
3. Humaidan P. Agonist trigger: what is the best approach? Agonist trigger and low dose hCG. Fertil Steril. 2012;97:529-30.
4. Humaidan P, Bredkjaer HE, Bungum L, et al. GnRH agonist (buserelin) or hCG for ovulation induction in GnRH antagonist IVF/ICSI cycles: a prospective randomized study. Hum Reprod 2005;20(5):1213-20.
5. Youssef M, Griesinger G. GnRH agonist versus HCG for oocyte triggering in antagonist ART cycles. A systematic review and meta analysis. Hum Reprod. 2009;24:1241-1530.

Chapter 72

1. Esteves SC, Roque M, Bedoschi GM, et al. Defining Low Prognosis Patients Undergoing Assisted Reproductive Technology: POSEIDON Criteria-The Why. Front Endocrinol (Lausanne). 2018;9:461.
2. Leung AS, Dahan MH, Tan SL. Techniques and technology for human oocyte collection. Expert Rev Med Devices. 2016;13:701-3.
3. Özaltin S, Kumbasar S, Savan K. Evaluation of complications developing during and after transvaginal ultrasound-guided oocyte retrieval. Ginekol Pol. 2018;89:1-6.
4. Sharma A, Borle A, Trikha A, et al. Anesthesia for in vitro fertilization. J Obstet Anaesth Crit Care. 2015;5:62-72.
5. Wang W, Zhang XH, Wang WH, et al. The time interval between hCG priming and oocyte retrieval in ART program: a meta-analysis. J Assist Reprod Genet. 2011;28:901-10.
6. Wongtran-Ngan S, Vutyavanich T, Brown J. Follicular flushing during oocyte retrieval in assisted reproductive techniques. Cochrane Database Syst Rev. 2010;9:CD004634.

Chapter 73

1. Jones HW, Acosta AA, Garcia JE, et al. On the transfer of conceptuses from oocytes fertilized in vitro. Fertil Steril. 1982;39:241-3.
2. Laufer N, DeCherney AH, Haseltine FP, et al. The use of high dose human menopausal gonadotropin in an in vitro fertilization program. Fertil Steril. 1983;40:734-41.
3. Leeton J, Trounson A, Jessup D, et al. The technique for human embryo transfer. Fertil Steril. 1982;38:156-61.
4. Practice Committee of Society for Assisted Reproductive Technology, Practice Committee of American Society for Reproductive Medicine. Guidelines on number of embryos transferred. Fertil Steril. 2008;90:S163-4.
5. Practice Committee of the American Society for Reproductive Medicine. Performing the embryo transfer: a guideline. Fertil Steril. 2017;107:882-96.

Chapter 74

1. Linden M, Buckingham K, Farquhar C, et al. Luteal phase support for assisted reproduction cycles. Cochrane Database Syst Rev. 2011;CD009154.
2. Toth TL, Vaughan DA. Optimizing luteal support in frozen embryo transfer cycles. Fertil Steril. 2018;109(2):242-3.

Chapter 76

1. Blockeel C. Estradiol valerate pretreatment in GnRH-antagonist cycles. Reprod Biomed Online. 2012;25(2):223-4.
2. Fatemi HM, Blockeel C, Devroey P. Ovarian stimulation: today and tomorrow. Curr Pharm Biotechnol. 2012;13(3):392-7.
3. Garcia-Velasco JA, Fatemi HM. To pill or not to pill in GnRH antagonist cycles: that is the question! Reprod Biomed Online. 2015;30(1):39-42.

Chapter 77

1. Ghobara T, Gelbaya TA, Ayeleke RO. Cycle regimens for frozen-thawed embryo transfer. Cochrane Database Syst Rev. 2017;7:CD003414.

2. Irani M, Robles A, Gunnala V, et al. Optimal parameters for determining the LH surge in natural cycle frozen-thawed embryo transfers. J Ovarian Res. 2017;10(1):70.
3. Testart J, Frydman R, Feinstein MC, et al. Interpretation of plasma luteinizing hormone assay for the collection of mature oocytes from women: definition of a luteinizing hormone surge-initiating rise. Fertil Streril. 1981;36(1):50-4.

Chapter 78

1. Glujovsky D, Pesce R, Fiszbajn G, et al. Endometrial preparation for women undergoing embryo transfer with frozen embryos or embryos derived from donor oocytes. Cochrane Lib. 2010;(1):CD006359.
2. Groenewoud ER, Cantineau AE, Kollen BJ, et al. What is the optimal means of preparing the endometrium in frozen-thawed embryo transfer cycles? A systematic review and meta-analysis. Hum Reprod Update. 2013;19(5):458-70.
3. Guerrero LA, Arenaz L, Diaz P, et al. Endometrial preparation with increasing versus fixed dosing of estradiol during frozen embryo transfer cycles. Fertil Steril. 2011;96(3):S143.
4. Nawroth F, Ludwig M. What is the 'ideal' duration of progesterone supplementation before the transfer of cryopreserved-thawed embryos in estrogen/progesterone replacement protocols? Hum Reprod. 2005;20:1127-34.
5. Richter KS, Bugge KR, Bromer JG, et al. Relationship between endometrial thickness and embryo implantation, based on 1,294 cycles of in vitro fertilization with transfer of two blastocyst-stage embryos. Fertil Steril. 2007;87:53-9.
6. Tournaye H, Sukhikh GT, Kahler E, et al. A Phase III randomized controlled trial comparing the efficacy, safety and tolerability of oral dydrogesterone versus micronized vaginal progesterone for luteal support in in vitro fertilization. Hum Reprod. 2017;32(5):1019-27.

Chapter 79

1. ASRM. Repetitive oocyte donation: A committee opinion. Fertil Steril. 2014;102(4):964-96.
2. Indian Council of Medical Research. (2017). ICMR guidelines ART practices in India 2017.
3. The Practice Committees of the American Society for Reproductive Medicine and the Society for Assisted Reproductive Technology. Mature oocyte cryopreservation: a guideline. Fertil Steril. 2013;99(1):37-43.

Chapter 80

1. Barad DH, Kim A, Kubba H, et al. Does hormonal contraception prior to in vitro fertilization (IVF) negatively affect oocyte yields? A pilot study. Reprod Biol Endocrinol. 2013;11:28.
2. Pereira N, Petrini AC, Zhou ZN, et al. Pretreatment of normal responders in fresh in vitro fertilization cycles: A comparison of transdermal estradiol and oral contraceptive pills. Clin Exp Reprod Med. 2016;43(4):228-32.

Chapter 81

1. Aitken RJ, Clarkson JS. Significance of reactive oxygen species and antioxidants in defining the efficacy of sperm preparation techniques. J Androl. 1988;9(6):367-76.
2. Björndahl L, Kvist U. Sequence of ejaculation affects the spermatozoon as a carrier and its message. Reprod Biomed Online. 2003;7(4):440-8.
3. Björndahl L, Mohammadieh M, Pourian M, et al. Contamination by seminal plasma factors during sperm selection. J Androl. 2005;26(2):170-3.

Chapter 82

1. Antinori M, Licata E, Dani G, et al. Intracytoplasmic morphologically selected sperm injection: a prospective randomized trial. RBM Online. 2008;16:835-41.
2. Balaban B, Yakin K, Alatas C, et al. Clinical outcome of intracytoplasmic injection of spermatozoa morphologically selected under high magnification: a prospective randomized study. RBM Online. 2011;22:472-76.
3. Bartoov B, Berkovitz A, Eltes F, et al. Real-time fine morphology of motile human sperm cells is associated with IVF-ICSI outcome. Androl. 2002;23(1):1-8.
4. Chang J, Jacobson JD, Corselli JU, et al. A simple zeta method for sperm selection based on membrane charge. 2006;85(2):481-6.
5. Cho BS, Schuster TG, Zhu X, et al. Passively driven integrated microfluidic system for separation of motile sperm. Anal Chem. 2003;75(7):1671-5.
6. Gianaroli L, Magli C, Collodel G. Sperm head's birefringence: a new criterion for sperm selection. Fertil Steril. 2008;90(1):104-12.
7. Henkel R. Sperm preparation: state-of-the-art—physiological aspects and application of advanced sperm preparation methods. Asian J Androl. 2012;14(2):260-9.

8. Huszar G, Jakab A, Sakkas D, et al. Fertility testing and ICSI sperm selection by hyaluronic acid binding: clinical and genetic aspects. Reprod Biomed Online. 2007;14:650-63.
9. Oliveira J, Petersen CG, Massaro FC, et al. Motile sperm organelle morphology examination (MSOME): intervariation study of normal sperm and sperm with large nuclear vacuoles. Reprod Biol Endocrinol. 2010;8:56.
10. Said TM, Land JA. Effects of advanced selection methods on sperm quality and ART outcome: a systematic review. Hum Reprod Update. 2011;17(6):719-33.

Chapter 84

1. Cohen J, Alikani M, Trowbridge J, et al. Implantation enhancement by selective assisted hatching using zona drilling of human embryos with poor prognosis. Hum Reprod. 1992;7:685-91.
2. Cohen J, Malter H, Fehilly C, et al. Implantation of embryos after partial opening of oocyte zona pellucida to facilitate sperm penetration. Lancet. 1988;2:162.
3. Fong CY, Bongso A, Ng SC, et al. Blastocyst transfer after enzymatic treatment of the zona pellucida, improving in-vitro fertilization and understanding implantation. Hum Reprod. 1998;13:2926-32.
4. Practice Committee of the American Society for Reproductive Medicine, Practice Committee of the Society for Assisted Reproductive Technology. Role of assisted hatching in in vitro fertilization, a guideline. Fertil Steril. 2014;102:348-51.
5. Rink K, Delacrétaz G, Salathé RP, et al. Non-contact microdrilling of mouse zona pellucida with an objective-delivered 1.48-microns diode laser. Lasers Surg Med. 1996;18:52-62.
6. Scott E, Moomjy M, Zaninovic N, et al. Human zona pellucida micromanipulation and monozygotic twinning frequency after IVF. Hum Reprod. 2000;15:890-5.

Chapter 85

1. Clemente-Ciscar M, Ruiz-Alonso M, Blesa D, et al. Endometrial receptivity analysis (ERA) using a next generation sequencing (NGS) predictor improves reproductive outcome in recurrent implantation failure (RIF) patients when compared to ERA arrays. Hum Reprod. 2018;33(Supp 1):8-18.
2. Díaz-Gimeno P, Horcajadas JA, Martínez-Conejero JA, et al. A genomic diagnostic tool for human endometrial receptivity based on the transcriptomic signature. Fertil Steril. 2011;95(1):50-60, 60.e1-15.
3. Díaz-Gimeno P, Ruiz-Alonso M, Blesa D, et al. The accuracy and reproducibility of the endometrial receptivity array is superior to histology as a diagnostic method for endometrial receptivity. Fertil Steril. 2013;99(2):508-17.
4. Findikli N, Gultomruk M, Boynukalin K, et al. Combinatorial use of endometrial receptivity array (ERA) and PGT-A can improve the clinical outcome in cases with previous ART failures. Hum Reprod. 2018;33(Supp1):84-5.
5. Hashimoto T, Koizumi M, Doshida M, et al. Efficacy of the endometrial receptivity array for repeated implantation failure in Japan: A retrospective, two-centers study. Reprod Med Biol. 2017;16(3):290-6.
6. Mahajan N. Endometrial receptivity array: Clinical application. J Hum Reprod Sci. 2015;8(3):121-9.

Chapter 87

1. Barrie A, Homburg R, McDowell G, et al. Examining the efficacy of six published time-lapse imaging embryo selection algorithms to predict implantation to demonstrate the need for the development of specific, in-house morphokinetic selection algorithms. Fertil Steril. 2017;107(3):613-21.
2. Basile N, Nogales Mdel C, Bronet F, et al. Increasing the probability of selecting chromosomally normal embryos by time-lapse morphokinetics analysis. Fertil Steril. 2014;101(3):699-704.
3. Campbell A, Fishel S, Bowman N, et al. Retrospective analysis of outcomes after IVF using an aneuploidy risk model derived from time-lapse imaging without PGS. Reprod Biomed Online. 2013;27(2):140-6.
4. Gardner DK, Meseguer M, Rubio C, et al. Diagnosis of human preimplantation embryo viability. Hum Reprod Update. 2015;21(6):727-47.
5. Meseguer M, Herrero J, Tejera A, et al. The use of morphokinetics as a predictor of embryo implantation. Hum Reprod. 2011;26(10):2658-71.
6. Montag MH, Pedersen KS, Ramsing NB. Time-lapse imaging of embryo development: Using morphokinetic analysis to select viable embryos. In: Quinn P (Ed). Culture Media, Solutions, and Systems in Human ART. Cambridge: Cambridge University Press; 2014. pp. 211-34.
7. Pribenszky C, Nilselid AM, Montag M. Time-lapse culture with morphokinetic embryo selection improves pregnancy and live birth chances and reduces early pregnancy loss: a meta-analysis. Reprod Biomed Online. 2017;35(5):511-20.
8. Wong CC, Loewke KE, Bossert NL, et al. Non-invasive imaging of human embryos before embryonic genome activation predicts development to the blastocyst stage. Nat Biotechnol. 2010;28:1115-21.

Chapter 88B

1. Absalan F, Ghannadi A, Kazerooni M, et al. Value of sperm chromatin dispersion test in couples with unexplained recurrent abortion. J Assist Reprod Genet. 2012;29:11-4.
2. Barad DH, Yu Y, Kushnir VA, et al. A randomized clinical trial of endometrial perfusion with granulocyte colony stimulating factor in in vitro fertilization cycles: impact on endometrial thickness and clinical pregnancy rates. Fertil Steril. 2014;101:710-15.
3. Bosteels J, Kasius J, Weyers S, et al. Hysteroscopy for treating subfertility associated with suspected major uterine cavity abnormalities. Cochrane Database Syst Rev. 2015;(2):CD009461.
4. Chang Y, Li J, Chen Y, et al. Autologous platelet-rich plasma promotes endometrial growth and improves pregnancy outcome during in vitro fertilization. Int J Clin Exp Med. 2015;8:1286-90.
5. Cohen J, Inge KL, Suzman M, et al. Videocinematography of fresh and cryopreserved embryos: a retrospective analysis of embryonic morphology and implantation. Fertil Steril. 1989;51:820-7.
6. Cohen J, Scott R, Alikani M, et al. Ooplasmic transfer in mature human oocytes. Mol Hum Reprod. 1998;4:269-80.
7. Das M, Holzer HE. Recurrent implantation failure: gamete and embryo factors. Fertil Steril. 2012;97:1021-7.
8. Davies S, Christopikou D, Tsorva E, et al. Delayed cleavage division and a prolonged transition between 2- and 4-cell stages in embryos identified as aneuploidy at the 8-cell stage by array-CGH. Hum Reprod. 2012;27:ii84-ii86.
9. De Vos A, Van Steirteghem A. Zona hardening, zona drilling and assisted hatching: new achievements in assisted reproduction. Cells Tissues Organs. 2000;166:220-7.
10. Díaz-Gimeno P, Horcajadas JA, Martínez-Conejero JA, et al. A genomic diagnostic tool for human endometrial receptivity based on the transcriptomic signature. Fertil Steril. 2011;95:50-60.e15.
11. Ferraretti AP, La Marca A, Fauser BC, et al. ESHRE consensus on the definition of 'poor response' to ovarian stimulation for in vitro fertilization: the Bologna criteria. Hum Reprod. 2011;26:1616-24.
12. Franasiak JM, Scott RT. Contribution of immunology to implantation failure of euploid embryos. Fertil Steril. 2017;107:1279-83.
13. Glujovsky D, Blake D, Bardach A, et al. Cleavage stage versus blastocyst stage embryo transfer in assisted reproductive technology (Review). Cochrane Database Syst Rev. 2016;(6):CD002118.
14. Habana A, Palter SF. Is tubal embryo transfer of any value? A meta analysis and comparison with the society for assisted reproductive technology database. Fertil Steril. 2001;76:293.
15. Hart R, Khalaf Y, Yeong CT, et al. A prospective controlled study of the effect of intramural uterine fibroids on the outcome of assisted conception. Hum Reprod. 2001;11:2411-7.
16. Hertig AT, Rock J, Adams EC. A description of 34 human ova within the first 17 days of development. Devel Dynam. 1956;98:435-93.
17. Hill MJ, Levens ED, Ryan ME, et al. The use of recombinant luteinizing hormone in patients undergoing assisted reproductive techniques with advanced reproductive age: a systematic review and meta-analysis. Fertil Steril. 2012;97:1108-14.
18. Jensen JR, Witz CA, Schenken RS, et al. A potential role for colony stimulating factor 1 in the genesis of the early endometriotic lesion. Fertil Steril. 2010;93:251-6.
19. Kahraman S, Bahce M, Samli H, et al. Healthy births and ongoing pregnancies obtained by preimplantation genetic diagnosis in patients with advanced maternal age and recurrent implantation failure. Hum Reprod. 2000;15:2003-7.
20. Kuliev A, Verlinsky Y. The role of preimplantation genetic diagnosis in women of advanced maternal age. Curr Opin Obs Gynecol. 2003a;15:233-8.
21. Kupesic PS. Ultrasound imaging of the endometrium. In: Simon C, Giudice LC (Eds). The Endometrial Factor: a Reproductive Precision Medicine Approach. Boca Raton: CRC Press; 2017. pp. 15-35.
22. Laufer N, Simon A. Recurrent implantation failure: current update and clinical approach to an ongoing challenge. Fertil Steril. 2012;97:1019-20.
23. Moffet A, Shreeve N. First do no harm: uterine natural killer (NK) cells in assisted reproduction. Hum Reprod. 2015;30:1519-25.
24. Montag M. Morphokinetics and embryo aneuploidy: has time come or not yet? Reprod Biomed Online. 2013;26:528-30.
25. Moreno I, Franasiak JM. Endometrial microbiota—new player in town. Fertil Steril. 2017;108:32-9.
26. Munne S, Sandalinas M, Escuredo T, et al. Improved implantation after preimplantation genetic diagnosis of aneuploidy. Reprod BioMed Online. 2003;7:91-7.
27. Nastri CO, Lensen SF, Gibreel A, et al. Endometrial injury in women undergoing assisted reproductive techniques. Cochrane Database Syst Rev. 2015;(3):CD009517.
28. Navot D, Scott RT, Droesch K, et al. The window of embryo transfer and the efficiency of human conception in vitro. Fertil Steril. 1991;55:114-8.
29. Penzias AS. Recurrent IVF failure: other factors. Fertil Steril. 2012;97:1033-8.
30. Pritts EA, Parker WH, Olive DL. Fibroids and infertility: an updated systematic review of the evidence. Fertil Steril. 2009;91:1215-23.
31. Sallam HN, Garcia-Velasco JA, Dias S, et al. Long-term pituitary down-regulation before in vitro fertilization (IVF) for women with endometriosis. Cochrane Database Syst Rev. 2006;(1):CD004635.
32. Scott RT, Snyder RR, Strickland DM, et al. The effect of interobserver variation in dating endometrial histology on the diagnosis of luteal phase defects. Fertil Steril. 1988;50:888-92.

33. Shapiro BS, Daneshmand ST, Garner FC, et al. Clinical rationale for cryopreservation of entire embryo cohorts in lieu of fresh transfer. Fertil Steril. 2014;102:3-9.
34. Simon A, Laufer N. Repeated implantation failure: clinical approach. Fertil Steril. 2012;97:1039-43.
35. Somigliana E, Vercellini P, Daguati R, et al. Fibroids and female reproduction: a critical analysis of the evidence. Hum Reprod Update. 2007;13:465-76.
36. Somigliana E, Vigano P, Busnelli A, et al. Repeated implantation failure at the crossroad between statistics, clinics and over-diagnosis. Reprod BioMed Online. 2018;36(1):32-8.
37. Strandell A, Lindhard A, Eckerlund I. Cost-effectiveness analysis of salpingectomy prior to IVF, based on a randomized controlled trial. Hum Reprod. 2005;20:3284-92.
38. Sunkara SK, Khairy M, El-Toukhy T, et al. The effect of intramural fibroids without uterine cavity involvement on the outcome of IVF treatment: a systematic review and meta-analysis. Hum Reprod. 2010;25:418-29.
39. Surrey ES, Minjarez DA, Stevens JM, et al. Effect of myomectomy on the outcome of assisted reproductive technologies. Fertil Steril. 2005;83:1473-9.
40. Surrey ES, Silverberg KM, Surrey MW, et al. Effect of prolonged gonadotropin-releasing hormone agonist therapy on the outcome of in vitro fertilization-embryo transfer in patients with endometriosis. Fertil Steril. 2002;78:699-704.
41. Swain JE. Could time-lapse embryo imaging reduce the need for biopsy and PGS? J Assist Reprod Genet. 2013;30:1081-90.
42. Urman B, Yakin K, Balaban B. Recurrent implantation failure in assisted reproduction: how to counsel and manage. B. Treatment options that have not been proven to benefit the couple. Reprod Biomed Online. 2005;11:382-91.
43. Wang P-H, Fuh J-L, Chao H-T, et al. Is the surgical approach beneficial to subfertile women with symptomatic extensive adenomyosis. Obstet Gynaecol. 2009;35:495-502.
44. Zini A, Bach PV, Al-Malki AH, et al. Use of testicular sperm for ICSI in oligozoospermic couples: how far should we go? Hum Reprod. 2017;32:7-13.

Chapter 89

1. ESHRE Early Pregnancy Guideline Development Group. Recurrent Pregnancy Loss: Guideline of the European Society of Human Reproduction and Embryology; 2017.

Chapter 90

1. Cenksoy P, Ficicioglu C, Yıldırım G, et al. Hysteroscopic findings in women with recurrent IVF failures and the effect of correction of hysteroscopic findings on subsequent pregnancy rates. Arch Gynecol Obstet. 2013;287(2):357-60.
2. Chang Y, Li J, Wei LN, et al. Autologous platelet-rich plasma infusion improves clinical pregnancy rate in frozen embryo transfer cycles for women with thin endometrium. Medicine (Baltimore). 2019;98(3):e14062.
3. Chen X, Chen SL. Successful pregnancy in recurrent thin endometrium with new uses for an old drug. J Fertil. 2013;1:110.
4. Dehghani Firouzabadi R, Davar R, Hojjat F, et al. Effect of sildenafil citrate on endometrial preparation and outcome of frozen-thawed embryo transfer cycles: a randomized clinical trial. Iran J Reprod Med. 2013;11(2):151-8.
5. Eftekhar M, Neghab N, Naghshineh E, et al. Can autologous platelet rich plasma expand endometrial thickness and improve pregnancy rate during frozen-thawed embryo transfer cycle? A randomized clinical trial. Taiwan J Obstet Gynecol. 2018;57(6):810-3.
6. Lebovitz O, Orvieto R. Treating patients with "thin" endometrium – an ongoing challenge. Gynecol Endocrinol. 2014;30(6):409-14.
7. Liu KE, Hartman M, Hartman A, et al. The impact of a thin endometrial lining on fresh and frozen-thaw IVF outcomes: An analysis of over 40,000 embryo transfers. Hum Reprod. 2018;33(10):1883-8.
8. Miwa I, Tamura H, Takasaki A, et al. Pathophysiologic features of "thin" endometrium. Fertil Steril. 2009;91(4):998-1004.
9. Mouhayara Y, Sharara Y. Review: Modern management of thin lining. Middle East Fertil Soc J. 2017;22:1-12.
10. Richter KS, Bugge KR, Bromer JG, et al. Relationship between endometrial thickness and embryo implantation, based on 1,294 cycles of in vitro fertilization with transfer of two blastocyst-stage embryos. Fertil Steril. 2007;87(1):53-9.
11. Tehraninejad E, Davari Tanha F, Asadi E, et al. G-CSF intrauterine for thin endometrium, and pregnancy outcome. J Family Reprod Health. 2015;9(3):107-12.
12. Zhang L, Xu WH, Fu XH, et al. Therapeutic role of granulocyte colony-stimulating factor (G-CSF) for infertile women under in vitro fertilization and embryo transfer (IVF-ET) treatment: A meta-analysis. Arch Gynecol Obstet. 2018;298(5):861-71.
13. Zhang T, Li Z, Ren X, et al. Endometrial thickness as a predictor of the reproductive outcomes in fresh and frozen embryo transfer cycles: A retrospective cohort study of 1512 IVF cycles with morphologically good-quality blastocyst. Medicine. 2018;97(4):e9689.

Chapter 91

1. Revelli A, Carosso A, Grassi G, et al. Empty follicle syndrome revisited: definition, incidence, aetiology, early diagnosis and treatment. Reprod Biomed Online. 2017;35(2):132-8.

Chapter 92

1. Chung K, Chndavarkar U, Opper N, et al. Reevaluating the role of dilation and curettage in the diagnosis of pregnancy of unknown location. Fertil Steril. 2011;96(3):659-62.
2. Conolly A, Ryan DH, Stuebe AM, et al. Reevaluation of threshold levels of serum B-hCG in early pregnancy. Obstet Gynaecol. 2013;121(1):65-70.
3. Della-Giustina D, Denny M. Ectopic pregnancy. Emerg Med Clin North Am. 2003;21:565-84.
4. Doubilet PM, Benson CB. Further evidence against the reliability of the human chorionic gonadotropin discriminatory level. J Ultrasound Med. 2011;30(12):1637-42.

Chapter 92B

1. ACOG Practice Bulletin. Clinical management guidelines for ectopic pregnancy, February 2018.
2. Hackmon R, Sakaguchi S, Koren G. Effect of methotrexate treatment of ectopic pregnancy on subsequent pregnancy. Can Fam Physician. 2011;57:37-9.
3. NHS. Ectopic pregnancy. Clinical Guidelines Register no 10121.

Chapter 93

1. ACOG. Multifetal pregnancy reduction – ACOG committee opinion – Number 719, September 2017.
2. Antsaklis A, Souka AP, Daskalakis G, et al. Pregnancy outcome after multifetal pregnancy reduction. J Matern Fetal Neonatal Med. 2004;16(1):27-31.
3. Belogolovkin V, Ferrar L, Moshier E, et al. Differences in fetal growth, discordancy, and placental pathology in reduced versus nonreduced twins. Am J Perinatol. 2007;10:575-9.
4. Chaveeva P, Peeva G, Pugliese SG, et al. Intrafetal laser ablation for embryo reduction from dichorionic triplets to dichorionic twins. Ultrasound Obstet Gynecol. 2017;50:632-4.
5. Evans MI, Andriole S, Britt DW. Fetal reduction: 25 years' experience. Fetal Diagn Ther. 2014;35:69-82.
6. Papageorghiou A, Liao AW, Skentou C, et al. Trichorionic triplet pregnancies at 10-14 weeks: Outcome after embryo reduction compared to expectant management. J Matern Fetal Neonatal Med. 2002;11:307-12.

Chapter 94

1. Jeng C, Shen J, Wang L, et al. The characteristics of vaginismus in an Asian society in selected abstracts of presentations during the XVII world congress of sexology. J Sex Res. 2006;43(1):2-37.

Chapter 95

1. Basson R, Schultz WW. Sexual sequelae of general medical disorders. The Lancet. 2007;369(9559):409-24.
2. Brotto L, Atallah S, Johnson-Agbakwu C, et al. Psychological and interpersonal dimensions of sexual function and dysfunction. J Sex Med. 2016;13(4):538-71.

Chapter 97

1. Bashir ST. Follicle growth and endocrine dynamics in women with spontaneous luteinized unruptured follicles versus ovulation. Hum Reprod. 2018;33(6):1130-40.
2. Check JH. Comparison of various therapies for the luteinized unruptured follicle syndrome. Int J Fertil. 1992;37(1):33-40.
3. Check JH. The use of granulocyte colony stimulating factor to enhance oocyte release in women with the luteinized unruptured follicle syndrome. Clin Exp Obstet Gynecol. 2016;43(2):178-80.
4. Eftekhar M. Role of granulocyte colony-stimulating factor in human reproduction. J Res Med Sci. 2018;23:7.
5. Koninckx PR. Clinical significance of the luteinized unruptured follicle syndrome as a cause of infertility. Eur J Obstet Gynecol Reprod Biol. 1982;13(6):355-68.
6. Qublan H, Amarin Z, Nawasreh M, et al. Luteinized unruptured follicle syndrome: Incidence and recurrence rate in infertile women with unexplained infertility undergoing intrauterine insemination. Hum Reprod. 2006;21(8):2110-3.

Chapter 98

1. Gaskins AJ, Chavarro JE. Diet and fertility: a review. Am J Obstet Gynecol. 2018;218(4):379-89.
2. Gaskins AJ, Williams PL, Keller MG, et al. Maternal physical and sedentary activities in relation to reproductive outcomes following IVF. Reprod Biomed Online. 2016;33(4):513-21.

3. Grodstein F, Goldman MB, Cramer DW. Infertility in women and moderate alcohol consumption. Am J Public Health. 1994;85:1021-2.
4. Hakim RB, Gray RH, Zacur H. Alcohol and caffeine consumption and decreased fertility. Fertil Steril. 1998;70:632-7.
5. Juhl M, Nyboe Andersen AM, Gronbaek M, et al. Moderate alcohol consumption and waiting time to pregnancy. Hum Reprod. 2001;16:2705-9.
6. Mikkelsen EM, Riis AH, Wise LA, et al. Alcohol consumption and fecundability: Prospective Danish cohort study. BMJ. 2016;354:i4262.
7. Mínguez-Alarcón L, Chavarro JE, Gaskins AJ. Caffeine, alcohol, smoking, and reproductive outcomes among couples undergoing assisted reproductive technology treatments. Fertil Steril. 2018;110:587-92.
8. World Health Organization. (2016). Obesity and overweight fact sheet 2016. [online] Available from http://www.who.int/mediacentre/factsheets/fs311/en/. [Last accessed March 6, 2017].

Chapter 99

1. Lensen S, Sadler L, Farquhar C. Endometrial scratching for subfertility: everyone's doing it. Hum Reprod. 2016;31:1241-4.
2. Lensen SF, Manders M, Nastri CO, et al. Endometrial injury for pregnancy following sexual intercourse or intrauterine insemination. Cochrane Database Syst Rev. 2016;(6):CD011424.
3. Mol BW, Barnhart KT. Scratching the Endometrium in IVF—Time to Stop. N Engl J Med. 2019;380:391-2.
4. Nastri CO, Lensen SF, Gibreel A, et al. Endometrial injury in women undergoing assisted reproductive techniques. Cochrane Database Syst Rev. 2015;22;(3):CD009517.
5. Vitagliano A, Noventa M, Saccone G, et al. Endometrial scratch injury before intrauterine insemination: is it time to re-evaluate its value? Evidence from a systematic review and meta-analysis of randomized controlled trials. Fertil Steril. 2017;109:84-96.

Chapter 100

1. de Ronde W, de Jong FH. Aromatase inhibitors in men: effects and therapeutic options. Reprod Biol Endocrinol. 2011;9:93.
2. Ho CC. Treatment of the hypogonadal infertile male-A review. Sex Med Rev. 2013;1(1):42-9.
3. Owen RC, Elkelany OO, Kim ED. Testosterone supplementation in men: a practical guide for the gynecologist and obstetrician. Curr Opin Obstet Gynecol. 2015;27(4):258-64.
4. Patel DP, Chandrapal JC, Hotaling JM. Hormone-based treatments in subfertile males. Curr Urol Rep. 2016;17(8):56.
5. Tadros N, Sabanegh ES. Empiric medical therapy with hormonal agents for idiopathic male infertility. Indian J Urol. 2017;33(3):194-8.

Index

A

Abortion
 incomplete 43
 missed 43
Acid-fast bacilli 100, 101, 103
Adenomyosis 94
Adhesions 43
 severity of 44
Adnexal mass 248
Adrenal hyperplasia, congenital 17, 60, 61, 218
Advanced sperm preparation 204
 techniques 204
Agglutination 116
Alcohol 267
Amenorrhea
 primary 10
 secondary 12
American Fertility Society 43, 84
American Society for Reproductive
  Medicine 37, 38, 112, 150
American Urological Association 112
Androgens 74
Andrology, gynecologist's view 111
Androstenedione 73
Anejaculation 124
 anorgasmic 124
 orgasmic 124
 situational 124
Antiandrogens 123
Antibody
 antinuclear 234
 antiphospholipid 235
Anticardiolipin antibodies 234
Anti-Müllerian hormone 10, 11, 18, 19, 27, 70, 107, 146, 147, 160-164, 168, 169, 174, 175, 188, 189, 200, 228, 260, 267, 269
Antioxidant supplements 268
Antithyroid drug 59
Anti-tubercular therapy 101, 102, 237
Antral follicle 18
 count 18, 23, 107, 141, 147, 160-164, 168, 175, 189, 228
Anxiety, impact of 4
Applebaum uterine scoring system 144
Aromatase inhibitors 71
Artificial insemination 202
 donor 150
Ascitic fluid, aspiration of 190
Asherman syndrome 43
 management of 44
Aspirin 74
Assisted hatching 211
 indications 21
 technique 210
 methods 210
Assisted reproductive technique 6, 11, 22, 26, 40, 52, 58, 70-72, 81, 84-89, 92, 94, 102, 103, 106, 109, 116, 121, 124, 125, 128, 129, 136, 144, 157-160, 164, 166, 168, 169, 174, 177, 185, 187, 188, 192, 193, 196, 198, 222, 240, 260, 268, 269
 bank 198
 cycle 162, 175, 214, 270
 sperm preparation for 202
 stimulation 168
 treatments 267
Assisted reproductive therapy 18
Asthenozoospermia 272
Autosomal dominant 218
Autosomal recessive 218
 diseases 150
Azoospermia 121
 clinical varieties of 121
 evaluation 121
 histopathological types of 122
 obstructive 207

B

Basal antral follicle count 18
Basal follicle-stimulating hormone 18
Batch in vitro fertilization 192
Batching embryo transfer, cycle preparation for 193
Becker muscular dystrophy 218
Beta human chorionic gonadotropin 196, 197, 250
Beta thalassemia 150, 218
Biopsy, endometrial 101
Body mass index 4, 57, 61, 68, 72, 130, 134, 146, 147, 164, 169, 174, 175, 189, 272

C

Caffeine 267
Cell
 2 gonadotropin theory 173
 phone, impact of 4
Center for Disease Control and Prevention 267
Charcot-Marie-tooth disease 218
Chemical hatching 210
Chest X-ray 100
Chlamydia antibody test 48
Chlamydia trachomatis 4, 34
Clinical pregnancy rate 152, 211
Clomiphene citrate 56, 57, 68-73, 134, 135, 158, 163, 170, 171, 262
 challenge test 19
Coenzyme Q10 109
Cognitive behavioral therapy 257
Coital frequency and timing 3
Color flow Doppler imaging 130
Comparative genomic hybridization 218
Complete blood count 27, 100
Computed tomography 81, 100
Conjugated estrogen 44
Contraception, previous methods of 3
Controlled ovarian stimulation 40, 72, 86, 162, 168, 172, 173
Conventional sperm preparation
  techniques 202
Corifollitropin alfa 71
Corpus luteum 153
Craniopharyngioma 62
Crown rump length 253
Cryopreservation 151
Cryptorchidism 123
Cumulus-oocyte complex 177
Cushing's disease 61
Cyclic adenosine monophosphate 173
Cyclical intestinal cramps 82
Cyclooxygenase 186
Cyproterone acetate 60
Cystic fibrosis 218
 transmembrane conductance regulator 160, 161
Cytomegalovirus 150

D

Deep dyspareunia 82
Deep vein thrombosis 191
Dehydroepiandrosterone 74, 75, 108, 109, 173
 sulfate 60, 61, 72, 73
Density-gradient centrifugation 202, 204
Deoxyribonucleic acid 128, 129, 151, 161, 202, 204, 227, 228, 273
 damage, majority of 128
 fragmentation
  index 113, 129, 149, 207, 230
  test 207
Diabetes 150
 mellitus, gestational 73
Diarrhea 250
Dichorionic diamniotic twins 253

Diethylstilbestrol 37
Dihydrotestosterone 60
Direct swim up 204
Distal hydrosalpinx and block 46
Distal tubal block 28
Donor
    insemination, clinical indications for 150
    profile 150
    screening 150
    selection, criteria for 198
    sourcing of 198
Dopamine agonists 64
Doppler flow 40
Duchenne Muscular dystrophy 218
Dye, intravasation of 46
Dysmenorrhea 80, 82
Dyspareunia 80

E

Ectopic pregnancy 48, 184, 249
    management of 249, 250
    previous 49
    surgical management 248
Ejaculatory duct obstruction 121
Electroejaculation 124
Electrophoretic system 204
Embryo transfer 7, 22, 23, 86, 87, 164, 169, 181, 183, 192, 231, 237, 238
    catheter 184
    history of 39
Embryo, time-lapse imaging of 222
Empty follicle syndrome 240, 241
Endometrial microbiome metagenomic analysis 33
Endometrial receptivity
    array 33, 214, 215
    factors affecting 227
Endometrial thickness 138, 237
    impact of 238
Endometrioma 106
Endometriosis 49, 79, 84, 86, 88
    deep infiltrating 158
    diagnosis of 80
    early 86
    fertility index 84, 87
        score 84
        staging 84
    laparoscopy staging 82
    role of endoscopy 88
Endometritis 34, 35
    acute 34
    chronic 34
Endometrium
    Doppler of 145
    evaluation, Doppler in 144
    progesterone receptors in 152
    thin 237
    trilaminar 24, 145

Enterobacteriaceae 34
Enterococcus faecalis 34
Epididymis 122
Epitestosterone 273
Erectile dysfunction 257
    diagnosis of 256
Erythrocyte sedimentation rate 100, 262
Estradiol 17, 138, 164, 169, 175, 189, 195, 269
    in controlled ovarian stimulation, role of 168
Ethambutol 102
Ethinyl estradiol 73
European Society for Gynecological Endoscopy 37
European Society of Human Reproduction and Embryology 37, 38, 106, 110, 234
Exercise 268

F

Fallopian tube 52
Familial adenomatous polyposis coli 218
Fatigue 82
Fatty acid, polyunsaturated 268
Ferriman-Gallwey score 60
Fertility
    low 19
    role of ultrasonography in 22
Fetal reduction 252
Fibroids 92
Fluorescence in situ hybridization 218
Folic acid 268
Follicle-stimulating hormone 10, 11, 13, 16, 19, 22, 26, 64, 70-72, 74, 75, 107, 108, 116-119, 122, 123, 136, 149, 164, 168, 169, 171-174, 185, 192, 200, 206, 210, 211, 228, 240, 260-262, 269
    ovarian response test, exogenous 19
    receptor 106
        polymorphism 260
Follicular Doppler 143
Follicular monitoring 140, 148
    Doppler in 142
Follicular output rate 106
Folliculogenesis 240
Fragile X syndrome 218
Free thyroxine 59
Free triiodothyronine 59
Freezing sperm 151
Freezing technique 150
Fresh embryo transfer 238
Frozen donor semen sample
    advantage of 150
    disadvantages of 150
Frozen embryo transfer 7, 73, 185, 193, 195, 196, 215, 239
    endometrial preparation for 194, 196

Frozen semen sample, thawing method of 150
Frozen-thawed embryo transfer 87
Full blood count 250, 251
Fundal polyp 42

G

Galactorrhea 62, 63
    evaluation of 63
    treatment of 63
    true 62
Gamete 227
Gardnerella vaginalis 34
Gene Xpert 101
Genital tuberculosis, female 102, 103
Georgetown Male Factor Infertility Study 128
Glands, endometrial 79
Glucose tolerance test 16
Goiter, multinodular 59
Gonadism, treatment of secondary 118
Gonadotropin 6, 11, 26, 56, 70, 73, 134, 136, 138, 141, 149, 163, 169, 260, 261, 269
    agonist stimulation test 19
    releasing hormone
        agonist 10, 86, 90, 94, 146, 153, 164, 185
        analogs 162
        antagonist 231
    stimulation 110
    external supplementation of 70
    high-dose 108
    ovulation induction with 136
    releasing hormone 11, 23, 74, 87-89, 92, 95, 118, 119, 122, 148, 153, 164, 166, 167, 171, 174, 175, 179, 187-189, 191, 240, 241, 260
Granulocyte colony stimulating factor 196, 197, 231, 235, 237, 239, 265
Gravid uterus 43
Growth hormone 108
    use of 74

H

Healthcare Products Regulatory Agency 152
Hematocrit 189, 190
Hemoconcentration 190
Hemophilia 218
Hemorrhage, postpartum 43
Heparin, unfractionated 234
Hepatitis
    B 150
        surface antigen 151, 161
    C 150
        virus 8, 151, 160, 161
High antral follicle count 188
Hirsutism 60
    causes of 60
    drug-induced 61

Hormone
  adrenocorticotropic 64
  replacement therapy 196
    cycle 194
    history of 39
    treatment 44
Human chorionic gonadotropin 6, 70, 71, 74, 75, 106, 108, 146-149, 152, 153, 163, 172, 174, 175, 179, 186-188, 194, 195, 200, 214, 234, 239-241, 249-251, 264, 265, 273
Human immunodeficiency virus 8, 100, 150, 151, 160, 161
Human menopausal gonadotropin 10, 70, 71, 121, 159, 163, 169-173, 200, 264, 273
Human T-cell lymphotropic virus 199
Huntington's disease 218
Hyaluronic acid binding sites 204
Hydrosalpinx 54
Hyperprolactinemia 16, 62-64
  idiopathic 64
Hypertension 150
Hypogonadism
  hypergonadotropic 121
  idiopathic hypogonadotropic 119
  male 118
  primary 118
  secondary 118
Hypomenorrhea 43
Hypo-osmotic swelling 116
Hyporesponders 172
Hypospermatogenesis 122
Hysterosalpingo-contrast sonography 8, 23
Hysterosalpingogram 26, 27, 48, 235
Hysterosalpingography 8, 28, 29, 33, 36-39, 43, 45, 51, 101
Hysteroscopic resection 38
Hysteroscopic transcervical resectoscopic myomectomy 28
Hysteroscopy 43, 93, 101
  diagnostic 33
  indications of 28
  role in infertility 28
Hysterosonography, three-dimensional 33

I

Immunoglobulin, intravenous 235
In vitro activation 110
In vitro fertilization 6, 7, 40, 50-52, 56, 57, 74, 86, 95, 101, 106, 108, 122, 128, 129, 147, 149, 155, 163, 177, 181, 188, 192, 196, 202, 203, 211, 218, 222, 227, 267, 269-271, 273
  clinic 198
  cycle 146
  female factor 158
  history of 39
  male factor 157
In vitro maturation 56, 57
Indian Council of Medical Research 151
Infections 122, 123
Infertile couple, history taking for 3
Infertility 43, 56, 92, 94
  causes of 79
  diet and lifestyle in 267
  duration of 3
  epidemiology of 1
  etiology of 79
  evaluation of 8, 112
  male 130
  psychological 264
  thyroid disorders in 58, 59
  unexplained 159
Intensive care unit 191
Intracytoplasmic morphologically selected sperm injection 117, 205
Intracytoplasmic sperm injection 51, 56, 57, 95, 116, 117, 122, 123, 128, 129, 157, 202, 203, 218, 224, 273, 274
  physiological 204, 205
  technique 206
Intrauterine adhesions 28, 43
Intrauterine contraceptive device 29, 43
Intrauterine device 43
  postoperative 38
Intrauterine growth restriction 252
Intrauterine insemination 6, 7, 11, 22, 23, 26, 27, 40, 50, 69-71, 85-89, 95, 116, 128, 129, 134, 135, 136, 138, 146-149, 152, 153, 157-159, 237, 270, 271, 273, 274
  cycle, trigger in 147
  endometritis during 114
  history of 39
  ovulation
    induction in 134, 136
    trigger in 146
Intrauterine procedure 43
Isoniazid 102

J

Jaundice, unexplained 150

K

Kallmann syndrome 119, 122
Klinefelter syndrome 123

L

Laparoscopic ovarian
  drilling 26
  surgery 56, 57
Laparoscopy 26, 48, 50, 80, 82, 101
  role in infertility 26
Laptop use, impact of 4
Laser hatching 211
Lesch-Nyhan syndrome 218
Letrozole 68, 134
  inhibits 68
Lippes loop 44
Liquefaction time 114
Live birth rate 238
Liver function test 250, 251
Low molecular weight heparin 187, 191, 239
Löwenstein-Jensen medium 100
Lupus anticoagulant 234
Luteal phase
  defect 152, 235
  deficiency 185
  support 152, 153, 185, 186
Luteinized unruptured follicle 265
  syndrome 264
Luteinizing hormone 10-13, 16, 17, 22, 26, 27, 64, 68, 70, 71, 73, 75, 108, 109, 117-119, 140, 142, 149, 164, 166, 168, 169, 172, 173, 189, 194-196, 214, 230, 241, 261, 264, 265
  endogenous 162, 164
  premature 148
  preovulatory 146, 174
  recombinant 74, 169, 173
  role of 172
  stimulation 260
    addition of 108
Lymphadenopathy, disseminated 150

M

MacKler's chamber 116
Macroadenomas 64
Magnetic resonance imaging 36, 37, 80, 81, 92, 93, 100, 234
Magnetic-activated cell sorting 129, 202, 204
  procedure 129
Male sexual dysfunction 258
Mantoux test 100
Marfan syndrome 218
Mature endometrium, features of 140
Mature follicle, features of 140
Medroxyprogesterone acetate 13, 44
Meningitis 122
Menses, normal 43
Menstrual cycle 169
Menstrual disturbances 43
Messenger ribonucleic acid 188
Methotrexate 250, 251
Microadenomas 64
Microdissection testicular sperm extraction 206
Microfluidics 129
Micronized progesterone, oral administration of 185
Microsurgical epididymal sperm aspiration 206, 207

Microsurgical testicular sperm extraction 206
Miscarriage rate 152
Mitochondrial deoxyribonucleic acid 110
Mitochondrion activation, autologous 110
Monochorionic pair 252
Motile sperm organelle morphology examination 202, 205
Müllerian duct 36
    anomalies 36
Multifetal pregnancy reduction 252, 253
Multiple pregnancy loss 126
Mycobacterium growth inhibitor tube 100
Mycobacterium tuberculosis 34, 100, 101
Mycoplasma 34
Myomas, submucous 28
Myotonic dystrophy 218

N

Natural killer cells 234, 270
Nausea 250
Needle aspiration biopsy 206, 207
Neisseria gonorrhoeae 34
Neodymium-doped yttrium aluminum garnet 28
Neonatal intensive care unit 253
Neural tube defect 268, 269
Nonapoptotic sperm, selection of 204
Nonobstructive azoospermia 206
    causes of 123
Nonsteroidal anti-inflammatory drugs 250, 264, 265
Nuchal translucency 253
Nuclear transfer 110
Nucleic acid amplification test, cartridge-based 101
Nutrition, effects of 4

O

Obesity 4, 267
Oligoasthenoteratozoospermia 157, 272-273, 274
    medical management of 272
Oligozoospermia 272
Oocyte
    donor 198
        controlled ovarian stimulation 200
        recruitment protocol 198
    functional capacity of 142
    pickup 6, 18, 22, 40, 86, 87, 171, 177, 187, 189, 192, 193, 241
        history of 39
        set up 176
    sharing 198
Optimal ovarian stimulation protocol 134
Oral contraceptive 164, 200
    pill 23, 60, 61, 72, 88, 168, 193, 261
        combined 61, 73, 192

Oral glucose
    challenge test 8
    tolerance test 8
Oral ovulogens 68, 134
Ovarian baseline scan 140
Ovarian endometrioma, endoscopy for 90
Ovarian fertility potential 19
Ovarian hyperstimulation 188
    syndrome 23, 57, 70, 86, 134, 136, 146, 158, 162, 163, 170, 174, 188, 191, 198, 260
        diagnosis of 188
        management of 190
        prevention of 166
Ovarian reserve testing 18
Ovarian stimulation
    mild 108, 170
    triggers for 174
Ovarian volume 19
Ovulation disorders 16
Ovulation induction 26, 27, 68, 70, 72, 74, 148, 164, 166
    adjuvants in 73, 74
Ovulation trigger 146, 174
Ovulatory dysfunction 56, 158
Ovulatory follicle 142
Ovulogen 6
Ovum capture inhibitor 79
Oxidative stress 4

P

Pain, anticipatory 256
Peak systolic velocity 143
Pelvic
    factor 79
    inflammatory disease 48, 49, 51, 53, 100, 158
    pain
        chronic 80, 82
        cyclic 43
    tuberculosis
        diagnosis 100
        management 102
Penile vibratory stimulation 124
Percutaneous epididymal sperm aspiration 116, 122, 123, 125, 206-208
Perineal muscles 256
Photosensitivity 250
Pituitary adenoma 62
Platelet rich plasma 44, 110, 196, 197, 239
    autologous 237
Polycystic ovarian
    disease 185
    syndrome 8, 56, 72, 134, 135, 149, 153, 162, 168, 172, 189, 227, 235, 240, 260, 268, 269
Polymerase chain reaction 100, 101, 103
Polyp
    endometrial 28, 40
    feeding vessels of 42

Polypectomy, hysteroscopic 40
Poor ovarian reserve 74, 106, 108
Poor ovarian response 105, 110
    diagnosis 106
    medical management 108
Poor sperm movement 272
Positron emission tomography 100
Potassium chloride 252, 253
Pouch of Douglas 80, 82, 84, 141, 179
Preantral follicles 18
Pregnancy
    probability of 144
    safety in 102
Pre-human chorionic gonadotropin scan 140
Preimplantation genetic
    diagnosis 159, 218, 220, 235
    screening 159, 230, 235
    testing 218, 219
Pre-in vitro fertilization evaluation 160
Primordial follicles 18
Progesterone 169, 183, 195
    intramuscular preparation 185
Prolactin 12, 16, 64
    level 17, 62
Prophylactic dose heparin 234
Propylthiouracil 58
Prostaglandins 265
Prostate, transurethral resection of 122, 123
Proximal tubal block 28, 50
Pulsatility index 141, 142, 145
Pyrazinamide 102

R

Radioactive iodine 58, 59
Random blood sugar 27
Randomized controlled trials 26, 270
Reactive oxygen species 128, 129, 151, 272
Real-time polymerase chain reaction 34
Recombinant follicle-stimulating hormone 163, 173, 273
Recurrent implantation failure 93, 227, 228, 230
    etiology for 227
    evaluation for 228
Recurrent pregnancy loss 43, 93, 112, 126, 234
    management 234
Renal function test 250
Renal hypoperfusion 190
Resistive index 141
Reversible liver impairment 250
Rifampicin 102, 103
Royal College of Obstetricians and Gynaecologists 49

S

Saline infusion sonography 33, 39, 40, 43, 45, 48, 92, 93
    history of 39

Salpingostomy 248
Sarcoidosis 122
Scrotal ultrasonography 130
Selective estrogen receptor modulator 68, 69
Selective serotonin reuptake inhibitor 258
Semen
    analysis 112, 114, 130, 160
        interpretation of 114, 116
    collection 202
    volume 272
Seminal plasma 151
Sertoli only cell syndrome 122
Serum anti-müllerian hormone 16
Serum beta human chorionic gonadotropin 248
Serum follicle-stimulating hormone 121, 130
Serum thyroid-stimulating hormone 58
Sex hormone-binding globulin 61, 258
Sexual violence 4
    history of 4
Sexually transmitted
    disease 150
    infections 4
Sickle cell anemia 218
Sildenafil citrate 124
Single cell gel electrophoresis assay 128
Single gene mutations 122
Single nucleotide polymorphism, types of 260
Single seminiferous tubule biopsy 206, 208
Sonohysterography 28
Sonosalpingography 48, 51
Sperm 128
    absence of 206
    apoptotic 204
    birefringence 205
    chromatin
        dispersion test 128, 129
        structure assay 128, 129
    concentration 272
    deoxyribonucleic acid 235
        damage, etiology of 128
        fragmentation values 129
    membrane maturity, selection based on 204
    parameters 148
    preparation techniques 202
    retrieval techniques 206, 207
    slow 204
    surface 204
Spermatogenesis, normal 122
Spinal muscular atrophy 218
Spiral artery power Doppler 140
Steelma-Pohley in vivo assay 70
Stem cell
    bone marrow-derived 110, 238
    ovarian transplant, autologous 110
    treatment 44

Steroidogenesis 240
Stomatitis 250
Stress, impact of 4
Surrogate human chorionic gonadotropin, administration of 142
Syphilis 150

T

Tamoxifen 68, 238
Tay-Sachs disease 150, 218
Teratozoospermia 272
Testes 122
Testicular atrophy 122
Testicular failure 118
Testicular sperm
    aspiration 122, 123, 125, 206-208
    extraction 116, 122, 206, 207
Testosterone 108, 122, 273
    replacement therapy 118
Thrombophilias 234
Thumb rest 184
Thyroid
    disorders 58
    peroxidase 59, 234
    stimulating hormone 12, 13, 16, 17, 27, 59, 62-64, 234, 235
Thyrotropin
    receptor antibody 59
    releasing hormone 59
Total motile sperm count 148
Transabdominal sonography 81
Transabdominal ultrasound 183
Transcervical uterine incision 28, 29
Transrectal ultrasound 123
Transvaginal sonography 28, 33, 40, 81, 94, 95, 169, 234
    three-dimensional 94, 95
Transvaginal ultrasound, history of 39
Trauma 122
Tubal adhesion 82
Tubal assessment 49
Tubal disease 50
Tubal disorders 158
Tubal evaluation 48
Tubal patency test 50
Tubal re-anastomosis 52
Tubal surgery, role of 50, 52
Tuberculosis 27, 100, 123
Tumor 122
    adrenal 61
    necrosis factor 79, 231
Turner syndrome 10

U

Ultrasonography 12, 19, 29, 39, 22, 38, 40, 50, 56, 86, 88, 89, 113, 126, 131, 160, 175, 189, 196, 197, 200
    history of 39

Ultrasound 92, 103, 113
Unconsummated marriage 256
Unruptured follicular syndrome 264, 265
Ureaplasma urealyticum 34
Urinary follicle-stimulating hormone 71
Urinary tract infection 115
Urine pregnancy test 12, 17, 241
Uterine
    anomalies 36, 38
    artery Doppler 140
    biophysical profile 144
    factor 31, 33, 158
    fibroids 92
    polyps 40
Uterus
    arcuate 46
    baseline scan of 140
    bicornuate 32
    normal 24, 32
    septate 28, 32, 38, 46
    three-D imaging of 32
    unicornuate 28, 46

V

Vaginal route of administration 185
Valsalva maneuver 130
Varicocele 130
    clinical grades of 130
Vas deferens 115, 122
Vasal aplasia 121
Vascular endothelial growth factor 188, 189, 239
Venereal disease research laboratory 160
Viagra 124
Viral orchitis 123
Vitamin
    B 268
    D 268
    D3 109
Vomiting 250
Vulval pain 256
Vulvodynia 256

W

Water-soluble preparation 185
White blood cell 189
World Health Organization 102
Worms, bag of 130

Y

Y chromosome deletions 123

Z

Zeta potential 204
    method 204
Zona pellucida 210

EU GSPR Authorised Reprsentative
Logos Europe, 9 rue Nicolas Poussin
1700, La Rochelle, France
Phone: +33 (0) 6 67 93 73 78
E-mail: contact@logoseurope.eu